Gynecologic Cancer Care: Innovative Progress

Editor

CAROLYN Y. MULLER

OBSTETRICS AND GYNECOLOGY CLINICS OF NORTH AMERICA

www.obgyn.theclinics.com

Consulting Editor
WILLIAM F. RAYBURN

March 2019 • Volume 46 • Number 1

ELSEVIER

1600 John F. Kennedy Boulevard • Suite 1800 • Philadelphia, Pennsylvania, 19103-2899

http://www.theclinics.com

OBSTETRICS AND GYNECOLOGY CLINICS OF NORTH AMERICA Volume 46, Number 1
March 2019 ISSN 0889-8545, ISBN-13: 978-0-323-65538-5

Editor: Kerry Holland
Developmental Editor: Kristen Helm

Obstetrics and Gynecology Clinics (ISSN 0889-8545) is published quarterly by Elsevier Inc., 360 Park Avenue South, New York, NY 10010-1710. Months of issue are March, June, September, and December. Periodicals postage paid at New York, NY, and additional mailing offices. Subscription price per year is $322.00 (US individuals), $685.00 (US institutions), $100.00 (US students), $404.00 (Canadian individuals), $865.00 (Canadian institutions), $225.00 (Canadian students), $459.00 (international individuals), $865.00 (international institutions), and $225.00 (international students). To receive student/resident rate, orders must be accompanied by name of affiliated institution, date of term, and the signature of program/residency coordinator on institution letterhead. Orders will be billed at individual rate until proof of status is received. Foreign air speed delivery is included in all *Clinics* subscription prices. All prices are subject to change without notice. POSTMASTER: Send address changes to *Obstetrics and Gynecology Clinics*, Elsevier Health Sciences Division, Subscription Customer Service, 3251 Riverport Lane, Maryland Heights, MO 63043. **Customer Service: Telephone: 1-800-654-2452 (U.S. and Canada); 314-447-8871 (outside U.S. and Canada). Fax: 314-447-8029. E-mail: journalscustomerservice-usa@elsevier.com (for print support); journalsonlinesupport-usa@elsevier. com (for online support).**

Reprints. For copies of 100 or more of articles in this publication, please contact the Commercial Reprints Department, Elsevier Inc., 360 Park Avenue South, New York, New York 10010-1710. Tel.: 212-633-3874; Fax: 212-633-3820; E-mail: reprints@elsevier.com.

Obstetrics and Gynecology Clinics of North America is also published in Spanish by McGraw-Hill Interamericana Editores S.A., P.O. Box 5-237, 06500, Mexico; in Portuguese by Reichmann and Affonso Editores, Rio de Janeiro, Brazil; and in Greek by Paschalidis Medical Publications, Athens, Greece.

Obstetrics and Gynecology Clinics of North America is covered in MEDLINE/PubMed (Index Medicus), Excerpta Medica, Current Concepts/Clinical Medicine, Science Citation Index, BIOSIS, CINAHL, and ISI/BIOMED.

Contributors

CONSULTING EDITOR

WILLIAM F. RAYBURN, MD, MBA
Associate Dean, Continuing Medical Education and Professional Development, Distinguished Professor and Emeritus Chair, Obstetrics and Gynecology, University of New Mexico School of Medicine, Albuquerque, New Mexico, USA

EDITOR

CAROLYN Y. MULLER, MD
Professor, Obstetrics and Gynecology, Chief, Gynecologic Oncology, University of New Mexico Comprehensive Cancer Center, Albuquerque, New Mexico, USA

AUTHORS

JILL ALLDREDGE, MD
University of California, Irvine, Orange, California, USA

DAVID P. BENDER, MD
Clinical Professor, Division of Gynecologic Oncology, Department of Obstetrics and Gynecology, The University of Iowa, University of Iowa Hospitals and Clinics, Iowa City, Iowa, USA

EVELYN CANTILLO, MD, MPH
Assistant Professor, Division of Gynecologic Oncology, Department of Obstetrics, Gynecology and Reproductive Sciences, University of Vermont College of Medicine, Burlington, Vermont, USA

YOVANNI CASABLANCA, MD
Director of the Gynecologic Cancer Center of Excellence, Department of Obstetrics and Gynecology, Uniformed Services University of the Health Sciences, Bethesda, Maryland, USA

PHILIP E. CASTLE, PhD, MPH
Professor, Department of Epidemiology and Population Health, Albert Einstein College of Medicine, Bronx, New York, USA

LOGAN COREY, MD
Resident, Department of Obstetrics and Gynecology, Ochsner Clinic Foundation, New Orleans, Louisiana, USA

JAMES C. CRIPE, MD
Division of Gynecologic Oncology, Department of Obstetrics and Gynecology, Washington University School of Medicine, Alvin J. Siteman Cancer Center, St Louis, Missouri, USA

LINDA R. DUSKA, MD, MPH
Professor, Division of Gynecology Oncology, Department of Obstetrics and Gynecology, University of Virginia, University of Virginia Medical Center, Charlottesville, Virginia, USA

LAURIE M. ELIT, MD, MSc, FRCSC
Division of Gynecologic Oncology, Department of Obstetrics and Gynecology, McMaster University, Juravinski Cancer Centre, Hamilton, Ontario, Canada

JENNA B. EMERSON, MD
Fellow, Program in Women's Oncology, Women & Infants Hospital, Warren Alpert Medical School at Brown University, Providence, Rhode Island, USA

RICARDO A. GOMEZ-MARTINEZ, MD
Gynecologic Oncology Fellow, The University of New Mexico, Albuquerque, New Mexico, USA

ELIZABETH LOKICH, MD
Assistant Professor of Obstetrics and Gynecology, Division of Gynecologic Oncology, Women & Infants Hospital, Warren Alpert Medical School at Brown University, Providence, Rhode Island, USA

CARA MATHEWS, MD
Assistant Professor, Program in Women's Oncology, Women & Infants Hospital, Warren Alpert Medical School at Brown University, Providence, Rhode Island, USA

MEGAN E. McDONALD, MD
Clinical Assistant Professor, Division of Gynecologic Oncology, Department of Obstetrics and Gynecology, The University of Iowa, University of Iowa Hospitals and Clinics, Iowa City, Iowa, USA

MARY M. MULLEN, MD
Division of Gynecologic Oncology, Department of Obstetrics and Gynecology, Washington University School of Medicine, Alvin J. Siteman Cancer Center, St Louis, Missouri, USA

AMANDA PIERZ, MS
Department of Epidemiology and Population Health, Albert Einstein College of Medicine, Bronx, New York, USA

REBECCA ANN PREVIS, MD, MS
Assistant Professor, Division of Gynecologic Oncology, Department of Obstetrics and Gynecology, Duke Cancer Institute, Duke University Medical Center, Durham, North Carolina, USA

LESLIE RANDALL, MD
University of California, Irvine, Orange, California, USA

CLARE J. READE, MD, MSc, FRCSC
Division of Gynecologic Oncology, Department of Obstetrics and Gynecology, McMaster University, Juravinski Cancer Centre, Hamilton, Ontario, Canada

CHRISTINE ROJAS, MD
Gynecologic Oncology Fellow, Gynecologic Cancer Center of Excellence, Murtha Cancer Center, Walter Reed National Military Medical Center, Bethesda, Maryland, USA

ANGELES ALVAREZ SECORD, MD
Professor, Division of Gynecologic Oncology, Department of Obstetrics and Gynecology,
Duke Cancer Institute, Duke University Medical Center, Durham, North Carolina, USA

JEANINE N. STAPLES, MD, MPH
Division of Gynecology Oncology, Department of Obstetrics and Gynecology, University
of Virginia, University of Virginia Medical Center, Charlottesville, Virginia, USA

PREMAL H. THAKER, MD, MS
Division of Gynecologic Oncology, Department of Obstetrics and Gynecology,
Washington University School of Medicine, Alvin J. Siteman Cancer Center, St Louis,
Missouri, USA

ANA VALENTE, MD
Resident, Department of Obstetrics and Gynecology, Ochsner Clinic Foundation,
New Orleans, Louisiana, USA

KATRINA WADE, MD
Gynecologic Oncologist, Department of Gynecologic Oncology, Ochsner Clinic
Foundation, New Orleans, Louisiana, USA

DANIEL WEINBERG, MD
Obstetrics and Gynecology Resident, The University of New Mexico, Albuquerque,
New Mexico, USA

Contents

Evaluating the quality of care received by gynecologic cancer patients in the real world is essential for excellent outcomes. The recent population-based literature looking at quality of care was reviewed for all gynecologic malignancies. Outcomes are generally highest when care is provided by high-volume providers in high-volume cancer centers. Provision of care according to clinical practice guidelines has also been demonstrated to improve outcomes in many situations. Disparities exist for marginalized groups in terms of the care they receive and subsequent outcomes. Health systems need to improve care for these populations.

This article provides an up-to-date summary of screening approaches and key strategies in prevention of gynecologic malignancies. The Pap smear is the only proven screening intervention in the field of gynecologic oncology. Women should receive treatment for precancerous conditions of the cervix, vulva, vagina, and endometrial lining. Women with inherited conditions should consider having a risk-reducing surgery once they have finished childbearing. The human papilloma virus vaccination should be offered to all girls and boys aged 11 to 12 years, and can also be given as early as age 9 through 45 years of age.

New technologies have advanced the science of tumor biology and genomics. Commercially available germline and somatic testing modalities have the downstream benefits of enabling prevention strategies in women with hereditary cancers and their family members in addition to identifying women who benefit most from novel targeted therapeutics. The matrix of available testing is complex and evolving. Women's health providers need to be versed in benefits and limitations of available testing. Genetic counselors play a pivotal role in interpretation of relevant mutations, and in avoiding common pitfalls, but their skill set is not sufficient to optimally integrate cancer genomics into clinical practice.

> Surgery is a cornerstone of gynecologic oncology. Minimally invasive techniques have been adopted rapidly, in lieu of open approaches, in cervical and endometrial cancer staging. In addition, nodal assessment has undergone significant changes with the introduction of SLN biopsies. The movement toward less is more has also been seen with perioperative and postoperative care and the advent of ERAS protocols, which attempt to maintain normal physiology with the goal of improving functional recovery. It is imperative that new technology be critically evaluated to ensure that oncologic outcomes are not compromised.

> Ovarian cancer treatment continues to evolve. Despite aggressive surgery and chemotherapy, most women will ultimately die from disease. Improvement in disease control are due to the incorporation of molecular targeted agents and the adoption of maintenance therapy. Maintenance therapy has been shown to enhance progression-free survival. Recent surgical trials have evaluated the role of neoadjuvant chemotherapy versus primary debulking at the time of diagnosis in advanced stage ovarian cancer. The role of lymph node dissection and secondary cytoreductive surgeries have also been evaluated. This article reviews contemporary trials of maintenance therapy and novel drug development.

> It is imperative to understand the underlying mechanisms of both endometrial carcinogenesis and recurrence in order to develop more effective prevention and treatment. This article reviews available molecular data, the interplay between endometrial cancer carcinogenesis with obesity and genetics, as well as current targeted therapies.

> Cervical cancer disproportionately burdens lower-resourced settings, in which nearly 90% of cervical cancer and cervical cancer–related deaths occur. Targeting human papillomavirus (HPV) by prophylactic HPV vaccination in young adolescent girls and HPV-based screening in mid-adult women offers the most cost-effective strategy to reduce cervical cancer burden worldwide and mitigate the health disparities in cervical cancer burden between low-resourced and high-resourced settings. Political and social will, along with the necessary financial investments, will be necessary to realize the opportunity for significant global reductions in the cervical cancer burden. Perfect cervical cancer prevention (total eradication) is practically and financially unrealistic.

symptom burden, and better quality of life for patients and caregivers. Consequently, this comprehensive approach is formally recognized and endorsed by the Society of Gynecologic Oncology, the National Comprehensive Cancer Network, and the American Society of Clinical Oncology. This article reviews the background, benefits, barriers, and most practical delivery models of palliative care. It also discusses management of common symptoms experienced by gynecologic oncology patients.

OBSTETRICS AND GYNECOLOGY CLINICS

ISSUE OF RELATED INTEREST

Hematology/Oncology Clinics of North America, December 2018 (Vol. 32, No. 6)
Ovarian Cancer
Ursula A. Matulonis, *Editor*
Available at: http://www.hemonc.theclinics.com/

THE CLINICS ARE AVAILABLE ONLINE!
Access your subscription at:
www.theclinics.com

Foreword

Gynecologic Cancer Care: Innovative Progress

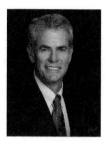

William F. Rayburn, MD, MBA
Consulting Editor

This issue of the *Obstetrics and Gynecology Clinics of North America* provides scientific and practice-changing updates in gynecologic oncology during the past 6 years. Once again, Carolyn Muller, MD has done a fine job as editor, coordinating and providing an excellent overview on the progress made in the specialty. It is clear that the field of gynecologic oncology continues to undergo remarkable evolution since our last issue on this subject in 2012.

Guidelines about early detection and screening of certain gynecologic malignancies have been refined and updated in this issue. Discussions about tumor markers, imaging, and risk-reduction surgery are balanced. It impresses me how cancer screening, prevention, and treatment, especially chemotherapy, and biologic targeted therapies and immunotherapy continue to change. Staging continues to be best handled with a gynecologic oncologist whenever possible.

We live in an era of rapid progress and utilization of technology to better understand the many mechanisms of cancer leading to a more "personalized" approach to management. Each of the sites of malignancy: ovaries, fallopian tubes, endometrium, cervix, and vulva, are given separate attention in this issue. Corresponding innovations in diagnosis and management are offered. After reviewing these articles, I am more hopeful of improved survival and less morbidity with the progress that has been made.

Outcomes of procedures when performed by a gynecologic oncologist have been shown to be better than when performed by other surgeons. The value of skilled minimally invasive and robot-assisted approaches in select patients encourages the attitude that "less may be more." Improved understandings set the foundation of developing actionable drug targets and neoadjuvant chemotherapy. Biologic targeted therapy is discussed in several articles, along with immune checkpoint blockade and other immunotherapy strategies.

Obstet Gynecol Clin N Am 46 (2019) xiii–xiv
https://doi.org/10.1016/j.ogc.2018.11.002
0889-8545/19/© 2018 Published by Elsevier Inc.

I especially enjoyed the articles that relate to personalized medicine in gynecologic cancer (fact or fiction) and palliative care. All three topics have appropriately gained more attention in recent years. Patient education cannot be stressed enough in plain spoken and written language. Information about therapeutic success, frequency and outcome of recurrent disease, any need for hereditary testing for cancer syndromes, and safety of medication is often difficult yet essential to discuss. In some cases, patients desire fertility preservation, especially young women with ovarian tumors of low-malignant potential.

This issue should activate the reader's attention about cutting-edge interests in gynecologic oncology. The articles are presented in a sophisticated, yet understandable manner that emphasizes how approaches are changing. I wish to thank Dr Muller and her excellent team of knowledgeable contributors in providing practical information and attempting to answer tough questions through evidence-based and well-planned approaches.

William F. Rayburn, MD, MBA
Department of Obstetrics and Gynecology
Office of Continuing Medical Education and
Professional Development
University of New Mexico School of Medicine
MSC10 5580, 1 University of New Mexico
Albuquerque, NM 87131-0001, USA

E-mail address:
wrayburn@salud.unm.edu

Preface

Innovation and Progress in Gynecologic Cancer Care: Faster than Ever

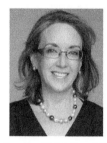

Carolyn Y. Muller, MD
Editor

Gynecologic cancers affect millions of women worldwide across all ages often leading to significant disruption in general health, quality of life, and, in many cases, early death. Despite continued challenges in access to care and health literacy and lack of equality in screening and prevention, we now live in an era of rapid progress and utilization of technology to better understand the numerous mechanisms of cancer in search for actionable drug targets that can identify the "Achilles heel" of a particular cancer. The rapidity of the progress made is astounding. In fact, 25 years ago (when I was in fellowship), we learned extreme radical open surgery and really only had three classes of drugs that were predominantly used in most of the gynecologic cancers: platinum, taxanes, and anthracyclines. Having a vaccine that can eradicate cancer was a topic for science fiction. Thankfully, contemporary practice is based on "less is more" surgically, seeing the advent of skilled minimally invasive and "robotic" surgical platforms. Chemotherapy, biologic-targeted therapy (PARP inhibitors, antiangiogenic blockade, tyrosine kinase inhibitors and monoclonal antibody therapy), and now immune checkpoint blockade and other immunotherapy strategies have changed the landscape of medical therapy for our patients. "Bench-to-bedside" collaborative science and the evolution of novel clinical trial design have led to more rapid FDA approval of beneficial drugs, and for the first time ever, a drug was approved based on a *molecular signal* from a novel designed "basket" trial. And the human papillomavirus (HPV) vaccine can indeed eradicate high-risk HPV-driven cancers if mass vaccination could ever be accomplished! Keeping up with the advances can be very challenging, and, in fact, two major updates have occurred after the content of this issue was fully typeset. I am happy to report that (1) the HPV vaccine has been approved for expanded use in adults aged 27 to 45, and (2) results of the randomized

Obstet Gynecol Clin N Am 46 (2019) xv–xvi
https://doi.org/10.1016/j.ogc.2018.11.001
0889-8545/19/© 2018 Published by Elsevier Inc.

phase 3 SOLO-1 trial showed the PARP inhibitor olaparib significantly improves progression-free survival (hazard ratio 0.30; 95% confidence interval, 0.23-0.41; $P<.0001$) in women with a BRCA mutation and advanced ovarian cancer when used as frontline maintenance therapy as reported at the late October ESMO meeting. This clearly will set a new standard of care for this group of patients with ovarian cancer!

This exceptional group of authors has provided a unique perspective on the innovation and progress in our field of Gynecologic Oncology as they cover where we are today and where we still need to go in the future. Our field encompasses more than surgery and chemotherapy now, complete with important expertise in palliative care and survivorship. The impact of genomics and technology is discussed as it relates to the advancement to personalized medicine (...are we there yet?) and technology in surgical management of our patients (....is less really more in all cases?). And the recent breakthroughs in the care of our patients will be outlined, more of which likely will occur even before the production of this issue. I hope you will find the updates in this issue exhilarating with extreme hope for better outcomes for our patients and the hope to eradicate cancer not only in North America but also worldwide. That passion is what drives all of us to continue to strive for the best for our patients with gynecologic cancer.

Carolyn Y. Muller, MD
Gynecologic Oncology
University of New Mexico
Comprehensive Cancer Center
1 University of New Mexico
MSC 07 4025
Albuquerque, NM 87131, USA

E-mail address:
cmuller@salud.unm.edu

Current Quality of Gynecologic Cancer Care in North America

Clare J. Reade, MD, MSc, FRCSC, Laurie M. Elit, MD, MSc, FRCSC*

KEYWORDS

- Quality of care • Population-based care • Gynecologic cancer outcomes
- Structure of care • Processes of care • Disparities

KEY POINTS

- Significant disparities exist for patients with gynecologic malignancies.
- Each health care system has challenges that must be addressed to improve access to high-quality care.
- Complex cancer care should be centralized into high-volume cancer centers in most cases.
- Gynecologic oncologists should provide care for women with gynecologic malignancies.

Quality of care[1] involves an assessment of both structure and processes of care in terms of their impact on patient outcomes. Structure describes the setting in which health care is delivered. Process describes the care actually provided to patients (eg, diagnostic testing). Outcomes of interest are generally of importance to both patients and health care providers (eg, overall survival). The authors previously summarized the population-based published data on the care of North American women with gynecologic malignancies.[2] The goal of this article is to review North American health systems and to update the health services literature as it pertains to gynecologic malignancies.

CONTEXT OF GYNECOLOGIC CANCER CARE

According to the World Health Organization (WHO), health is a fundamental human right. Access to essential, quality health services should not be denied for unfair reasons, especially those with economic or social roots.[3] Often, it is those individuals lacking in political, social, or economic power (eg, racial and ethnic minorities) who

Disclosure Statement: None of the authors have any commercial or financial conflicts of interest to declare. This study did not receive support from any funding source.
Division of Gynecologic Oncology, Department of Obstetrics and Gynecology, McMaster University, Juravinski Cancer Centre, 699 Concession Street, Hamilton, Ontario L8V 5C2, Canada
* Corresponding author.
E-mail address: elitlor@hhsc.ca

Obstet Gynecol Clin N Am 46 (2019) 1–17
https://doi.org/10.1016/j.ogc.2018.09.001
0889-8545/19/© 2018 Elsevier Inc. All rights reserved.

experience the most health inequities.[3] As part of the Sustainable Development Goals, all United Nations (UN) member states have agreed to try to achieve universal health coverage (UHC) by 2030. In 2018, at least half of the world's population does not have coverage of essential health services.[4] Within North America, access to health services is better than many places around the world; however, there are ongoing challenges in the provision of health care.

In Mexico, there is a combination of private health care and government-funded programs. Most employees have health care coverage through their work, provided by the Institute of Social Security. Persons enrolled in this program pay monthly premiums based on their income, and both the employer and government also contribute to the cost. This program covers approximately half of the Mexican population. For citizens who are unemployed and uninsured, basic health care coverage for all citizens has been available since 2004 under the Seguro Popular, a government program. Families enrolled in this program pay an annual fee that varies depending on ability to pay, and those with very low income do not pay any fee. **Table 1** shows characteristics of health care spending for Mexico.

Health care in Canada is provided by the provinces, and organized as a universal single-payer system.[8] The federal government plays a role by contributing funding and by providing direct health care to certain groups (eg, First Nations populations). All citizens receive hospital and physician care without having to provide direct payment. However, drugs used outside of hospital and ancillary health care such as vision care are covered only for certain populations (eg, seniors). The issue with access to care in Canada remains a combination of wait times (eg, diagnostic testing), and the cost of new targeted agents, which may not be funded by the provinces.

In the United States, health care is provided by both the private and public sector through a complex web of government programs and private health insurance. Many employees receive health insurance as a benefit of employment, and private health insurance can also be purchased on the open market. Government programs such as Medicaid, Medicare, and the Children's Health Insurance Program provide insurance for low-income populations, seniors, and children. In 2015, 56% of Americans had health insurance coverage through an employer; 15% had purchased insurance directly, and public programs covered 21% of residents. Nine percent of Americans were uninsured.[9] The proportion of uninsured Americans has declined significantly since the introduction of the Affordable Care Act, which made health insurance more accessible and subsidized rates for low-income individuals.

A recent report on health care quality by the OECD makes several recommendations to improve the quality of health care systems.[10] At the systems level, there needs to be a

Table 1
Profile of country health care spending

Country	Uninsured	Percentage of Gross Domestic Product Spent on Health	Government Spending on Health	Public Spending on Health	Total per Capita Spending on Health	Life Expectancy at Birth (y)
Mexico	18%	51.7%	51.7%	$249 USD	$428 USD	77.2[5]
Canada	—	10.6%	70.3% $3122.43	—	$4442.06	82.4[6]
United States	8.6%[9]	17.2%	49.1% $9892.30	—	$4860.10	78.8[7]

focus on shared care models to promote comprehensive and coordinated care. Health care systems should engage patients and measure health outcomes important to patients. Patient safety is a priority, and requires ongoing data collection and analysis to learn from adverse events, and external evaluation is important for driving continuous quality improvement. Transparency is important, with information infrastructures linked to quality improvement tools, and the ability to connect patient data across providers and pathways of care. This is all applicable to cancer care in North America, and implementation of these principles has the potential to improve population care.

Ovarian Cancer

Incidence and mortality from ovarian cancer are described in **Table 2**.

The incidence of ovarian cancer (see **Table 2**) has remained relatively stable, with a slight decrease over the last 20 years. Despite advances in treatment, overall mortality rates have not improved. This in part is because most patients are diagnosed with advanced disease. With the exception of prophylactic salpingectomy or salpingo-oophorectomy as a risk-reducing strategy, there are no effective population-based screening tests to detect earlier stage disease.

From January 1, 2011, to December 31, 2017, the published English-language literature on gynecologic cancers showed 10 unique studies that reported on structural variables in relation to clinical outcomes for ovarian cancer (**Table 3**). Of these, 4 studies showed an improvement in overall survival, and 2 others showed impact on mortality prior to discharge or death within 90 days. Physician surgical volumes, hospital ovarian cancer volumes, physician type (ie, specialization), and hospital type (eg, teaching or community) were the structural variables described.

Studies showed an association between high physician volumes for surgery and improved outcomes. Hospitals treating a high volume of women with ovarian cancer and teaching hospitals or academic centers had improved patient survival,[11,12] along with other benefits such as lower in-hospital postoperative mortality rate[13] and lower rates of failure to rescue.[13]

Studies addressing physician type showed that if surgery was by a gynecologic oncologist, the patients had better survival, along with more compliant guideline care, more optimal debulking, appropriate staging, and increased use of adjuvant chemotherapy and combination chemotherapy.[13] General surgeons continue to have higher in-hospital mortality, complications, and longer length of stay.[13] It is likely that general surgeons see a higher proportion of emergent cases due to bowel obstruction or cases where the primary cancer diagnosis is difficult to define because of the extent of disease. A detailed understanding of the disease process is an important factor in providing optimal care, in addition to surgical skill. Moving ovarian cancer

Table 2				
Ovarian cancer incidence and mortality rates				
	Incidence		Mortality	
Country	Number of Cases in 2018	Age-Standardized Rate (per 100,000)[a]	Number of Deaths in 2018	Age-Standardized Rate (per 100,000)
Mexico	4,759	6.8	2,765	4.0
Canada	2,716	7.9	1,847	4.4
United States	24,469	8.5	14,008	4.1

[a] The standard population used for the age-standardized rate is the world standard population.
Data from Ferlay J, Soerjomataram I, Mery L, et al. GLOBOCAN 2018: Cancer Today 2018 IARC. Available at: http://gco.iarc.fr/today. Accessed October 25, 2018.

Table 3
Structure variables that influence health care outcomes

Study	Country	Data Source	Number of Patients	Did Structural Variables Impact Survival?	Did Structural Variables Impact Surrogate Outcomes?	Which Surrogate Outcomes Were Used?
Bristow et al,[15] 2011	United States	Maryland Health Services Cost Review	2487	No; surgeon volumes	Yes	Optimal debulking, Surgical staging
Bristow et al,[16] 2013	United States	National Cancer Database	47,160	Yes; hospital volumes		
Dahm-Kahler et al,[14] 2016	Sweden	Swedish Quality Registry	817	Yes; centralized care		
Dehaeck et al,[17] 2013	Canada	BC Cancer Control	854	No; surgeon type		
Eggink et al,[12] 2016	Netherlands	Managed clinical network of 11 hospitals, University of Groningen	7987	Yes; high-volume hospitals		
Leandersson et al,[18] 2017	Sweden	Retrospective cohort	1108	No; teaching hospitals	Yes	Optimal debulking, Length of stay, Readmission, Complications
Mandato et al,[19] 2013	Italy	Audit of Emilia-Romagna 40-hospital system	614	Yes; Surgical volumes, Specialist care		
Shakeel et al,[13] 2017	Canada	Canadian Institute of Health Information	16,089	Surgeon volumes, Hospital type, Hospital volumes, Care provider type	Yes	Mortality prior to discharge, Complications, Failure to rescue, Length of stay
Urban et al,[20] 2016	United States	Surveillance, Epidemiology, and End Results (SEER)	9491	No; surgeon type	Yes	Death within 90 d of surgery
Warren et al,[21] 2017	United States	SEER	4427	No; surgeon type, hospital volumes	Yes	Guideline care

care to high-volume centers (HVCs) where gynecologic oncologists are on staff has shown superior survival outcomes in 2 studies.[12,13]

Processes of care involve the provision of specific procedures (eg, debulking surgery) and therapy (eg, multiagent chemotherapy) known to improve outcomes. **Table 4** lists the 9 population-based studies of women with ovarian cancer from 5 countries, and 7 showed specific process variables impacting survival. Interestingly, Warren[21] clearly showed that guideline-specific care does improve over time when care is centralized; however, 2 year survival rate did not improve. Their data showed that only 40% of women with ovarian cancer in the centralized model received guideline care. Thus, although improving adherence to evidence-based processes improves survival, further work is required to understand why gynecologic oncologists are not uniformly providing such care. A novel area explored since the authors' last report is the importance of surgery at the time of first recurrence.[22] Secondary cytoreduction is not yet a component of guideline care for ovarian cancer.

Disparities in care and outcomes have been linked to race and ethnic classification, socio-economic status (SES), age,[23] educational level, geography, and health system factors.[24] However, if for example, black American women received surgery by a high-volume surgeon in an HVC[15] or on a Gynecologic Oncology Group trial,[25] they had better outcomes and more comprehensive surgical care.[15] It appears that "equal care yields equal outcomes," independent of race. When disparities exist, the quality of ovarian cancer care may be in variance with National Comprehensive Cancer Network (NCCN) guidelines, and this affects survival. It is important to define patient, provider, health care system, and societal factors leading to these disparities so that targeted interventions can be designed to reduce and eliminate them.

Uterine Cancer

Uterine cancer incidence and mortality rates are described in **Table 5**.

Uterine cancer is the most common gynecologic malignancy in NA. The most recent country-specific data on the incidence and mortality of uterine cancer are presented in **Table 5**. Globocan demonstrate an increasing age-standardized incidence of uterine cancer for all countries. The age-standardized mortality has increased slightly in all three countries.[2] There are wide variations in patterns of treatment for high-risk endometrial cancer patients across centers.[29] This is likely due to the fact that despite endometrial cancer's relatively high incidence, there are still areas of significant controversy in the treatment of this disease, including the role of lymphadenectomy and the type and extent of adjuvant therapy.

There were 2 population-based studies looking at structural variables in endometrial cancer and the impact on outcomes (**Table 6**). For nonendometrioid histologies, care at an HVC increased the rate of chemotherapy use and also improved survival. However, for endometrial cancer in general, whether surgery is done at an HVC or low-volume center (LVC) did not make a difference in survival. This likely reflects the fact that most endometrial cancers are low-grade localized cancers, and simple hysterectomy and bilateral salpingo-oophorectomy are adequate treatment for those patients.

Table 7 reviews recently published population-based studies evaluating process and outcomes. Several studies reported improved survival with the use of adjuvant radiotherapy, which is in contrast to results of randomized trials. However, the largest of the population-based studies reported that the group receiving radiotherapy had lower noncancer mortality, indicating this was a healthier group of patients. These authors conclude the reason other population-based studies demonstrated an improved overall survival with radiotherapy was simply the reduced noncancer mortality rates in this healthier population.[29] However, multiple studies reported that the use of adjuvant

Table 4
Process variables found to improve survival at a population level

Study	Country	Data Source	Number of Patients	Did Process Variables Impact Survival?	Did Process Variables Impact Surrogate Outcomes?	Which Surrogate Outcomes Were Used?
Bristow et al,[15] 2011	United States	Single hospital	433	Yes; computed tomography (CT), cytoreduction		
Bristow et al,[16] 2013	United States	National cancer database	47,160	Yes; NCCN guideline care		
Chatterjee et al,[26] 2016	United States	Retrospective data	21,758	Yes; CT	No	
Dahm-Kahler et al,[11] 2017	Sweden	Retrospective data	4381	Yes; neoadjuvant chemotherapy (NACT) + interval debulking surgery (IDS), single drug platinum		
Dehaeck et al,[17] 2013	Canada	Prospective cohort	854	Yes; Optimal debulking, combination chemotherapy		
Eskander et al,[27] 2014		Retrospective cohort	5152	Yes; 30 d readmission	Yes	1 y mortality
Lee et al,[28] 2015	Korea	Retrospective data	266	No; lymphadenectomy, guideline adherence	Yes	Recurrence-free survival
Van de Laar et al,[22] 2016	Netherlands	Retrospective cohort	1146	Yes; secondary cytoreduction without preoperative chemotherapy		
Warren et al,[21] 2017	United States	Patterns of care	3409 in 2002, 3018 in 2011	No	Yes	Guideline-adherent staging, debulking surgery, and multiagent chemotherapy

Table 5
Uterine cancer incidence and mortality rates

	Incidence		Mortality	
Country	Number of Cases in 2018	Age-Standardized Rate (per 100,000)[a]	Number of Deaths in 2018	Age-Standardized Rate (per 100,000)
Mexico	7,266	10.6	1,128	1.6
Canada	8,180	23.6	1,247	2.7
United States	57,004	20.1	10,647	3.0

[a] The standard population used for the age-standardized rate is the world standard population
   Data from Ferlay J, Soerjomataram I, Mery L, et al. GLOBOCAN 2018: Cancer Today 2018 IARC.
Available at: http://gco.iarc.fr/today. Accessed October 25, 2018.

radiotherapy and/or CT did improve survival for women with aggressive histologies and for women with advanced-stage disease. Women with aggressive histologies have a much worse prognosis, and in these patients, it is certainly possible there is a real survival benefit from adjuvant therapy.

In the United States, endometrial cancer incidence is rising across all ethnic groups, with rates rising most in black and Asian women.[30] African Americans continue to have a lower rate of survival, possibly related to an increase in aggressive histologies, differing biologic factors,[31] and socioeconomic disparities that contribute to both poorer health in general, and less access to health care.[32] Some studies suggest that when factors such as socioeconomic status and health care coverage are controlled for, outcomes are similar for African American patients.[33] However, most studies indicate there is a real increase in aggressive histologies and differences in tumor biologic factors in black women,[31] and this contributes to poorer survival.[34]

Cervical Cancer

Incidence and mortality rates of cervical cancer are described in **Table 8**.

Cervical cancer is the most common gynecologic malignancy worldwide. Screening programs have led to lower rates in high income countries, and vaccination programs are expected to significantly lower incidence rates even further. In Canada and the USA, the incidence and mortality rates from cervical cancer were stable between 2008 and 2018; however, incidence decreased in Mexico over the same time frame (see **Table 8**).

The recent population-based literature reiterates findings known from the past. Two studies evaluated structural variables in cervix cancer treatment, and found that uninsured patients had worse outcomes, and patients treated by high-volume physicians for their brachytherapy had better outcomes (**Table 9**). In terms of process outcomes, high-quality radiation, with few treatment delays, and including concurrent chemotherapy and intracavitary brachytherapy is associated with improved survival

Table 6
Structural variables in relation to outcomes for uterine cancer

Study	Country	Data Source	Number of Patients	Did Structure Impact Survival?	Did Structure Impact Surrogate Outcomes?
Doll et al,[35] 2016	United States	Retrospective database	2053	Yes	Yes
Wright et al,[36] 2012	United States	Retrospective database	4137	N/A	No

Table 7
Process variables in relation to outcomes for uterine cancer

Study	Country	Data Source	Number of Patients	Did Process Impact Survival?	Which Process Variables Affected Survival?
Papathemelis et al,[37] 2017	Germany	Retrospective database	284	Yes	Surgical staging
Holloway et al,[38] 2017	Canada	Retrospective database	57	Yes	Adjuvant CT
Matsuo et al,[39] 2017	United States	Retrospective database (SEER)	323	Yes	Adjuvant radiotherpay
Wong et al,[40] 2017	United States	Retrospective database (national cancer database)	61,697	Yes	Adjuvant radiotherapy
Mahdi et al,[41] 2016	United States	Retrospective database (SEER)	317	Yes	Adjuvant radiotherapy
Manzerova et al,[42] 2016	United States	Retrospective database (SEER)	2342	Yes	Adjuvant radiotherapy
Gockley et al,[43] 2016	United States	Retrospective database (national cancer database)	3212	Yes / No	Adjuvant CT or CT + radiotherapy / Adjuvant treatment for early stage clear cell
Mahdi et al,[45] 2015	United States	Retrospective database (SEER)	1838	Yes	Adjuvant CT + radiotherapy
Wright et al,[44] 2016	United Stats	Retrospective database (national cancer database)	15,648	No	Ovarian conservation in young women
Acharya et al,[46] 2015	United States	Retrospective database (SEER)	460	Yes	Brachytherapy
Rauh-Hain et al,[47] 2015	United States	Retrospective database (national cancer database)	13,752	Yes	Adjuvant CT+
Rauh-Hain et al,[48] 2015	United States	Retrospective database (national cancer database)	10,609	Yes	Adjuvant CT or CT + radiotherapy
Garg et al,[49] 2014	United States	Retrospective database (SEER)	462	No	Adjuvant CT
Mell et al,[29] 2013	United States	Retrospective database (SEER)	58,172	No	Adjuvant radiotherapy
Hanna et al,[50] 2012	Canada	Retrospective database	9411	Yes	Adjuvant radiotherapy
Boll et al,[51] 2011	Netherlands	Retrospective database	2099	No	Adjuvant radiotherapy

Table 8
Cervical cancer incidence and mortality rates

Country	Incidence		Mortality	
	Number of Cases in 2018	Age-Standardized Rate (per 100,000)[a]	Number of Deaths in 2018	Age-Standardized Rate (per 100,000)
Mexico	7,869	11.0	4,121	5.8
Canada	1,434	7.7	586	1.7
United States	14.065	6.5	5,266	1.9

[a] The standard population used for the age-standardized (ASR) rate is the world standard population.
    Data from Ferlay J, Soerjomataram I, Mery L, et al. GLOBOCAN 2018: Cancer Today 2018 IARC. Available at: http://gco.iarc.fr/today. Accessed October 25, 2018.

(**Table 10**). Interestingly, the addition of chemotherapy to radiotherapy for adjuvant treatment of cervical cancer patients with the intermediate, so-called 'Sedlis' criteria, did not improve survival at a population level.

Cervical cancer highlights health care and socioeconomic disparities. In the United States, black women have a higher incidence of cervical cancer, and also have double the rate of mortality compared with non-Hispanic white women.[31] In part this is related to lower rates of follow-up with colposcopy and treatment for abnormal cytology, which could account for the higher rate of more advanced disease. In the United States, women with low socioeconomic status and no health insurance coverage had lower rates of knowledge about the human papilloma virus (HPV) and the HPV vaccines,[52] and black and Hispanic adolescent girls are less likely to complete the HPV vaccination schedule. Adolescents living below the poverty line are less likely to complete the vaccination schedule, regardless of race.[31] When access to health care is equally available, and other aspects of socioeconomic status are equal (eg, members of the US Armed Forces), outcomes for women with cervical cancer are unaffected by race. Additional disparities exist for patients with cervical cancer who are older,[51,52] or who live far away from a comprehensive cancer center. Lowering the incidence and mortality from cervical cancer will likely depend, in large part, on increasing access to preventive health care and high-quality treatment. The US Department of Health and Human Services has listed improving access to health care as a major component of the Healthy People 2020 initiative.[53]

Vulvar Cancer

Table 11 Shows the incidence rates for vulvar cancer.[68]

There were 2 studies that addressed structural variables; however, survival was not assessed (**Table 12**). Surgeon type affected whether a groin node dissection

Table 9
Structural variables in relation to outcomes for cervical cancer

Study	Country	Data Source	Number of Patients	Did Structure Impact Survival?	Did Structure Impact Surrogate Outcomes?
Churilla et al,[54] 2016	United States	Retrospective database (SEER)	11,714	Yes	Yes
Lee et al,[55] 2014	Taiwan	Retrospective database	818	Yes	Not available

Table 10
Process variables in relation to outcomes for cervical cancer

Study	Country	Data Source	Number of Patients	Did Process Impact Survival?	Which Process Variables Affected Survival?
Chiew et al,[56] 2017	Australia	Retrospective database	208	Yes	Adherence to guidelines
Jhawar et al,[57] 2017	United States	Retrospective database (national cancer database)	3051	Yes	High-quality radiotherapy
Zhou et al,[58] 2017	United States	Retrospective database (SEER)	2773	Yes	Appropriate surgery
Mahmoud et al,[59] 2016	United States	Retrospective database (national cancer database)	869	No	CT to radiotherapy for intermediate risk factors
Mayadev et al,[60] 2018	United States	Retrospective database (California Cancer Registry)	4783	Yes	Brachytherapy
Haque et al,[61] 2018	United States	Retrospective database (national cancer database)	1691	No	Hysterectomy after chemoradiation
Shen et al,[62] 2016	Taiwan	Retrospective database	9081	Yes	Treatment delays
Tergas et al,[63] 2016	United States	Retrospective database (national cancer database)	7209	Yes	Radiotherapy duration >10 wk
Trifiletti et al,[64] 2015	United States	Retrospective database (national cancer database)	3053	Yes	CT to radiotherapy
Kang et al,[65] 2015	Canada	Retrospective database	1085	Yes	CT to radiotherapy
Lim & Sia,[66] 2012	Australia	Retrospective database	69	Yes	Brachytherapy
Mahmud et al,[67] 2011	Canada	Retrospective database	714	Yes	Brachytherapy

Table 11				
Incidence and rates of vulvar cancers in Canada and Surveillance, Epidemiology, and End Results from 2003 to 2007				
Country	Period	Number of Cancers	Crude Rate	ASR
Mexico	—	—	—	—
Canada	2003–2007	2044	2.5	1.4
United States	2003–2007	4909	2.5	1.4

Modified from Bruni L, Barrionuevo-Rosas L, Albero G, et al. ICO/IARC information centre on HPV and cancer (HPV Information Centre). Human papillomavirus and related diseases in the world. Summary Report 27 July 2017; with permission.

was completed.[69] Sentinel node surgery was more likely in teaching hospitals and HVCs.[70] There were 3 studies that addressed process variables and their impact on survival. Groin surgery decreased the rate of groin recurrence but had no impact on survival.[71] Those who had groin radiation did have a lower survival, but radiotherapy was likely a confounder for more aggressive disease as opposed to a direct cause. These data showed the importance of pathology review on treatment decision making.[72]

SEER shows that per 100,000 women, 2.7 white women and 1.8 black women will develop vulvar cancer.[60] In their prior report,[2] the authors showed that there were racial disparities in relative survival. There was no new data on this topic in this review. Rauh-Hain[74] reviewed the 1988 to 2009 SEER data and showed that age influenced the rates of appropriate surgery. In particular, women over 80 years old are less likely to receive a groin node dissection. Five-year survival in older women (52.5%) is worse than in younger women (87.5%).

SUMMARY

Population-based data are valuable sources for identifying variations in care and determining whether structure and/or process related issues impact on survival. High-quality data from all data sources and adjustment for confounding variables wherever possible are important to make conclusions that are true and not biased. As a result, there is a movement toward centralization of gynecologic cancer care delivery in HVCs. It is clear that HVCs are key to minimizing failure to rescue in the perioperative period[17] and guideline adherence. The value of centralized care is clear in ovarian cancer. Additional research is required to assess its value in the care of women with aggressive endometrial cancer histologies and for cervix and vulvar cancers. It appears that patients with early stage low-grade endometrial cancer may not benefit substantially from centralization of care, in terms of oncologic outcomes.

It appears that processes of care are different in women who are older, from a minority, and from lower income strata. These women suffer a disproportionate amount of the gynecologic cancer-related mortality and often do not receive evidence-based care. Understanding the reason for gaps between care that is recommended and what is actually delivered is important[25] and should be an area of inquiry in the future.

A look at the 3 North American health care systems shows there are issues with women having access to high-quality, timely care. Society must decide if people have a right to health care. Countries must decide if they will strive to meet the

Table 12
Structure and process variables in relation to outcomes for vulvar cancer

Study	Country	Data Source	Number of Patients	Did Structure Variables Impact Survival?	Did Structure Variables Impact Surrogate Outcomes?	Did Process Variables Impact Survival?
Barbera et al,[72] 2017	Canada	Ontario Cancer Registry	1038	Not addressed	Not addressed; pathology review	Not addressed; change in treatment decision
Cham et al,[70] 2016	United States	Prospective database >500 US hospitals	2273	Not addressed; volume of surgeries, teaching centers	Yes; sentinel node surgery	
Gien et al,[69] 2015	Canada	Ontario Cancer Registry	1038	Not evaluated; surgeon type, hospital volumes	Yes	Yes
Gien et al,[71] 2017	Canada	Ontario Cancer Registry	1038	Not evaluated	Not evaluated; groin surgery, groin radiation	No
Mahner et al,[73] 2013	Germany	Prospective observational study CaRE1	1618		Radiotherapy	Yes
Rottmann et al,[75] 2016	Germany	Munich Cancer Registry	1113			No

sustainable development goal of UHC, where every individual should receive the health care they need without risking financial hardship.[76] Whether this kind of broad equitable access can be achieved for women with gynecologic cancers in North America remains to be seen.

ACKNOWLEDGMENTS

The authors would like to thank Nicole Gervais for her contribution to this article.

REFERENCES

1. Donabedian A. Evaluating the quality of medical care. Milbank Q 2005;83(4): 691–729.
2. Reade C, Elit L. Trends in gynecologic cancer care in north america. Obstet Gynecol Clin North Am 2012;39(2):107–29.
3. World Health Organization. Equity. 2018. Available at: http://www.who.int/healthsystems/topics/equity/en/. Accessed January 11, 2018.
4. World Health Organization. Universal health coverage (UHC). 2018. Available at: http://www.who.int/en/news-room/fact-sheets/detail/universal-health-coverage-(uhc). Accessed January 11, 2018.
5. Pan American Health Organizations, World Health Organization. Health in the Americas. Country report: Mexico. 2015. Available at: https://www.paho.org/salud-en-las-americas-2017/?page_id=137. Accessed January 11, 2018.
6. Pan American Health Organizations, World Health Organization. Health in the Americas. Country report: Canada. 2015. Available at: https://www.paho.org/salud-en-las-americas-2017/?page_id=101. Accessed January 11, 2018.
7. Pan American Health Organizations, World Health Organization. Health in the Americas. Country report: United States of America. 2015. Available at: https://www.paho.org/salud-en-las-americas-2017/?page_id=165. Accessed January 11, 2018.
8. Organization for Economic Co-operation and Development. Health systems characteristics. 2016. Available at: http://www.oecd.org/health/characteristics.htm. Accessed January 11, 2018.
9. The Commonwealth Fund. The U.S. health care system. 2017. Available at: http://international.commonwealthfund.org/countries/united_states/. Accessed June 3, 2018.
10. Organization for Economic Co-operation and Development. Caring for quality in health: lessons learnt from 15 reviews of health care quality. 2017.
11. Dahm-Kahler P, Borgfeldt C, Holmberg E, et al. Population-based study of survival for women with serous cancer of the ovary, fallopian tube, peritoneum or undesignated origin - on behalf of the swedish gynecological cancer group (SweGCG). Gynecol Oncol 2017;144(1):167–73.
12. Eggink FA, Mom CH, Kruitwagen RF, et al. Improved outcomes due to changes in organization of care for patients with ovarian cancer in the Netherlands. Gynecol Oncol 2016;141(3):524–30.
13. Shakeel S, Elit L, Akhtar-Danesh N, et al. Care delivery patterns, processes, and outcomes for primary ovarian cancer surgery: a population-based review using a national administrative database. J Obstet Gynaecol Can 2017;39(1):25–33.
14. Dahm-Kahler P, Palmqvist C, Staf C, et al. Centralized primary care of advanced ovarian cancer improves complete cytoreduction and survival - a population-based cohort study. Gynecol Oncol 2016;142(2):211–6.

15. Bristow RE, Ueda S, Gerardi MA, et al. Analysis of racial disparities in stage IIIC epithelial ovarian cancer care and outcomes in a tertiary gynecologic oncology referral center. Gynecol Oncol 2011;122(2):319–23.
16. Bristow RE, Powell MA, Al-Hammadi N, et al. Disparities in ovarian cancer care quality and survival according to race and socioeconomic status. J Natl Cancer Inst 2013;105(11):823–32.
17. Dehaeck U, McGahan CE, Santos JL, et al. The impact of geographic variations in treatment on outcomes in ovarian cancer. Int J Gynecol Cancer 2013;23(2): 282–7.
18. Leandersson P, Granasen G, Borgfeldt C. Ovarian cancer surgery - a population-based registry study. Anticancer Res 2017;37(4):1837–45.
19. Mandato VD, Abrate M, De Iaco P, et al. Clinical governance network for clinical audit to improve quality in epithelial ovarian cancer management. J Ovarian Res 2013;6(1):19.
20. Urban RR, He H, Alfonso R, et al. Ovarian cancer outcomes: predictors of early death. Gynecol Oncol 2016;140(3):474–80.
21. Warren JL, Harlan LC, Trimble EL, et al. Trends in the receipt of guideline care and survival for women with ovarian cancer: a population-based study. Gynecol Oncol 2017;145(3):486–92.
22. van de Laar R, Kruitwagen RF, IntHout J, et al. Surgery for recurrent epithelial ovarian cancer in the Netherlands: a population-based cohort study. Int J Gynecol Cancer 2016;26(2):268–75.
23. Jordan S, Steer C, DeFazio A, et al. Patterns of chemotherapy treatment for women with invasive epithelial ovarian cancer–a population-based study. Gynecol Oncol 2013;129(2):310–7.
24. Institute of Medicine. The unequal burden of cancer: an assessment of NIH research and programs for ethnic minorities and the medically underserved. Washington, DC: The National Academies Press; 1999. Available at: https://www.nap.edu/catalog/6377/the-unequal-burden-of-cancer-an-assessment-of-nih-research.
25. Winter WE III, Maxwell GL, Tian C, et al. Prognostic factors for stage III epithelial ovarian cancer: a gynecologic oncology group study. J Clin Oncol 2007;25(24): 3621–7.
26. Chatterjee S, Chen L, Tergas AI, et al. Utilization and outcomes of chemotherapy in women with intermediate-risk, early-stage ovarian cancer. Obstet Gynecol 2016;127(6):992–1002.
27. Eskander RN, Chang J, Ziogas A, et al. Evaluation of 30-day hospital readmission after surgery for advanced-stage ovarian cancer in a medicare population. J Clin Oncol 2014;32(36):4113–9.
28. Lee JY, Kim TH, Suh DH, et al. Impact of guideline adherence on patient outcomes in early-stage epithelial ovarian cancer. Eur J Surg Oncol 2015;41(4): 585–91.
29. Mell LK, Carmona R, Gulaya S, et al. Cause-specific effects of radiotherapy and lymphadenectomy in stage I–II endometrial cancer: a population-based study. J Natl Cancer Inst 2013;105(21):1656–66.
30. Cote ML, Ruterbusch JJ, Olson SH, et al. The growing burden of endometrial cancer: a major racial disparity affecting black women. Cancer Epidemiol Biomarkers Prev 2015;24(9):1407–15.
31. Collins Y, Holcomb K, Chapman-Davis E, et al. Gynecologic cancer disparities: a report from the health disparities taskforce of the society of gynecologic oncology. Gynecol Oncol 2014;133(2):353–61.

32. Long B, Liu FW, Bristow RE. Disparities in uterine cancer epidemiology, treatment, and survival among african americans in the united states. Gynecol Oncol 2013;130(3):652–9.

33. Rauh-Hain JA, Buskwofie A, Clemmer J, et al. Racial disparities in treatment of high-grade endometrial cancer in the medicare population. Obstet Gynecol 2015;125(4):843–51.

34. Mahdi H, Han X, Abdul-Karim F, et al. Racial disparity in survival of patients with uterine serous carcinoma: Changes in clinical characteristics, patterns of care and outcomes over time from 1988 to 2011. Gynecol Oncol 2016;143(2):334–45.

35. Doll KM, Meng K, Gehrig PA, et al. Referral patterns between high-and low-volume centers and associations with uterine cancer treatment and survival: a population-based study of medicare, medicaid, and privately insured women. Am J Obstet Gynecol 2016;215(4):447.e1-13.

36. Wright JD, Hershman DL, Burke WM, et al. Influence of surgical volume on outcome for laparoscopic hysterectomy for endometrial cancer. Ann Surg Oncol 2012;19(3):948–58.

37. Papathemelis T, Scharl S, Kronberger K, et al. Survival benefit of pelvic and para-aortic lymphadenectomy in high-grade endometrial carcinoma: a retrospective population-based cohort analysis. J Cancer Res Clin Oncol 2017;143(12):2555–62.

38. Holloway CL, Alexander C, Walter C, et al. Stage IIIC endometrial cancer: Relapse and survival outcomes in women treated with pelvic or extended field para-aortic nodal radiation therapy. Am J Clin Oncol 2017;40(5):458–63.

39. Matsuo K, Machida H, Ragab OM, et al. Patient compliance for postoperative radiotherapy and survival outcome of women with stage I endometrioid endometrial cancer. J Surg Oncol 2017;116(4):482–91.

40. Wong AT, Rineer J, Schwartz D, et al. Patterns of adjuvant radiation usage and survival outcomes for stage I endometrial carcinoma in a large hospital-based cohort. Gynecol Oncol 2017;144(1):113–8.

41. Mahdi H, Moulton L, Nutter B, et al. The impact of combined radiation and chemotherapy on outcome in uterine clear cell carcinoma compared with chemotherapy alone. Clin Oncol 2016;28(12):776–82.

42. Manzerova J, Sison CP, Gupta D, et al. Adjuvant radiation therapy in uterine carcinosarcoma: a population-based analysis of patient demographic and clinical characteristics, patterns of care and outcomes. Gynecol Oncol 2016;141(2):225–30.

43. Gockley AA, Rauh-Hain JA, Anders AM, et al. Patterns of care, predictors, and outcomes of adjuvant therapy for early- and advanced-stage uterine clear cell carcinoma: a population-based analysis. Int J Gynecol Cancer 2016;26(4):697–704.

44. Wright JD, Jorge S, Tergas AI, et al. Utilization and outcomes of ovarian conservation in premenopausal women with endometrial cancer. Obstet Gynecol 2016;127(1):101–8.

45. Mahdi H, Nutter B, Abdul-Karim F, et al. The impact of combined radiation and chemotherapy on outcome in uterine papillary serous carcinoma compared to chemotherapy alone. J Gynecol Oncol 2015;27(2):e19.

46. Acharya S, Perkins SM, DeWees T, et al. Brachytherapy is associated with improved survival in inoperable stage I endometrial adenocarcinoma: a population-based analysis. Int J Radiat Oncol Biol Phys 2015;93(3):649–57.

47. Rauh-Hain JA, Diver E, Meyer LA, et al. Patterns of care, associations and outcomes of chemotherapy for uterine serous carcinoma: analysis of the national cancer database. Gynecol Oncol 2015;139(1):77–83.
48. Rauh-Hain JA, Starbuck KD, Meyer LA, et al. Patterns of care, predictors and outcomes of chemotherapy for uterine carcinosarcoma: a national cancer database analysis. Gynecol Oncol 2015;139(1):84–9.
49. Garg G, Yee C, Schwartz K, et al. Patterns of care, predictors, and outcomes of chemotherapy in elderly women with early-stage uterine carcinosarcoma: a population-based analysis. Gynecol Oncol 2014;133(2):242–9.
50. Hanna T, Richardson H, Peng Y, et al. A population-based study of factors affecting the use of radiotherapy for endometrial cancer. Clin Oncol 2012;24(8):e113–24.
51. Boll D, Verhoeven RH, van der Aa MA, et al. Adherence to national guidelines for treatment and outcome of endometrial cancer stage I in relation to co-morbidity in southern netherlands 1995-2008. Eur J Cancer 2011;47(10):1504–10.
52. Radecki BC, Finney Rutten LJ, Victoria F, et al. Awareness and knowledge of human papillomavirus (HPV), HPV-related cancers, and HPV vaccines in an uninsured adult clinic population. Cancer Med 2016;5(11):3346–52.
53. Dumas L, Ring A, Butler J, et al. Improving outcomes for older women with gynaecological malignancies. Cancer Treat Rev 2016;50:99–108.
54. Churilla T, Egleston B, Dong Y, et al. Disparities in the management and outcome of cervical cancer in the united states according to health insurance status. Gynecol Oncol 2016;141(3):516–23.
55. Lee M, Tsai S, Lee C, et al. Higher caseload improves cervical cancer survival in patients treated with brachytherapy. Radiat Oncol 2014;9(1):234.
56. Chiew KL, Shanley C, Duggan Kirsten J, et al. Assessing guideline adherence and patient outcomes in cervical cancer. Asia-Pac J Clin Oncol 2017;13(5):e373–80.
57. Jhawar S, Hathout L, Elshaikh MA, et al. Adjuvant chemoradiation therapy for cervical cancer and effect of timing and duration on treatment outcome. Int J Radiat Oncol Biol Phys 2017;98(5):1132–41.
58. Zhou J, Wu S, Sun J, et al. The effect of local treatment modalities in patients with early-stage adenocarcinoma of the uterine cervix: a population-based analysis. Int J Surg 2017;41:16–22.
59. Mahmoud O, Hathout L, Shaaban SG, et al. Can chemotherapy boost the survival benefit of adjuvant radiotherapy in early stage cervical cancer with intermediate risk factors? A population based study. Gynecol Oncol 2016;143(3):539–44.
60. Mayadev J, Klapheke A, Yashar C, et al. Underutilization of brachytherapy and disparities in survival for patients with cervical cancer in California. Gynecol Oncol 2018;150(1):73–8.
61. Haque W, Verma V, Butler EB, et al. Utilization of hysterectomy following chemoradiation for IB2/IIA2 cervical cancer in the national cancer data base. Anticancer Res 2018;38(5):3175–9.
62. Shen S, Hung Y, Kung P, et al. Factors involved in the delay of treatment initiation for cervical cancer patients: a nationwide population-based study. Medicine 2016;95(33):e4568.
63. Tergas AI, Neugut AI, Chen L, et al. Radiation duration in women with cervical cancer treated with primary chemoradiation: a population-based analysis. Cancer Invest 2016;34(3):137–47.
64. Trifiletti DM, Swisher-McClure S, Showalter TN, et al. Postoperative chemoradiation therapy in high-risk cervical cancer: Re-evaluating the findings of

gynecologic oncology group study 109 in a large, population-based cohort. Int J Radiat Oncol Biol Phys 2015;93(5):1032–44.

65. Kang Y, O'Connell DL, Lotocki R, et al. Effect of changes in treatment practice on survival for cervical cancer: results from a population-based study in Manitoba, Canada. BMC Cancer 2015;15(1):642.

66. Lim A, Sia S. Outcomes of chemoradiotherapy in cervical cancer—the western Australian experience. Int J Radiat Oncol Biol Phys 2012;82(4):1431–8.

67. Mahmud A, Brydon B, Tonita J, et al. A population-based study of cervix cancer: Incidence, management and outcome in the Canadian province of Saskatchewan. Clin Oncol 2011;23(10):691–5.

68. Bruni L, Barrionuevo-Rosas L, Albero G, et al. Human papillomavirus and related diseases in the world. Summary report 27 July 2017. Table 8. 2017.

69. Gien LT, Sutradhar R, Thomas G, et al. Patient, tumor, and health system factors affecting groin node dissection rates in vulvar carcinoma: a population-based cohort study. Gynecol Oncol 2015;139(3):465–70.

70. Cham S, Chen L, Burke WM, et al. Utilization and outcomes of sentinel lymph node biopsy for vulvar cancer. Obstet Gynecol 2016;128(4):754–60.

71. Gien LT, Sutradhar R, Thomas G, et al. Does a groin node dissection in vulvar cancer affect groin recurrence and overall survival?: Results from a population-based cohort study. Gynecol Oncol 2017;144(2):318–23.

72. Barbera L, Gien LT, Sutradhar R, et al. The added value of pathology review in vulvar cancer: Results from a population-based cohort study. Int J Gynecol Pathol 2017;36(2):107–10.

73. Mahner S, Eulenburg C, Staehle A, et al. Prognostic impact of the time interval between surgery and chemotherapy in advanced ovarian cancer: analysis of prospective randomised phase III trials. Eur J Cancer 2013;49(1):142–9.

74. Rauh-Hain J, Clemmer J, Clark R, et al. Management and outcomes for elderly women with vulvar cancer over time. BJOG 2014;121(6):719–27.

75. Rottmann M, Beck T, Burges A, et al. Trends in surgery and outcomes of squamous cell vulvar cancer patients over a 16-year period (1998–2013): a population-based analysis. J Cancer Res Clin Oncol 2016;142(6):1331–41.

76. UN General Assembly. Resolution adopted by the General Assembly on 25 September 2015. 2015. Available at: http://www.un.org/en/development/desa/population/migration/generalassembly/docs/globalcompact/A_RES_70_1_E.pdf. Accessed February 6, 2018.

Cancer Screening and Prevention Highlights in Gynecologic Cancer

Jeanine N. Staples, MD, MPH*, Linda R. Duska, MD, MPH

KEYWORDS

- Vaccine • HPV • Screening • Prevention

KEY POINTS

- Women should receive treatment for precancerous conditions of the cervix, vulva, vagina and endometrial lining.
- Women with inherited conditions should consider having a risk-reducing surgery once they have finished childbearing.
- Use of oral contraceptive pills significantly reduces the risk of endometrial cancer and ovarian cancer in both low- and high-risk populations.
- The target age for human papilloma virus vaccination is 11 to 12 years for girls and boys, but the vaccine can be given as early as age 9 through 45 years of age.

INTRODUCTION

In 2018, an estimated 110,070 cases of gynecologic cancers will be diagnosed among women in the United States, including malignancies of the uterus, cervix, ovary, vagina and vulva.[1] Gynecologic malignancies represent 13% of all cancers diagnosed among women in the United States and contribute to 32,120 annual deaths.[1] One in 162 women will be diagnosed with cervical cancer in her lifetime[1]; 1 in 78 women will be diagnosed with ovarian cancer,[2] and 1 in 35 women will be diagnosed with uterine cancer.[1] Identifying high-risk populations and ensuring appropriate screening and preventative measures are critical to decreasing the morbidity and mortality associated with these malignancies.

ENDOMETRIAL CANCER
Epidemiology and Risk Factors

Endometrial cancer is the most common gynecologic malignancy in developed countries, including the United States.[1] An estimated 63,230 women will be

Disclosure: The authors have no disclosures.
Division of Gynecology Oncology, Department of Obstetrics and Gynecology, University of Virginia, University of Virginia Medical Center, PO Box 800712, Charlottesville, VA 22908, USA
* Corresponding author.
E-mail address: js6qf@hscmail.mcc.virginia.edu

diagnosed with uterine cancer in the United States in 2018, and 11,350 will die from the disease.[1] More than 90% of cases arise from the endometrium, and the remaining cases develop within the corpus.[3] The age-standardized incidence is 26.0 cases per 100,000 women with a cumulative lifetime risk of 2.9%.[4] Over the last decade, the number of new uterine cancer cases has risen on average 1.3% per year, with an annual increase in death rate of approximately 1.6%.[4] Worldwide, endometrial cancer accounts for an estimated 320,000 new cases and 76,000 deaths annually.[5] The highest incidence rates are seen in Northern America and northern and western Europe.[4]

Endometrial carcinoma can be classified into 2 different histologic subtypes, with distinct genetic, molecular, and clinico-pathological features. Endometrioid adenocarcinomas (type 1) represent the vast majority (80%–90%) of endometrial cancers.[6] This subtype is most often confined to the uterus at presentation. leading to a more favorable prognosis.[6] Type 2 endometrial cancers include high-grade endometrioid adenocarcinomas, as well as serous, clear cell, carcinosarcoma, or otherwise undifferentiated carcinomas. Type 2 cancers tend to be high-grade, deeply invasive tumors and account for about 40% of deaths from endometrial cancer.[7] **Table 1** describes the major differences between these 2 subtypes.

Type I cancers are associated with unopposed estrogen exposure; thus risk factors include anything that perpetuates this clinical scenario.[9] **Table 2** describes the risk and protective factors associated with type 1 endometrial cancer.

In a meta-analysis of 24 epidemiologic studies evaluating risk factors for type 2 tumors, the authors found that parity, oral contraceptive use, cigarette smoking, age at menarche, and diabetes were associated with type 1 and type 2 tumors to a similar extent.[12] However, body mass index (BMI) had a greater effect on type 1 tumors

Table 1
Characteristics of type 1 and type 2 endometrial carcinomas

Characteristic	Type 1 (85%)	Type 2 (15%)
Histology	Endometrioid grades 1–2	Endometrioid grade 3, serous, clear cell, carcinosarcoma, otherwise undifferentiated carcinomas
Genetic alteration	Loss of PTEN function, KRAS, CTNNB1 and PIK3CA and MLH1 promoter hypermethylation	P53, Her-2/neu overexpression and amplification, inactivation of p16, loss of E-cadherin
Background histology	Hyperplasia	Atrophy
Preceding histology	Atypical hyperplasia Endometrial intraepithelial neoplasia (EIN)	Endometrial intraepithelial carcinoma (EIC)
Association with estrogen stimulation	+++	+
Differentiation	Well to moderate	Poor
Growth	Slow-growing	Rapid progression
Invasion	Superficial	Deep
Typical patient	Perimenopausal, obese	Older women, thin
Clinical course	Indolent	Aggressive
Stage at diagnosis	Early	Later
Prognosis	Good	Poor

Data from Refs.[6–8]

Table 2	
Risk factors for endometrial cancer	
Risk Factor	**Relative Risk**
Genetic predisposition (MLH1 or MSH2 mutation)	14–21
Long-term exogenous estrogen use	10–20
High cumulative doses of tamoxifen	3–7
Polycystic ovarian syndrome	>5
Estrogen-producing tumors	>5
Obesity	2–5
Nulliparity	3
Late age of menopause	2–3
Older age	2–3
History of infertility	2–3
History of diabetes, hypertension, or gallbladder disease	1.3–3
White race	2
Menstrual irregularity	1.5
Endometrial hyperplasia without atypia	1.01–1.03
Atypical endometrial hyperplasia	14–45
Protective Factor	**Relative Risk**
Long-term use of oral contraceptives	0.3–05
Cigarette smoking	0.5
Breast feeding	0.7

Data from Refs.[9–12]

than on type 2 tumors. Furthermore, risk factor patterns for high-grade endometrioid tumors and type 2 tumors were similar.

Inherited Genetic Risk

About 5% of endometrial cancers are hereditary.[13] Most inherited cases are caused by hereditary nonpolyposis colorectal cancer (HNPCC), also known as Lynch syndrome. Lynch syndrome is inherited in an autosomal-dominant fashion with incomplete penetrance caused by a germline mutation in one of the mismatch repair genes, including MLH1, MSH2, MSH6, or PMS2.[14] It is characterized by a high lifetime incidence of colorectal cancer and gynecologic malignancies. Several studies have highlighted that for women, the risk of endometrial cancer actually exceeds the risk for colon cancer.[14,15] Moreover, among women, more than half of Lynch-associated malignancies present with a gynecologic cancer as their sentinel cancer.[16] Women with Lynch syndrome have a 50% to 70% lifetime risk of developing endometrial cancer and a 9% to 12% lifetime risk of developing ovarian cancer.[17,18]

Endometrial Cancer Screening Tests

There is no standard screening test for endometrial cancer in asymptomatic women. In symptomatic women or for women who are high risk, endometrial tissue sampling and transvaginal ultrasonography may be used for evaluation of malignancy.

Endometrial curettage has historically been the preferred method for obtaining a tissue sample. Use of the office endometrial biopsy offers a less expensive and less invasive alternative, with detection rates of 99.6% and 91% for endometrial cancer in postmenopausal and premenopausal women, respectively.[19]

Screening for Low-Risk Individuals

For asymptomatic women in the general population without risk factors, there is no evidence to support endometrial cancer screening. Studies show that screening asymptomatic low-risk women with ultrasound leads to false-positive test results, resulting in unwarranted biopsies.[20] For asymptomatic women with incidentally discovered endometrial thickening on ultrasound, The American College of Obstetricians and Gynecologists (ACOG) recommends against routine further investigation.[20] Decisions about further investigations should be made on a case-by-case basis in asymptomatic women with increased endometrial thickening and risk factors such as obesity, diabetes, or late menopause.[20] Women taking tamoxifen should be counseled about the increased risk of endometrial cancer and symptoms to monitor. They do not, however, require additional monitoring beyond routine gynecologic care.[21] Tissue sampling should only be performed in the following asymptomatic patients: (1) women with granulosa cell tumor (or other estrogen-secreting tumor) in whom hysterectomy has not been performed,[22] (2) patients with epithelial ovarian cancer who desire fertility-sparing treatment,[23] and (3) individuals with Lynch syndrome who have an intact uterus.[13]

Screening for High-Risk Individuals

Recommendations for screening among patients with Lynch syndrome are based on expert opinion. Even in this high-risk population, surveillance by transvaginal ultrasonography, hysteroscopy, and endometrial biopsy is of unproven benefit.[24] The age at initiation of cancer surveillance is also controversial. The risk of endometrial cancer rises significantly after the age of 40, with a mean diagnosis at age 46 in patients with Lynch syndrome.[25] Thus, the Cancer Genetics Consortium gynecologic cancer screening guidelines for women with Lynch syndrome include annual endometrial sampling and transvaginal ultrasonography at age 30 to 35 years or 5 to 10 years prior to the earliest age of first diagnosis of Lynch-associated cancer of any kind in the family.[26] Similarly, ACOG recommends endometrial biopsy every 1 to 2 years, beginning at age 30 to 35 years.[13] Ultrasound likely does not improve efficacy of screening for endometrial cancer when used in combination with sampling. Rather, the main role of ultrasound in women with Lynch syndrome is ovarian cancer screening.[13]

Prevention

In low-risk women, reducing risk factors and introducing protective factors into lifestyle may lower the risk of endometrial cancer development. Women should be counseled on risk factors and encouraged to maintain a healthy weight, active lifestyle, and optimal blood pressure and diabetes control. For women taking hormone replacement therapy to control menopausal symptoms, unopposed estrogen should never be started in women with a uterus in situ. Rather, a combination of estrogen and progesterone is preferred. Also, treatment for atypical hyperplasia is crucial in preventing progression to endometrial cancer.

The use of combined oral contraceptive pills, depo medroprogesterone acetate, and the levonorgestrel intrauterine device (IUD) have all been shown to decrease risk of developing endometrial cancer.[27–29] The cancer and steroid hormone case-control studies demonstrated a 50% reduction in the risk of endometrial and ovarian cancer associated with the use of oral contraceptive pills (OCPs).[27] Women who reported use of OCPs for at least 1 year had an age-adjusted risk of 0.6 (95% confidence interval [CI] 0.3–0.9), which persisted for at least 15 years following cessation of use. The protective effect was independent of the type of histology, and independent of the dosage and type of progestogen. Furthermore, the Norwegian Women and Cancer study showed that the levonorgestrel-releasing intrauterine system (LNG-IUS) reduces endometrial cancer risk by 78%.[29]

For individuals with Lynch syndrome, prophylactic hysterectomy and bilateral salpingo-oophorectomy should be discussed at age 40 or once child bearing is complete.[26] Cost-effectiveness analyses of management strategies for women with Lynch syndrome support use of prophylactic surgery rather than other surveillance and prevention methods.[30]

Lastly, identification of high-risk individuals is important for implementing the screening and preventative measures mentioned previously. The Bethesda Guidelines were developed in 1997 and revised in 2004 to provide recommendations for which individuals should be considered for testing.[31] Limitations to the Bethesda Guidelines include low specificity and the exclusion of endometrial cancer as a sentinel cancer. To address this, The Society of Gynecologic Oncologists released a statement in 2007 to recommend genetic risk assessment in women who meet the criteria outlined in **Box 1**.

Germline DNA testing or direct tumor testing are the 2 methods of testing for a faulty mismatch repair system. Furthermore, universal tumor testing with microsatellite instability testing or tumor testing using immunohistochemistry has proven to be cost effective and highly sensitive for Lynch syndrome screening in patients with colorectal cancer and endometrial cancer.[32,33]

UTERINE SARCOMAS

Uterine sarcomas account for 9% of all cancers of the uterine corpus, yet contribute to a significant number of uterine cancer deaths.[34] The subtypes include leiomyosarcomas

---

Box 1
The 2004 Bethesda Guidelines to identify individuals with colorectal or endometrial cancer for whom genetic risk assessment is recommended (with modifications to include endometrial cancer as a sentinel cancer)

- Patients with endometrial or colorectal cancer diagnosed before age 50 years

- Patient with endometrial or ovarian cancer with a synchronous or metachronous colon or other Lynch/HNPCC-associated tumor[a] at any age

- Patients with colorectal cancer with tumor-infiltrating lymphocytes, peritumoral lymphocytes, Crohn-like lymphocytic reaction, mucinous/signet-ring differentiation, or medullary growth pattern diagnosed before age 60 years

- Patients with endometrial or colorectal cancer and a first-degree relative with a Lynch/HNPCC-associated tumor[a] diagnosed before age 50 years

- Patients with colorectal or endometrial cancer diagnosed at any age with 2 or more first-degree or second-degree relatives with Lynch/HNPCC- associated tumors, regardless of age

[a] Lynch/HNPCC-related tumors: colorectal, endometrial, stomach, ovarian, pancreas, ureter and renal pelvis, biliary tract, and brain tumors, sebaceous gland adenomas and keratoacanthomas in Muir-Torre syndrome, and carcinoma of the small bowel.

Adapted from Lancaster JM, Powell CB, Kauff ND, et al, Society of Gynecologic Oncologists Education Committee. Society of Gynecologic Oncologists Education Committee statement on risk assessment for inherited gynecologic cancer predispositions. Gynecol Oncol 2007;107(2):161; with permission.

(most common), endometrial stromal sarcomas, undifferentiated uterine sarcomas, and adenosarcomas.[35] Carcinosarcomas were historically classified as uterine sarcomas, however are now considered carcinomas, although they do have stromal differentiation. Risk factors include excess estrogen exposure, tamoxifen use, African-American race, and prior pelvic radiation.[36] Similar to endometrial carcinomas, OCPs and smoking appear to be protective.[36] Preoperative diagnosis of uterine sarcoma is often difficult because of the overlapping symptomatology seen with benign uterine fibroids, including abnormal uterine bleeding, pelvic pain, pressure, bloating, and distention.

The sensitivity of an office endometrial biopsy to detect leiomyosarcoma is lower than that for endometrial carcinomas.[36] Unfortunately, many sarcomas are not diagnosed until time of surgery. Power morcellation, a process that involves cutting up the specimen within the abdomen, has come under recent scrutiny because of the potential to unknowingly disseminate an otherwise contained occult malignancy. The US Food and Drug Administration (FDA) concluded that the risk of morcellating an unsuspected uterine sarcoma is 1 in 352, and the risk of morcellating an unsuspected uterine leiomyosarcoma is 1 in 498.[37] However, in a more rigorous meta-analysis of 133 studies published in 2015, the authors determined that the prevalence of leiomyosarcoma among women having surgery for presumed fibroids was actually 1 in 1960, or 0.051%.[38]

OVARIAN CANCER
Epidemiology and Risk Factors

In the United States, ovarian cancer is the tenth most common cancer among women, yet the fifth leading cause of cancer death.[1] Ovarian cancer is the cause of more deaths than any other female genital tract cancer. An estimated 22,240 new cases will be diagnosed in 2018, and 14,070 women will die from the disease. Based on 2013 to 2015 SEER data, approximately 1.3% of women will be diagnosed with ovarian cancer at some point during their lifetime.[4] Worldwide, ovarian cancer accounts for an estimated 239,000 new cases and 152,000 deaths annually.[5] The highest rates are seen in eastern and central Europe.[5]

Malignant ovarian tumors originate from 1 of 3 cell types: epithelial cells, stromal cells, and germ cells. Malignant germ cell tumors are more commonly seen in girls younger than age 20 years, whereas epithelial cancers of the ovary are primarily seen in women older than age 50.[39] Epithelial ovarian carcinomas account for 75% of all ovarian tumors and represent 90% to 95% of ovarian malignancies.[39] Epithelial tumors may arise from the ovarian surface epithelium but also may arise from fallopian tube or the peritoneum.[39] The more aggressive subtypes of epithelial ovarian cancer (high-grade serous and undifferentiated carcinomas) represent approximately 75% of all ovarian carcinomas and are responsible for 90% of deaths caused by ovarian cancer.[40] Women are commonly diagnosed with stage 3 or 4 disease (70%), for which 5-year survival rates are around 39% and 16%, respectively.[3] Efforts to develop early detection strategies using serum CA125 and ultrasound have been prioritized for the last 2 decades.

Epidemiologic research has long implicated hormonal and reproductive factors in the pathogenesis of ovarian cancers. The incessant ovulation theory hypothesizes that the number of ovulatory cycles increases the rate of cellular division associated with the repair of the surface epithelium after each ovulation, thereby increasing spontaneous mutations.[41] Thus, early age at menarche, late age at menopause, and nulliparity have all been shown to increase the risk of ovarian cancer.[42] **Table 3** describes other risk and protective factors associated with epithelial ovarian cancer.

Because of the heterogeneity of epithelial ovarian cancers, certain exposures have varying risks on the different subtypes. For example, smoking confers an increased

Table 3
Risk factors for ovarian cancer

Risk Factor	Relative Risk
Genetic predisposition	
Lynch syndrome	2–7
BRCA1	12–30
BRCA2	5–15
STK11	42
Family history of ovarian cancer	3–4
Family history of breast cancer	1–2
Personal history of breast cancer	3–4
Endometriosis	1–2
Early age at menarche	1–2
Late age of menopause	1–2
Older age	2–3
Obesity	1–2
Hormone replacement therapy	1–3
White race	2
Nulliparity	1–2
Infertility	1–2
Protective Factor	**Relative Risk**
Oral contraceptive use	0.4–0.6
Breastfeeding	0.6
Tubal ligation	0.4–0.7
Salpingectomy (bilateral, unilateral)	0.50, 0.65
Salpingo-oophorectomy	0.05

Data from Refs.[27,42–48]

risk for mucinous subtype, but a weak protective effect against endometrioid and clear cell subtypes.[42] Endometriosis increases risk of low-grade serous ovarian cancer (LGSOC), endometrioid and clear cell.[42] Tubal ligation confers a strong protection for endometrioid and clear cell and a weak protection on mucinous and high-grade serous ovarian cancer (HGSOC), with no protection against low-grade serous ovarian cancer (LGSOC).[42] Hormone therapy yields a moderate-strong risk for HGSOC. Lastly, BMI increases the risk of mucinous cancers.[42]

Inherited Genetic Risk

An estimated 23% of ovarian cancer diagnoses are linked to genetic predisposition.[49] Most hereditary breast and ovarian cancers are caused by mutations in the BRCA1 and BRCA2 genes.[49] Other genetic mutations associated with hereditary ovarian cancer include BRIP1, RAD51 C, RAD51D, and the genes associated with Lynch Syndrome (MSH2, MLH1, MSHH6, PMS2, and EPCAM).[49]

Women with BRCA1 mutation have a risk of ovarian cancer (including tubal and primary peritoneal) of approximately 39% to 46% by age 70 years, and 10% to 27% for BRCA2 mutations.[50,51] Ovarian cancer associated with BRCA1 and BRCA2 mutations usually is a high-grade EOC,[50,51] and a large percentage of cases may actually develop from the fallopian tube.[52]

Ovarian Cancer Screening Tests

The need for reliable serum biomarkers for early detection of ovarian cancer remains a long awaited priority. Despite its poor specificity, CA-125 is the most evaluated serum marker for ovarian cancer screening. CA-125 is a protein produced by more than 90% of advanced epithelial ovarian cancers.[53] It is currently US Food and Drug Administration (FDA) recommended to monitor response to therapy in patients with epithelial ovarian cancer and to detect residual or recurrent disease in patients who have undergone first-line therapy and would be considered for second-look procedures.[53] When stratified by disease stage, elevated levels were found in more than 90% of patients with advanced-stage ovarian cancer but in only 50% of patients with stage 1 disease.[54] In addition, elevated levels of CA125 are more strongly associated with serous, rather than mucinous tumors.[55]

Transvaginal ultrasound has consistently proven to be the most promising imaging method for routine screening of ovarian cancer.

Screening for Low-Risk Individuals

For women with a risk near that of the general population, ovarian cancer screening is not recommended. There are no screening tests for ovarian cancer that have proven effective in screening low-risk asymptomatic women, including pelvic ultrasonography and measurement of CA-125. An annual gynecologic examination with pelvic examination is recommended for preventive health care.[56]

In the largest randomized controlled trial to date,[57] the United Kingdom Collaborative Trial of Ovarian Cancer Screening (UKCTOCS) randomized 202,638 women to 1 of 3 arms:

1. No treatment
2. Multimodal screening, consisting of annual C-125 (interpreted using a risk of ovarian cancer algorithm) with transvaginal ultrasound as a second-line test
3. Annual screening with transvaginal ultrasound alone

Although there was no difference in the rate of ovarian cancer diagnosis, the authors reported a stage shift with annual multimodal screening using the longitudinal CA-125 risk of ovarian cancer algorithm. However, there was no definitive mortality reduction with either screening strategy compared with no screening. Although encouraging, there is not yet evidence to support general population screening.

Screening for Individuals with Inherited Risk Caused by Known Genetic Mutations

There are no data demonstrating that screening improves early detection in women who carry high-risk genetic mutations; however, these women should be referred to genetic counseling and begin screening for ovarian cancer at a relatively early age.[58] In the absence of high-quality data, the National Comprehensive Cancer Network recommends screening with CA-125 measurement and pelvic ultrasound every 6 or 12 months for women with Lynch syndrome, starting at age 30 or 35, although evidence is insufficient to show that these methods improve survival rates.[26,58] For women with BRCA mutations or who have a personal or family history of ovarian cancer, routine ovarian cancer screening with measurement of serum CA-125 level or transvaginal ultrasonography generally is not recommended. The American College of Obstetrics and Gynecology states that transvaginal ultrasonography or measurement of serum CA-125 level may be reasonable only for short-term surveillance in women at high risk of ovarian cancer.[59] This can be starting at age 30 to 35 years until the time they choose to pursue risk-reducing bilateral salpingo-oophorectomy, which is the only proven intervention to reduce ovarian cancer-specific mortality.

Prevention

Identifying women with inherited high-risk mutations is crucial in risk reduction. It is ideal to perform testing in the family member who is most likely to test positive for a mutation, namely the individual affected with cancer. **Box 2** outlines recommendations from the Society of Gynecologic Oncology regarding who should be referred for counseling and consideration of genetic testing.

In contrast to Hereditary Breast and Ovarian Cancer syndrome, assessment for Lynch may be performed through tumor testing of affected individuals.[13] Loss of mismatch repair proteins identified through immunohistochemistry can direct targeted germline genetic testing.[13] Affected individuals should inform family members immediately. Genetic testing should include pretest education and counseling regarding the risks, benefits, and limitations of testing. Furthermore, post-test counseling should include education on risk-reduction strategies.[13]

Risk-reducing bilateral salpingo-oophorectomy is the most effective ovarian cancer risk-reduction strategy for women with known BRCA mutations. Meta-analysis results show that risk-reducing bilateral salpingo-oophorectomy reduces the risk of ovarian cancer, fallopian tube cancer, or peritoneal cancer by approximately 80% in women with known mutations in BRCA1 or BRCA2.[60] In addition, risk-reducing bilateral

---

Box 2
Patients with increased likelihood of having an inherited predisposition to breast and ovarian cancer who should receive genetic counseling and be offered genetic testing

An individual affected with any of the following:

- High-grade EOC/tubal/peritoneal cancer
- Breast cancer in a patient no more than 45 years old
- Breast cancer with close relative with breast cancer at no more than 50 years old or close relative with EOC/tubal/peritoneal cancer at any age
- Breast cancer in a patient no more than 50 years old with a limited family history
- Breast cancer with at least 2 close relatives with breast cancer at any age
- Breast cancer with at least 2 close relatives with pancreatic cancer or aggressive prostate cancer (Gleason score ≥ 7)
- Two breast primaries, with the first diagnosed prior to age 50
- Triple negative breast cancer at an age of no more than 60 years
- With breast cancer and Ashkenazi Jewish ancestry
- Pancreatic cancer with at least 2 close relatives with breast, EOC/tubal/peritoneal, pancreatic, or aggressive prostate cancer

An individual with no personal history of cancer but with the following:

- First-degree or several close relatives who meet one of the above criteria
- Close relative carrying a known BRCA1 or BRCA2 mutation
- Close relative with male breast cancer

Adapted from Lancaster JM, Powell CB, Chen LM, et al. Society of Gynecologic Oncology Statement on risk assessment for inherited gynecologic cancer predispositions. Gynecol Oncol 2015;136(1):5; with permission.

salpingo-oophorectomy has been shown to decrease overall mortality in women with a BRCA1 or BRCA2 mutation.[61] The ACOG recommends that risk-reducing salpingo-oophorectomy, which includes removal of the ovaries and fallopian tubes in their entirety, be offered by age 40 years for women with BRCA 1 or BRCA 2 mutations.[59] Bilateral salpingectomy alone in high-risk women is not currently recommended for ovarian cancer risk reduction, although current investigation is underway.

Among low-risk women, however, bilateral tubal ligation is associated with a decreased risk of ovarian cancer.[45] The magnitude of risk reduction may be greater for invasive endometrioid and clear cell ovarian cancers than for serous cancers. Thus, an important potential prevention strategy includes consideration of salpingectomy after childbearing is complete at the time of elective pelvic surgery or hysterectomy. In a nationwide Scandinavian study including over 5.7 million women, the authors found a significantly lower risk for ovarian cancer among those with previous salpingectomy (hazard ratio [HR] = 0.65).[46] Those who underwent bilateral salpingectomy saw a 50% decrease in risk compared with women who underwent a unilateral procedure (HR 0.35 vs 0.71). The mounting evidence that salpingectomy may lower the risk of ovarian cancer has led to several national and international societies to recommend consideration of opportunistic salpingectomy at the time of benign gynecologic surgery.[62]

Furthermore, use of the oral contraceptive pill (OCP) has consistently been demonstrated to have a significant risk-reducing effect on the development of ovarian cancer by 40% to 60% in both low- and high-risk individuals.[27,63] It should, however, be noted that there are conflicting data whether OCP increases breast cancer risk among BRCA mutation carriers.[63]

CERVICAL CANCER
Epidemiology and Risk Factors

Cervical cancer is the most common gynecologic malignancy in the world, with an estimated 528,000 new cases and 266,000 deaths annually.[5] Around 85% of the global burden occurs in undeveloped countries. Increased rates in these areas are a reflection of a lack of screening and vaccination programs. In the United States, an estimated 13,240 women will be diagnosed with cervical cancer in 2018, and 4170 will die from the disease.[1] The age-standardized incidence of cervical cancer is 7.4 cases per 100,000 women per year with a cumulative lifetime risk of 0.6%.[5]

There are 2 major subtypes of cervical cancer. Squamous cell carcinoma accounts for approximately 70% of invasive cervical cancer, whereas adenocarcinoma and its variants account for about 25%.[64] Neuroendocrine carcinomas and other rare cell types comprise the remaining 3% to 5% of cases. Despite the decrease in squamous cell carcinoma seen over the past 5 decades, the incidence of cervical adenocarcinoma has been increasing, especially in younger women.[64] Adenocarcinoma is associated with a greater probability of distant recurrence, and poorer overall survival.[65]

The most important risk factor for the development of invasive cervical cancer is infection with human papillomavirus (HPV). Other risk factors include cigarette smoking, lower socioeconomic status, multiple sexual partners, early age of first intercourse, high parity, coinfection with other sexually transmitted diseases, or presence of immunocompromised conditions (HIV or pharmacologic).[66]

Natural Course of Cervical Cancer

At least 200 genotypes of HPV have been described, including, about 40 that affect the genital area. Of these, 15 have been shown to have oncogenic properties, including subtypes 16, 18, 31, 33, 35, 39, 45, 51, 52, 56, 58, 59, 68, 73, and 82.[67] Infection with an oncogenic subtype in the HPV family is a necessary factor for the development of invasive cervical cancer. HPV can be detected in 99.7% of cervical cancers.[68] In addition, HPV is associated with 90% of anal cancers, approximately 70% of vaginal, vulvar, and oropharyngeal cancers, and 60% of penile cancers.[69] Most HPV infections are transient, with little risk of progression. In fact, more than 90% of new HPV infections are cleared within 2 years of infection, with clearance typically occurring within the first 6 months after infection. Persistent cervical infection with high-risk HPV strongly predicts subsequent risk of high-grade dysplasia or cancer.[70]

Cervical Cancer Screening Tests

The current available methods for cervical cancer screening are the Pap test and HPV testing. The histologic diagnosis of cervical dysplasia or carcinoma requires an actual tissue biopsy. The Pap test consists of collection of exfoliated cells from the transformation zone of the cervix and transferred to either a liquid preservative (liquid-based technique) or directly to a slide and fixed (conventional technique). Either conventional or liquid-based Pap tests are acceptable for cervical cancer screening, but liquid-based cytology may increase the yield of adequate specimens in individuals with obscuring blood or inflammation.[71] Furthermore, the liquid-based method of collection has the advantage of allowing a single specimen to be used to perform cytology, HPV testing, and testing for gonorrhea and chlamydial infection.

There are several FDA-approved tests available for the detection of cervical HPV. Most test for the 13 or 14 of the most common high-risk genotypes. Current indications for HPV testing include (1) women with ASC-US cytology result (reflex testing), or (2) as an adjunct to cytology for cervical cancer screening in women aged 30 to 65 years and older (cotesting).[72]

Screening for the General Population

In the United States, among immunocompetent asymptomatic women, screening should be initiated at age 21, even if the individual reports sexual abstinence. The ASCCP recommends that women should be screened every 3 years with Pap test alone until age 30.[73] Women starting at age 30 years may continue with Pap test alone every 3 years (acceptable) or initiate cotesting (Pap test and HPV testing) every 5 years if both tests are negative. Cotesting is preferred in this population.

Screening by any modality should be discontinued after age 65 in women with evidence of adequate negative prior screening test results, including no history of CIN2 or higher.[73] Screening women older than 65 is associated with an increased risk for potential harms, including false-positives and invasive procedures, so the US Preventative Services Task Force concludes that the harms of screening this age group are likely to exceed benefits.[74] Adequate negative prior screening test results are defined as 3 consecutive negative cytology results or 2 consecutive negative cotest results within the previous 10 years, with the most recent test performed within the past 5 years. ASCCP guidelines should be used to triage abnormal cytology and histology. Screening for special populations is summarized in **Box 3**.

Prevention

HPV vaccination is the key approach to primary prevention of cervical cancer. In 2006, the FDA approved the first preventative HPV vaccine, marketed by Merck & Company under the trade name Gardasil, a quadrivalent vaccine (4vHPV) offering protection against HPV types 6, 11, 16, and 18. Initially, it was only approved for girls to women

---

Box 3
Cervical cancer screening among special populations

- History of abnormal Pap: Women with a history of CIN 2 or higher should continue to undergo age-based screening for 20 years after the initial post-treatment surveillance period.[74,75]

- Pregnant: Pap smears should only be performed in pregnancy if indicated under current screening guidelines. Colposcopy may be deferred in pregnancy for ASCUS and LSIL lesions, but should be used to triage more serious abnormalities. Cervical biopsies should be performed to exclude invasive cervical cancer.

- Previous hysterectomy: In women who have had a hysterectomy with removal of the cervix and have never had CIN 2 or higher, routine cytology screening and HPV testing should be discontinued.[73] Women who had a high-grade lesion before hysterectomy with removal of the cervix are at risk for recurrent HSIL or carcinoma at the vaginal cuff years after the procedure.[75] Continued screening for 20 years is recommended in women who still have a cervix or a history of CIN 2 or higher.

- DES: Women who were exposed to diethylstilbestrol in utero are at increased risk for clear cell adenocarcinoma of the cervix and vagina.[76] Although no official guidelines exist for DES daughters, the National Cancer Institute advises annual cervical screening along with a 4-quadrant vaginal smear, in which samples are taken from all sides of the vagina.[76]

- Individuals with HIV/acquired immunodeficiency syndrome (AIDS): Screening should commence within 1 year of the onset of sexual activity regardless of mode of HIV transmission, but no later than 21 year old.[72,73] Women aged 21 to 29 years should have a Pap test at the time of initial HIV diagnosis. Provided the initial Pap test for a young (or newly diagnosed) woman with HIV is normal, the next Pap test should be in 12 months. Some experts recommend a Pap test at 6 months after the baseline test. If the results of the 3 consecutive Pap tests are normal, follow-up Pap tests should be every 3 years. Cotesting is not recommended for women with HIV younger than 30 years of age. Screening in women with HIV should continue throughout a woman's lifetime.

- Otherwise immunocompromised: No studies or major society recommendations exist to guide cervical cancer screening in women who are immunocompromised because of non-HIV causes. Annual cytology traditionally has been performed in these women, but it is reasonable to extrapolate the recommendations for women with HIV infection to this group.[77]

---

aged 9 to 26 years of age; then approval was extended to boys of the same age in 2010. In 2010, a bivalent vaccine (2vHPV), Cervarix was approved, offering protection against HPV types 16 and 18, for use in girls and women 9 to 25 but not in boys. Finally, in 2014 a nonvalent vaccine (9vHPV), Gardasil 9, was approved in the United States, with protection against HPV types 6, 11, 16 18, 31, 33, 45, 52, and 58. Each of these vaccines is administered in a 3-dose schedule. The second dose is administered at least 1 to 2 months after the first dose, and the third dose at least 6 months after the first dose. If the vaccine schedule is interrupted, the vaccination series does not need to be restarted. On October 7, 2016, the FDA approved adding a 2-dose schedule for Gardasil for adolescents ages 9 through 14 years. On October 5th, 2018 the FDA approved the Gardasil 9 vaccine to extend the age range for the use of the vaccine to include women and men from 27 to 45 years of age. The CDC has not yet changed recommendations to reflect this most recent FDA approval.

Women who have received the HPV vaccine should be screened according to the same guidelines as women who have not been vaccinated.[73] The vaccine does not provide immunity against all HPV types responsible for cervical cancers, and some vaccine recipients may have already been infected with high-risk HPV.[78] Clinical trials examining efficacy of the 9vHPV revealed that at least 97.9% of participants seroconverted to all 9 vaccine-preventable HPV types by 4 weeks after the last dose.[78] Six additional studies found similar results for 4vHPV and 2vHPV.[79] Through 10 years of follow-up from clinical trials, no evidence of waning protection after a 3-dose series of HPV vaccine has been found.[80] Current Advisory Committee on Immunization Practices recommendations are described in **Box 4**.

VULVAR AND VAGINAL CANCER
Epidemiology and Risk Factors

Vulvar cancer accounts for approximately 5% of all gynecologic cancers worldwide.[1] In the United States, an estimated 6190 women will be diagnosed with vulvar cancer in 2018, and 1200 will die from the disease.[1] Vaginal cancer is even more rare, accounting for only 1% to 3% of gynecologic malignancies.[1] An estimated 5170 women will be diagnosed with vaginal cancer in 2018, and 1100 will die from the disease.[1] The annual incidence of vulvar and vaginal malignancies are approximately 2.5 cases and 1 case in 100,000 women, respectively.[4] Vulvar and vaginal cancers share many of the risk factors associated with cervical cancer (See Daniel Weinberg and Ricardo A. Gomez-Martinez's article, "Vulvar Cancer," in this issue).

Screening and Prevention

In asymptomatic low-risk individuals, there is no evidence to support screening for vulvar or vaginal cancer. However, thorough examination of the vulva and vagina should be performed when individuals are seen for routine Pap smears. Women who are no longer receiving regular Pap smears should have a thorough examination by their primary care providers at time of annual well woman appointment. In addition, being aware of signs and symptoms is important in early evaluation and diagnosis; these are further discussed in Drs Daniel Weinberg and Ricardo A. Gomez-Martinez's article, "Vulvar Cancer," in this issue.

Immunization with the HPV vaccine (quadrivalent or 9-valent) has been shown to be 97% to 100% effective against precancerous vulvar and vaginal lesions in women not previously infected with HPV.[81] Similar to CIN, vulvar and vaginal intraepithelial neoplastic lesions are important cancer precursors to evaluate and treat. Furthermore, appropriate treatment of vulvar dermatologic disorders, especially of lichen sclerosis,

---

Box 4
Human papillomavirus Advisory Committee on Immunization Practices vaccine recommendations

- Routine HPV vaccination at age 11 or 12 years (can be given as early as 9 years).

- Vaccination for girls and women through age 26 years and for boys and men through age 21 who were not adequately vaccinated previously. Transgender persons and men who have sex with men should be vaccinated through age 26 years if they were not adequately vaccinated previously.

- For persons initiating vaccination before their 15th birthday, the recommended immunization schedule is 2 doses of HPV vaccine (0, 6–12 month schedule).

- For persons initiating vaccination after their 15th birthday, the recommended immunization schedule is 3 doses of HPV vaccine (0, 1–2, 6 month schedule).

- If the vaccination schedule is interrupted, the series does not need to be restarted. The number of recommended doses is based on age at administration of the first dose.

From Meites E, Kempe A, Markowitz LE. Use of a 2-dose schedule for human papillomavirus vaccination - updated recommendations of the advisory committee on immunization practices. MMWR Morb Mortal Wkly Rep 2016;65:1405–8.

may reduce the risk of cancer.[82] In addition, delaying first sexual intercourse until the late teens, avoiding sexual intercourse with multiple partners, practicing safe sexual practices, and smoking cessation can help prevent these cancers.

REFERENCES

1. Siegel RL, Miller KD, Jemal A. Cancer statistics, 2018. CA Cancer J Clin 2018;68: 7–30.
2. Key statistics for ovarian cancer. American Cancer Society. Available at: http:// www.cancer.org/cancer/ovarian-cancer/about/key-statistics.html. Accessed May 1, 2018.
3. American Cancer Society. Cancer facts & figures 2018. Atlanta (GA): American Cancer Society; 2018.
4. Noone AM, Howlader N, Krapcho M, et al, editors. SEER cancer statistics review, 1975-2015. Bethesda (MD): National Cancer Institute; 2016.
5. Ferlay J, Soerjomataram I, Dikshit R, et al. Cancer incidence and mortality world-wide: sources, methods and major patterns in GLOBOCAN 2012. Int J Cancer 2015;136:E359–86.
6. Bokhman JV. Two pathogenetic types of endometrial carcinoma. Gynecol Oncol 1983;15:10.
7. Hamilton CA, Cheung MK, Osann K, et al. Uterine papillary serous and clear cell carcinomas predict for poorer survival compared to grade 3 endometrioid corpus cancers. Br J Cancer 2006;94:642.
8. Jordan LB, Abdul-Kader M, Al Nafussi A. Uterine serous papillary carcinoma: his-topathologic changes within the female genital tract. Int J Gynecol Cancer 2001; 11:283.
9. Brinton LA, Lacey JV Jr, Devesa SS, et al. Epidemiology of uterine corpus cancer. In: Gershenson DM, McGuire WP, Gore M, et al, editors. Gynecologic cancer: controversies in management. New York: Churchill Livingstone; 2004. p. 190.
10. Kandoth C, Schultz N, Cherniack AD, et al, Cancer Genome Atlas Research Network. Integrated genomic characterization of endometrial carcinoma. Nature 2013;497:67–73.
11. Zhan B, Liu X, Li F, et al. Breastfeeding and the incidence of endometrial cancer: a meta-analysis. Oncotarget 2015;6(35):38398–409.
12. Setiawan VW, Yang HP, Pike MC, et al. Type I and II endometrial cancers: have they different risk factors? J Clin Oncol 2013;31(20):2607–18.
13. Committee on Practice Bulletins-Gynecology, Society of Gynecologic Oncology. ACOG practice bulletin No. 147: Lynch syndrome. Obstet Gynecol 2014;124: 1042–54. Reaffirmed 2016.
14. Dunlop MG, Farrington SM, Carothers AD, et al. Cancer risk associated with germline DNA mismatch repair gene mutations. Hum Mol Genet 1997;6:105–10.
15. Aarnio M, Sankila R, Pukkala E, et al. Cancer risk in mutation carriers of DNA-mismatch-repair genes. Int J Cancer 1999;81:214–8.
16. Lu KH, Dinh M, Kohlmann W, et al. Gynecologic cancer as a "sentinel cancer" for women with hereditary nonpolyposis colorectal cancer syndrome. Obstet Gyne-col 2005;105(3):569–74.
17. Koornstra JJ, Mourits MJ, Sijmons RH, et al. Management of extracolonic tumours in patients with Lynch syndrome. Lancet Oncol 2009;10:400.
18. Barrow E, Robinson L, Alduaij W, et al. Cumulative lifetime incidence of extraco-lonic cancers in Lynch syndrome: a report of 121 families with proven mutations. Clin Genet 2009;75:141.

19. Dijkhuizen FP, Mol BW, Brölmann HA, et al. The accuracy of endometrial sampling in the diagnosis of patients with endometrial carcinoma and hyperplasia: a meta-analysis. Cancer 2000;89(8):1765–72.

20. American College of Obstetricians and Gyneoclogists. ACOG committee opinion No. 426: the role of transvaginal ultrasonography in the evaluation of postmeno-pausal bleeding. Obstet Gynecol 2009;113:462–4.

21. American College of Obstetricians and Gyneoclogists. Committee opinion No. 601: tamoxifen and uterine cancer. Obstet Gynecol 2014;123:1394–7.

22. Ottolina J, Ferrandina G, Gadducci A, et al. Is the endometrial evaluation routinely required in patients with adult granulose cell tumors of the ovary? Gynecol Oncol 2015;136(2):230–4.

23. Rema P, Ahmed I. Fertility sparing surgery in gynecologic cancer. J Obstet Gynaecol India 2014;64(4):234–8.

24. Auranen A, Joutsiniemi T. A systematic review of gynecological cancer surveillance in women belonging to hereditary nonpolyposis colorectal cancer (Lynch syndrome) families. Acta Obstet Gynecol Scand 2011;90(5):437–44.

25. Zhou XP, Kuismanen S, Nystrom-Lahti M, et al. Distinct PTEN mutational spectra in hereditary non-polyposis colon cancer syndrome-related endometrial carcinomas compared to sporadic microsatellite unstable tumors. Hum Mol Genet 2002;11(4):445–50.

26. National Comprehensive Cancer Network (NCCN). NCCN clinical practice guidelines in oncology. Available at: http://www.nccn.org/professionals/physician_gls/f_guidelines.asp. Accessed February 27, 2016.

27. The Cancer and Steroid Hormone Study. Combination oral contraceptive use and the risk of endometrial cancer. The Cancer and Steroid Hormone Study of the Centers for Disease Control and the National Institute of Child Health and Human Development. JAMA 1987;257:796–800.

28. Depot-medroxyprogesterone acetate (DMPA) and risk of endometrial cancer. The WHO Collaborative Study of Neoplasia and Steroid Contraceptives. Int J Cancer 1991;49:186–90.

29. Jareid M, Thalabard JC, Aarflot M, et al. Levonorgestrel-releasing intrauterine system use is associated with a decreased risk of ovarian and endometrial cancer, without increased risk of breast cancer. Results from the NOWAC Study. Gynecol Oncol 2018;149:127–32.

30. Yang KY, Caughey AB, Little SE, et al. A cost-effectiveness analysis of prophylactic surgery versus gynecologic surveillance for women from hereditary nonpolyposis colorectal cancer (HNPCC) Families. Fam Cancer 2011;10:535.

31. Umar A, Boland CR, Terdiman JP, et al. Revised Bethesda guidelines for hereditary nonpolyposis colorectal cancer (Lynch syndrome) and microsatellite instability. J Natl Cancer Inst 2004;96:261–8.

32. Mills AM, Liou S, Ford JM, et al. Lynch syndrome screening should be considered for all patients with newly diagnosed endometrial cancer. Am J Surg Pathol 2014; 38(11):1501–9.

33. Ladabaum U, Wang G, Terdiman J, et al. Strategies to identify the Lynch syndrome among patients with colorectal cancer: a cost-effectiveness analysis. Ann Intern Med 2011;155:69–79.

34. Ueda SM, Kapp DS, Cheung MK, et al. Trends in demographic and clinical characteristics in women diagnosed with corpus cancer and their potential impact on the increasing number of deaths. Am J Obstet Gynecol 2008;198(2):218.e1-6.

35. Acharya S, Hensley ML, Montag AC, et al. Rare uterine cancers. Lancet Oncol 2005;6(12):961–71.

36. Schorge JO, Schaffer JI, Halvorson LM, et al. Uterine sarcoma. In: Schorge JO, Schaffer JI, Halvorson LM, et al, editors. Williams gynecology. Columbus (OH): The McGraw-Hill Companies; 2008. p. 706–16.

37. US Food and Drug Administration. Medical devices safety communications. Updated laparoscopic uterine power morcellation in hysterectomy and myomectomy: FDA safety communication. 2014.

38. Pritts E, Vanness D, Berek J, et al. The prevalence of occult leiomyosarcoma at surgery for presumed uterine fibroids: a meta-analysis. Gynecol Surg 2015; 12(3):165–77.

39. Lacey JV, Sherman ME. Ovarian neoplasia. In: Robboy SL, Mutter GL, Prat J, editors. Robboy's pathology of the female reproductive tract. 2nd edition. Oxford (England): Churchill Livingstone Elsevier; 2009. p. 601–31. Available at: https://www.chartrrg.com/wp-content/uploads/2014/07/FDA-Warning.pdf. Accessed May 1, 2018.

40. Guth U, Huang DJ, Bauer G, et al. Metastatic patterns at autopsy in patients with ovarian carcinoma. Cancer 2007;110:1272–80.

41. Casagrande JT, Louie EW, Pike MC, et al. "Incessant ovulation" and ovarian cancer. Lancet 1979;2:170–3.

42. Reid BM, Permuth JB, Sellers TA. Epidemiology of ovarian cancer: a review. Cancer Biol Med 2017;14(1):9–32.

43. Kurian AW, Hughes E, Handorf EA, et al. Breast and ovarian cancer penetrance estimates derived from germline multiple-gene sequencing results in women. JCO Precis Oncol 2017;1:1–12.

44. Kim HS, Kim TH, Chung HH, et al. Risk and prognosis of ovarian cancer in women with endometriosis: a meta-analysis. Br J Cancer 2014;110:1878–90.

45. Cibula D, Widschwendter M, Májek O, et al. Tubal ligation and the risk of ovarian cancer: review and meta-analysis. Hum Reprod Update 2011;17(1):55–67.

46. Falconer H, Yin L, Grönberg H, et al. Ovarian cancer risk after salpingectomy: a nationwide population-based study. J Natl Cancer Inst 2015;107(2):dju410.

47. Rebbeck TR, Lynch HT, Neuhausen SL, et al. Prophylactic oophorectomy in carriers of BRCA1 or BRCA2 mutations. N Engl J Med 2002;346:1616–22.

48. Walker GR, Schlesselman JJ, Ness RB. Family history of cancer, oral contraceptive use, and ovarian cancer risk. Am J Obstet Gynecol 2002;186:8–14.

49. Walsh T, Casadei S, Lee MK, et al. Mutations in 12 genes for inherited ovarian, fallopian tube, and peritoneal carcinoma identified by massively parallel sequencing. Proc Natl Acad Sci U S A 2011;108(44):18032–7.

50. Ford D, Easton DF, Stratton M, et al. Genetic heterogeneity and penetrance analysis of the BRCA1 and BRCA2 genes in breast cancer families. The Breast Cancer Linkage Consortium. Am J Hum Genet 1998;62:676–89.

51. Antoniou A, Pharoah PD, Narod S, et al. Average risks of breast and ovarian cancer associated with BRCA1 or BRCA2 mutations detected in case series unselected for family history: a combined analysis of 22 studies. Am J Hum Genet 2003;72:1117–30.

52. Crum CP, Drapkin R, Kindelberger D, et al. Lessons from BRCA: the tubal fimbria emerges as an origin for pelvic serous cancer. Clin Med Res 2007;5:35–44.

53. Meyer T, Rustin GJ. Role of tumour markers in monitoring epithelial ovarian cancer. Br J Cancer 2000;82:1535–8.

54. Nustad K, Bast RC Jr, Brien TJ, et al. Specificity and affinity of 26 monoclonal antibodies against the CA 125 antigen: first report from the ISOBM TD-1 workshop. International Society for Oncodevelopmental Biology and Medicine. Tumour Biol 1996;17:196–219.

55. Hogdall EV, Christensen L, Kjaer SK, et al. CA125 expression pattern, prognosis and correlation with serum CA125 in ovarian tumor patients. From The Danish "MALOVA" Ovarian Cancer Study. Gynecol Oncol 2007;104:508–15.

56. ACOG statement on USPSTF draft recommendations on pelvic exams. 2016. Available at: https://www.acog.org/About-ACOG/News-Room/Statements/2016/ACOG-Statement-on-USPSTF-Draft-Recommendations-on-Pelvic-Exams. Accessed May 1, 2018.

57. Jacobs IJ, Menon U, Ryan A, et al. Ovarian cancer screening and mortality in the UK Collaborative Trial of Ovarian Cancer Screening (UKCTOCS): a randomised controlled trial. Lancet 2016;387(10022):945–56.

58. National Comprehensive Cancer Network. Genetic/familial high-risk assessment: breast and ovarian. V.1.2010. NCCN clinical practice guidelines in oncology. Fort Washington (PA): NCCN; 2010.

59. American College of Obstetricians and Gynecologists, ACOG Committee on Practice Bulletins–Gynecology, ACOG Committee on Genetics, Society of Gynecologic Oncologists. ACOG practice bulletin No. 103: hereditary breast and ovarian cancer syndrome. Obstet Gynecol 2009;113:957–66.

60. Rebbeck TR, Kauff ND, Domchek SM. Meta-analysis of risk reduction estimates associated with risk-reducing salpingo-oophorectomy in BRCA1 or BRCA2 mutation carriers. J Natl Cancer Inst 2009;101:80–7.

61. Domchek SM, Friebel TM, Neuhausen SL, et al. Mortality after bilateral salpingo-oophorectomy in BRCA1 and BRCA2 mutation carriers: a prospective cohort study. Lancet Oncol 2006;7:223–9.

62. Tamussino K. Should national societies recommend opportunistic salpingectomy? J Gynecol Oncol 2017;28(4):e53.

63. Friebel TM, Domchek SM, Rebbeck TR. Modifiers of cancer risk in BRCA1 and BRCA2 mutation carriers: systematic review and meta-analysis. J Natl Cancer Inst 2014;106:dju091.

64. Adegoke O, Kulasingam S, Virnig B. Cervical cancer trends in the United States: a 35-year population-based analysis. J Womens Health (Larchmt) 2012;21(10):1031–7.

65. Jung EJ, Byun JM, Kim YN, et al. Cervical adenocarcinoma has a poorer prognosis and a higher propensity for distant recurrence than squamous cell carcinoma. Int J Gynecol Cancer 2017;27(6):1228–36.

66. International Collaboration of Epidemiological Studies of Cervical Cancer. Comparison of risk factors for invasive squamous cell carcinoma and adenocarcinoma of the cervix: collaborative reanalysis of individual data on 8,097 women with squamous cell carcinoma and 1,374 women with adenocarcinoma from 12 epidemiological studies. Int J Cancer 2007;120:885–91.

67. Kumar V, Abbas AK, Fausto N, et al. "Chapter 19 the female genital system and breast". Robbins basic pathology. 8th edition. Philadelphia: Saunders; 2007.

68. Walboomers JM, Jacobs MV, Manos MM, et al. Human papillomavirus is a necessary cause of invasive cervical cancer worldwide. J Pathol 1999;189:12–9.

69. Centers for Disease Control and Prevention. HPV-associated cancer statistics. 2017. Available at: https://www.cdc.gov/cancer/hpv/statistics/index.htm. Accessed May 1, 2018.

70. Kjaer SK, Frederiksen K, Munk C, et al. Long-term absolute risk of cervical intraepithelial neoplasia grade 3 or worse following human papillomavirus infection: role of persistence. J Natl Cancer Inst 2010;102:1478–88 (Level II-3).

71. AbdullGaffar B, Kamal MO, Khalid M, et al. Lubricant, mucus, and other contaminant materials as a potential source of interpretation errors in ThinPrep cervical cytology. J Low Genit Tract Dis 2010;14(1):22–8.
72. Committee on Practice Bulletins—Gynecology. Practice Bulletin No. 168: cervical cancer screening and prevention. Obstet Gynecol 2016;128(4):e111–30. Reaffirmed 2018.
73. Saslow D, Solomon D, Lawson HW, et al, ACS-ASCCP-ASCP Cervical Cancer Guideline Committee. American Cancer Society, American Society for Colposcopy and Cervical Pathology, and American Society for Clinical Pathology screening guidelines for the prevention and early detection of cervical cancer. CA Cancer J Clin 2012;62:147–72.
74. Screening for cervical cancer: recommendations and rationale. U.S. Preventative Services Task Force. Am Fam Physician 2003;67(8):1759–66.
75. Soutter WP, Sasieni P, Panoskaltsis T. Long-term risk of invasive cervical cancer after treatment of squamous cervical intraepithelial neoplasia. Int J Cancer 2006; 118:2048–55.
76. National Cancer Institute (2006) DES: questions and answers. US Department of Health and Human Services. 2006. Available at: http://www.cancer.gov/cancertopics/factsheet/Risk/DES. Accessed May 1, 2018.
77. Nguyen ML, Flowers L. Cervical cancer screening in immunocompromised women. Obstet Gynecol Clin North Am 2013;40(2):339–57.
78. Iversen O-E, Miranda MJ, Ulied A, et al. Immunogenicity of the 9-valent HPV vaccine using 2-dose regimens in girls and boys vs a 3-dose regimen in women. JAMA 2016;316:2411–21.
79. CDC. Grading of recommendations assessment, development and evaluation (GRADE) of a 2-dose schedule for human papillomavirus (HPV) vaccination. Atlanta (GA): US Department of Health and Human Services, CDC; 2016. Available at: https://www.cdc.gov/vaccines/acip/recs/grade/hpv-2-dose.html.
80. Meites E, Kempe A, Markowitz LE. Use of a 2-dose schedule for human papillomavirus vaccination - Updated recommendations of the advisory committee on immunization practices. MMWR Morb Mortal Wkly Rep 2016;65:1405–8.
81. Petrosky E, Bocchini JA Jr, Hariri S, et al, Centers for Disease Control and Prevention (CDC). Use of 9-valent human papillomavirus (HPV) vaccine: updated HPV vaccination recommendations of the advisory committee on immunization practices. MMWR Morb Mortal Wkly Rep 2015;64:300–4.
82. Lee A, Bradford J, Fischer G. Long-term management of adult vulvar lichen sclerosus: a prospective cohort study of 507 women. JAMA Dermatol 2015;151: 1061–7.

Germline and Somatic Tumor Testing in Gynecologic Cancer Care

Jill Alldredge, MD*, Leslie Randall, MD

KEYWORDS

• Gynecologic cancer • Genomics • Germline • Somatic • Tumor testing

KEY POINTS

- Tumors may harbor somatic or germline mutations with clinically relevant implications for cancer prognosis, risk-reduction strategies, and screening.
- Genetic sequencing and functional tumor testing have evolved rapidly to support individualized care but have important pitfalls to be aware of.
- Genetic counselors are an essential resource and should be used early when patients have at-risk cancers, strong family history, or tumor testing suggestive of a germline mutation.
- Providers should be well versed in the constellation of cancers that may raise concern for hereditary cancer syndromes.
- In women with known hereditary cancer syndromes, adherence to screening recommendations and use of risk-reduction strategies are essential for patients.

INTRODUCTION

Heritable (germline) and nonheritable (somatic) mutational and epigenetic events, such as gene promoter methylation, which significantly impact cancer biology are common in gynecologic cancers, especially in ovarian and endometrial cancers. This places gynecologic health care providers in the unique and important position of identifying women who have or are at risk for these genomic changes. For the oncologist, these distinct subtypes enable personalized cancer treatment including improved prognostication, access to treatment with targeted therapies, and triage of patients and blood relatives to genetic testing and preventative surgery. This review discusses the translation of tumor genetics into clinical action for patients with gynecologic cancer.

Disclosure Statement: Neither author has any financial conflicts of interest to disclose.
University of California, Irvine, 333 The City Boulevard, Suite 1400, Orange, CA 92868, USA
* Corresponding author.
E-mail address: jalldred@uci.edu

UNDERSTANDING TUMOR PATHOPHYSIOLOGY

Mutations in key cell-cycle regulators result in uncontrolled cellular growth or impaired cellular death. This is typically caused by loss of tumor suppressor gene function or an upregulation of oncogenes, often requiring "two-hits" to result in malignant growth. The four key mutation types that result in malignancy include:

1. Point mutations: single-nucleotide variants causing missense or nonsense DNA
2. Complex mutations: frameshift insertions or deletions
3. Exon or gene copy number: large duplications or deletions changing functional domain of proteins
4. Structural variants: translocations or inversions from point-breaks resulting in fused proteins or nonfunctional proteins

These tumor mutations can occur sporadically or in an inherited fashion. Sporadic, or acquired, mutations may occur in either somatic (peripheral) cells or germ (gonadal) cells. If a mutation occurs in a somatic tissue, it may remain silent or be expressed as tumor growth. This phenotypic expression as tumor growth occurs if concurrent mutational changes or tumor microenvironmental pressures result in additional loss of cell-cycle regulation. These mutations are also thought of as random, or noninherited.

If a mutation occurs in germ cells, it may lead to tumor growth by a similar mechanism to that described previously, or remain silent and be passed down to the next generation. Inherited or germline mutations occur in germ cells, and thus allow a deleterious mutation to be transmitted to progeny in an autosomal-dominant fashion. In this progeny, all cells in the body are affected by the mutation, including somatic and germ cells (**Fig. 1**).

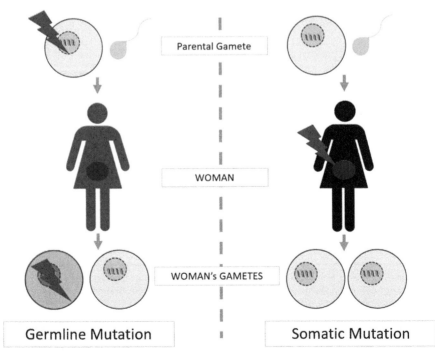

Fig. 1. Understanding germline and somatic mutations.

THE EVOLUTION OF GENETIC TESTING

The discovery of BRCA1 and BRCA2 gene mutations were landmark discoveries in the 1990s and heralded a new era of understanding for cancer genetics. With the sequencing of the human genome and genetic profiling of cancers over the past decade, the Cancer Genome Atlas and other comprehensive analyses have provided many additional insights into the genomic aberrations that elevate cancer risk.[1–4]

There are many approaches for interrogating a tumor or patient for relevant genetic mutations and phenotypic expression patterns that may be clinically relevant, reviewed in **Table 1**. Molecular testing can assess any of the four major gene alterations in cancer listed previously. Current molecular profiling paradigms typically use polymerase chain reaction, RNA or DNA sequencing technology, mass spectrometry, or fluorescence in situ hybridization to assess variants. Testing can range from a simple single-gene point mutation evaluation to a full sequencing of 20,000 genes. Emerging technology, called next-generation sequencing (NGS), allows assessment of all protein coding exosomes, the whole genome, or a customized panel of areas of interest. NGS permits evaluation of millions of base pairs simultaneously and is more time and cost-effective than prior techniques.[5]

In the absence of a germline mutation, several mutations isolated within the tumor itself can help to guide management decisions, particularly BRCA or loss of homologous recombination. As the understanding of genomics expands, there are hundreds of identifiable somatic mutations within a tumor. However, those currently considered to be most actionable in gynecologic oncology include BRCA1 and BRCA2; other HRD genes including ATM, BRIP1, RAD51C, and RAD51D; mismatch repair genes MLH1, MSH2, MSH6, PMS2, and EPCAM; ARID1A; BRAF; CDKN2A; CTNNB1; FBXW7; FGFR2; FGFR3; FOXL2; HRAS; KRAS; NRAS; PIK3CA; PPP2R1A; and PTEN among many others.[6,7] Several of these genes have matched, targeted therapeutic strategies.

In addition to the presence or absence of a mutation, it is also important to consider penetrance. Penetrance describes those with a specific mutation who exhibit signs or

Table 1			
Testing strategies to assess tumor behavior			
Source	**Study Technique**	**Data Abstracted**	**Example**
Tumor	Immunohistochemistry	Protein expression Immune microenvironment	Mismatch repair testing: MLH1, MLH2, PMS2, MLH6 T-cell recruitment, PD-L1
	Epigenetic modification	Hypermethylation	MLH1 hypermethylation
	Functional	Mass spectrometry Proteomics FISH	Prognostic biomarkers
	Molecular	PCR RNA/DNA sequencing	Somatic BRCA
Blood	Molecular	PCR RNA/DNA sequencing	Germline BRCA/Lynch
	Circulating tumor DNA	RNA/DNA sequencing Tumor burden quantification	Germline BRCA/Lynch
Saliva	Molecular	PCR RNA/DNA sequencing	Germline BRCA/Lynch

Abbreviations: FISH, fluorescent in situ hybridization; PCR, polymerase chain reaction; PD-L1, programmed death ligand-1.
Data from Refs.[6,8–12]

symptoms of a genetic disorder; it is the phenotypic expression of a mutation. Some genes mutations, and their associated hereditary cancer syndrome, are thought of as high, moderate, or low penetrance based on the inheritance pattern and associated cancer risk. For example, with *BRCA1* mutation, some allelic variations in the *BRCA1* mutation have a higher likelihood of cancer than others. Similarly, cancer risk overall with *BRCA1* is significantly higher than that of *DICER1*, which is considered low penetrance. Syndromes characterized by high-penetrance mutations are more amenable to aggressive preventative measures and active risk-reduction strategies (**Fig. 2**).

GENETIC TESTING IN OVARIAN CANCER
Hereditary Breast and Ovarian Cancer Syndrome

The BRCA-Fanconi anemia DNA repair pathway controls DNA repair via homologous recombination. Numerous important genes regulate this pathway, with *BRCA1* and *BRCA2* being the most commonly mutated. These two mutations, with their risk of breast cancer, define hereditary breast and ovarian cancer syndrome. Ovarian cancer is attributable to a *BRCA1* or *BRCA2* mutation in 24% of the 22,280 new cases of ovarian cancer each year in the United States, with 18% being germline mutation.[13,14]

Women with *BRCA1* have a 65% to 85% risk of breast cancer and a 39% to 46% risk of ovarian cancer.[14] Risk-reducing salpingo-oophorectomy is advised in women with *BRCA1* at age 35 to 40 and in *BRCA2* at age 40 to 45. Retrospective data show that the risk of uterine cancer in women with *BRCA1* and *2* mutations is not increased compared with the general population. However, in those women with *BRCA1* who develop uterine cancer, the risk of an aggressive, serous uterine cancer

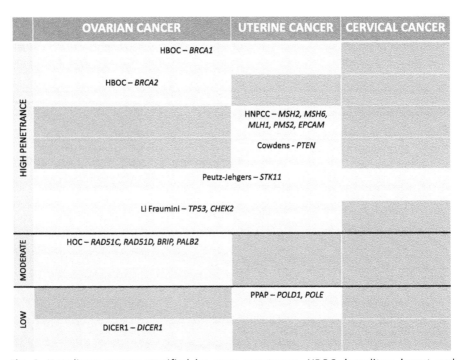

Fig. 2. Hereditary cancers stratified by gene penetrance. HBOC, hereditary breast and ovarian cancer; HNPCC, hereditary nonpolyposis colon cancer; HOC, hereditary ovarian cancer; PPAP, polymerase proofreading-associated polyposis.

is elevated at 4.7% between ages 45 and 70. This has elicited controversy regarding the role of risk-reducing hysterectomy in this population and should be discussed with patients at the providers discretion.[15] Women with *BRCA2* have a 45% to 85% risk of breast cancer and a 10% to 27% risk of ovarian cancer.[14] Additionally, these women carry an elevated risk of melanoma and pancreatic malignancies for which clear risk reduction and screening strategies do not current exist.

Hereditary Ovarian Cancer Syndromes

Numerous mutations within the BRCA pathway of double-stranded DNA repair confer an increased risk of ovarian cancer in 2.5% of patients, including *RAD51C*, *RAD51D*, and *BRIP1*. These are characterized as non-BRCA homologous recombination deficiencies (HRDs) and are termed hereditary ovarian cancer syndrome.[14,16–19] Additionally, *PALB2* and *BARD1* genes are responsible for a protein that binds *BRCA1* and *BRCA2* at the site of DNA damage and their role in ovarian cancer risk is not yet fully understood; however, the Cancer Genome Atlas project supports that *PALB2* is the most frequently mutated after *BRCA1* and *BRCA2*.[2,19] This is from a loss of homologous recombination phenotype leading to a "BRCA-ness" phenotype in some women.[20] Several other mutations in this pathway, such as *CHEK2*, have been linked to breast cancer and have been identified in women with ovarian cancer; however, the causal relationship remains unclear.[19] *RAD51C*, *RAD51D*, and *BRIP1* mutations are of moderate penetrance and merit consideration of risk-reduction bilateral salpingo-oophorectomy at age 40 to 45, following completion of childbearing.

Germline Testing in Ovarian Cancer

The numerous options available for genomic testing in ovarian cancer should be prioritized by the potential impact on clinical care. The testing paradigm in nonmucinous epithelial ovarian cancer, inclusive of fallopian tube and peritoneal primaries, is to begin with serum- or saliva-based germline testing in all women. Position papers from the Society for Gynecologic Oncology and a 2017 multidisciplinary summit on genetics services recommend germline testing in all women with these diagnoses.[21,22] Early germline testing informs prognosis, defines the patient's risk of secondary malignancy, and identifies families that are eligible for cascade testing to determine candidacy for risk reduction strategies, such as prophylactic surgery.[23] Early germline testing has recently been an important eligibility criterion for frontline PARP inhibitor trials of olaparib (SOLO-1, NCT01844986) and veliparib (GOG 3005, NCT02470585), and could become standard of care if these studies show a benefit with the use of frontline PARP inhibitors.

Germline testing should include *BRCA1* and *BRCA2* testing at a minimum, but expanded gene panels offer the added benefit of simultaneously testing for mutations in the other relevant HRD and mismatch repair genes.[24] An alternative strategy of performing panel testing only on women who are germline *BRCA* wild-type is impractical and cost-prohibitive, so the decision to panel test should be made when the first test is ordered. Several panels are available but no guidance currently exists regarding their use. Therefore, individual practitioners must choose which test to use based on the following principles: the test should be affordable; include actionable, relevant genes listed in **Fig. 3**; and have a low variant of uncertain significance (VUS) rate.[25] **Table 2** reviews rare nonepithelial ovarian cancer histologies and their unique approach.

VUS results are problematic because they are not immediately actionable, creating uncertainty for patients, family members, and physicians.[30] The VUS rate of an individual brand of test might be difficult to discern from the testing company, but in general, the more genes tested and the less dedicated the laboratory is to NGS germline testing by virtue of volume, experience, or sophistication, the higher is the VUS rate.

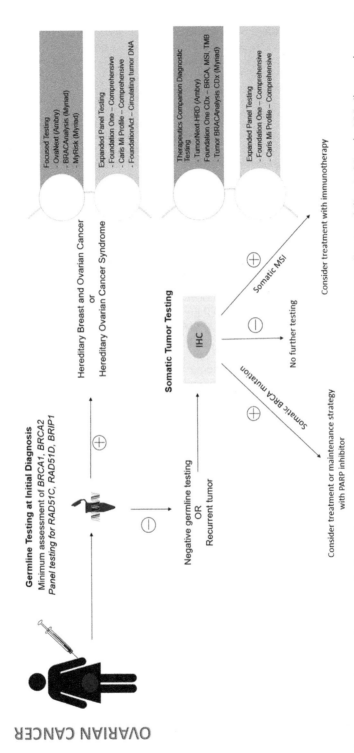

Fig. 3. Approach to testing strategies in ovarian cancer. IHC, immunohistochemistry; MSI, microsatellite instability; PARP, poly-ADP ribose polymerase; TMB, tumor mutational burden.

Table 2 Testing in rare ovarian cancer types		
Ovarian Tumor	**Implicated Gene**	**Comments**
Small cell ovarian hypercalcemic type	SMARCA4	Mutation with high sensitivity and specificity for this aggressive cancer[28]
Peutz-Jeghers syndrome Annular sex-cord/stromal	STK11	Test if family history and clinical findings (perioral pigmentation) supportive of syndrome.[29]
Sertoli-Leydig cell tumor	DICER1	Rare syndrome includes pleuropulmonary blastoma, nodular goiters, and cystic nephromas[26,27]

Laboratories use their internal databases and public databases, such as ClinVar to help classify variants, and most variants are classified as benign.[31] Of those that remain uncertain, findings are considered in the context of the family history as to whether they are likely to be clinically relevant. In the absence of compelling family history, women with VUS results have cancer risk equivalent to that of the general population. Therefore, women with VUS testing results are not candidates for risk-reducing programs and cascade testing is not indicated for their family members.

Somatic Testing in Ovarian Cancer

For ovarian cancer, somatic or tumor testing is most applicable in the recurrent setting. The number and variety of testing options available is daunting, and it is helpful to have a functional framework regarding the information provided by an individual test and its clinical applicability. Testing options are listed in **Fig. 3** and range from Food and Drug Administration (FDA) cleared companion diagnostics for treatment-intent PARP inhibitors that detect tumor BRCA mutations only, to complimentary diagnostics for maintenance-intent PARP inhibitors, to broad-spectrum NGS mutational analysis of multiple genes known to drive tumor biology that might select patients for other novel therapies. Microsatellite instability (MSI) testing is also relevant to ovarian cancer.

For women with germline BRCA wild-type ovarian cancer who are candidates for PARP inhibitor therapy as treatment in the third line or greater, Foundation Focus CDx BRCA is FDA-cleared as the companion diagnostic to rucaparib for this indication. This test only provides information on the status of the BRCA1 and BRCA2 genes and is unable to distinguish germline from somatic mutations. Assays that also examine normal tissue, such as Ambry TumorNext-HD, can make this determination.

A second indication for somatic testing includes determination of changes in DNA that, like BRCA mutations, cause HRD and, thus, the BRCA-ness phenotype.[20] Testing for HRD or loss of DNA heterozygosity can predict benefit from PARP inhibitors in the maintenance setting, although all women who are candidates for PARP maintenance, that is, platinum-sensitive and in partial or complete response to their last platinum-based chemotherapy, have been found to derive benefit from this treatment strategy.[32–34]

Lastly, expanded panel somatic testing is perhaps the most versatile option. Currently, this testing is best used for women who have platinum-resistant disease or who have exhausted other treatment options. Expanded somatic testing can detect mutations in the actionable genes previously mentioned and identify women for novel matched therapies, and serves as the basis of personalized medicine in oncology treatment. Mutation-matched drugs are often best accessed on clinical trials, such as the MATCH study, which was recently conducted by the National Cancer Institute (NCT02465060). This "basket" trial investigated several targeted agents in patients harboring specific mutations in chemorefractory tumors, regardless of the tumor type. As more is learned about chemotherapy-resistant rarer tumors, such as clear cell, endometrioid, and low-grade serous ovarian cancers, the use of mutational-matched drugs will move into earlier lines of therapy, perhaps becoming an alternative to the chemotherapies used today.

Finally, many expanded panel somatic tests include an assessment of MSI. Although only 1% of ovarian cancers harbor germline MSI and only 10% harbor somatic MSI, this finding does have important implications for therapeutic selection.[35] An immune checkpoint inhibitor, pembrolizumab, is now FDA-approved specifically for unresectable or MSI-high solid tumors, independent of tumor location.[36] These agents are emerging as an essential component of therapy for recurrent ovarian cancers, and are being actively studied in the upfront and maintenance settings.

GENETIC TESTING IN ENDOMETRIAL CANCER
Hereditary Nonpolyposis Colorectal Cancer Syndrome

Hereditary nonpolyposis colorectal cancer is also well known as Lynch syndrome. It is characterized by colorectal and endometrial, ovarian, gastric, renal, and skin malignancies. Approximately 15% of these cancers have MSI, often in the form of epigenetic silencing of *MLH1* or *MSH2* via hypermethylation; however, somatic and germline mutations can also exist in the four primary mismatch repair genes: *MSH2*, *MSH6*, *MLH1*, and *PMS2*.

Mutations within the *MLH1* and *MSH2* genes carry an elevated risk of numerous malignancies, including 25% to 60% uterine cancer; 52% to 82% colon cancer; 4% to 25% ovarian cancer; 6% to 13% gastric cancer; and approximately 5% risk of hepatobiliary, central nervous system, pancreatic, small bowel, and urothelial cancers. Conversely, *PMS2* and *MLH6* mutations carry a risk of 10% to 22% of colon cancer, 15% to 26% for uterine cancer, and less than 5% for all other cancer listed previously including ovarian cancer.[14] Because of its high penetrance, hereditary nonpolyposis colorectal cancer merits risk reduction with hysterectomy and salpingo-oophorectomy at age 40 to 45.

Cowden Syndrome

The *PTEN* gene, which encodes the phosphatase and tensin homolog protein, is a tumor suppressor gene that, when mutated, causes an elevated risk of uterine cancer at 19% to 28%.[14] Beginning at age 30 to 35, women should undergo annual transvaginal ultrasound and endometrial biopsy. Given this high penetrance mutation with elevated uterine cancer risk, consideration should be given to hysterectomy on completion of childbearing.

Women also carry an elevated risk of breast cancer of 50% and intensive and early screening are advised with annual examination, mammogram, and MRI. Follicular thyroid cancer risk is up to 38% and warrants annual thyroid ultrasound. Renal cell carcinoma risk of 5% should prompt consideration of annual renal ultrasound starting at age 40 and colon cancer risk of 9% requires colonoscopy every 5 years beginning at age 35.

Somatic Testing in Uterine Cancers

The 2014 Society for Gynecologic Oncology position statement and a 2017 multidisciplinary summit on genetics services recommend genetic testing (**Fig. 4**) in women with endometrial cancer.[21,22,37] There are four highly penetrant primary genes responsible for mismatch repair: *MSH2*, *MLH1*, *PMS2*, and *MSH6*. Any mutation in these genes or somatic loss of expression is known as MSI. Normal expression of all mismatch repair proteins is known as microsatellite-stable.

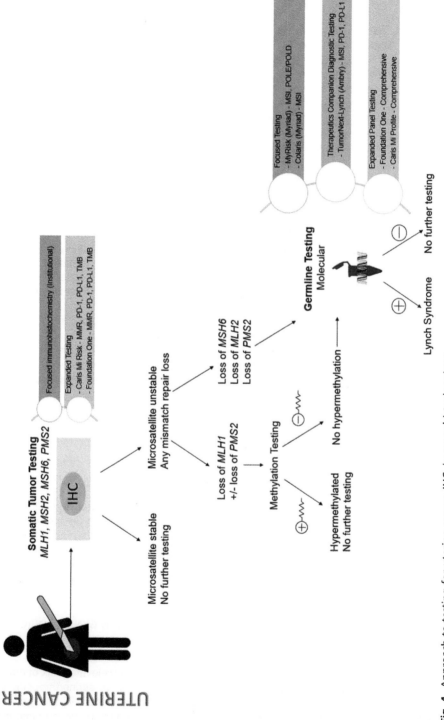

Fig. 4. Approach to testing for uterine cancer. IHC, immunohistochemistry.

In contrast to ovarian cancer, initial testing in endometrial cancer is tissue-based using either biopsy or preferably, hysterectomy tissue.[38] According to the 2017 consensus guidelines, immunohistochemistry (IHC) for the mismatch repair proteins should be performed for women at risk by personal or family history, or in all women younger than age 60. Loss of expression has excellent sensitivity and specificity greater than 90%.[39]

The inactivation of mismatch repair genes can be caused by germline or somatic mutation, or epigenetic silencing. The first step after IHC has detected a loss of mismatch repair protein expression for *MLH1*, *PMS2*, or both *MLH1* and *PMS2* is evaluation for epigenetic hypermethylation of the *MLH1* promoter, which allows functional silencing of these proteins but does not herald an underlying somatic or germline mutation. In the setting of negative IHC or MLH1 hypermethylation, further referral for germline testing should only be considered in situations of personal or family cancer histories, which confer a high clinical suspicion.

Germline Testing in Uterine Cancers

In the setting of loss of *MLH2*, *PMS2* alone, or *MLH6*, or a lack of hypermethylation of *MLH1* or *PMS2*, molecular testing should be performed. Molecular testing is performed on DNA from fresh, frozen, or paraffin-embedded tissue using polymerase chain reaction–based testing of five specific markers. If a germline mutation is identified, this characterizes Lynch syndrome and recommendations for cascade testing of family members, and risk reduction strategies, are undertaken.[22] If germline testing is negative, no further testing is required.

Although MSI-high represents a more favorable prognosis for colon cancer, this has not been confirmed in uterine cancer.[40] MSI does have important applications for therapeutic targeting. Immune checkpoint inhibitor, pembrolizumab, for unresectable or MSI-high solid tumors is used in this setting.[36] In uterine cancer, molecular targeting of vascular endothelial growth factor, *PIK3CA*, and *HER2* mutations as a result of somatic tumor testing can also guide therapeutic choices for these women given emerging data for these agents.

GENETIC TESTING IN CERVICAL AND VULVAR CANCER

Currently the role of somatic tumor testing is not well established for cervical or vulvar cancer and outside of rare clinical situations, such as cervical adenoma malignum, germline testing is not warranted.

Immunohistochemical or molecular evidence of MSI is of increasing relevance, because 5% to 11% of cervical cancers may express this phenotype and would be candidates for targeted checkpoint-inhibitor therapy as described previously.[41] In cervical and vulvar cancers, the role of somatic tumor testing remains limited otherwise; however, tyrosine-kinase inhibitors remain under investigation in the upfront and recurrent settings and the use of somatic tumor biomarkers to guide these therapeutic choices is needed.[42]

MODERATE TO LOW PENETRANCE SYNDROMES OF INTEREST IN GYNECOLOGIC ONCOLOGY
Peutz-Jeghers Syndrome

This syndrome, characterized by *STK11* mutation, results in an elevated risk of malignancy of several rare gynecologic malignancies.[29,43] *SKT11*, or serine/threonine kinase 11, is a tumor suppressor gene and a germline mutation in this gene is inherited in an autosomal-dominant fashion. Germline mutations result in pigmented skin and mucosal macules, gastrointestinal polyps, and elevated cancer risk. Sex cord stromal tumor of the ovary with annular tubules risk is elevated to 18% to 21% and uterine cancer risk is elevated to 9%, which merits an annual pelvic examination and consideration of pelvic ultrasound starting at age 18. There is also an elevated risk of cervical adenoma malignum at 10%. Although national guidelines suggest initiating Pap surveillance at age 21, this population warrants imitation of screening at age 18 to 20. There are currently no risk-reducing strategies that are supported.

In addition to gynecologic cancers, women are also at risk of breast cancer in 45% to 50% meriting significantly more frequent and intensive breast screening and consideration of risk-reducing mastectomy. Risk of colon cancer may be 39% and stomach cancer 29%, with increased surveillance using colonoscopy and esophago-gastroduodenoscopy every 2 to 3 years beginning by age 18.[29,43]

Li-Fraumeni Syndrome

The lifetime risk of cancer with this devastating syndrome approaches 90% to 100% by age 70. This results from mutation of the *CHEK2* tumor suppressor gene and TP53 oncogene, with resultant uncontrolled cellular growth. The most common malignancies include breast cancer at 50%; osteosarcoma and soft tissue sarcomas; and brain, adrenal, and hematologic cancers. This confers an elevated risk of ovarian and uterine cancers; however, no current screening guidelines or risk reduction strategies exist in this regard.[14,44]

Polymerase Proofreading-Associated Polyposis Syndrome

Polymerase proofreading-associated polyposis syndrome represents mutations in two DNA polymerases: *POLD1* and *POLE*.[14,45,46] This germline mutation results in a loss of proofreading capability and accumulation of mutations, manifesting as MSI with an elevated risk of uterine and colonic malignancies.[47] Assessment for mutations of these genes should be performed during routine genetic evaluation of those being tested for Lynch syndrome. The Cancer Genome Atlas additionally identified a subgroup of uterine cancers with an ultramutated phenotype that have a favorable prognosis.[2]

MOLECULAR TESTING PLATFORMS

There are several commercially available genetic sequencing platforms being used by genetic counselors and physicians, such as Foundation One, Personal Genome Diagnostics, Ambry, Caris, and Myriad. Each of these offers a preset panel of genes to be evaluated, ranging from 2 to 50 genes, and each has its inherent strengths and limitations.[8] Although single gene testing for only *BRCA1* and *BRCA2* is an option, standard practice at this time is multigene penal testing, which may identify mutations in up to 4% of patients in whom single gene testing would have missed their hereditary cancer (**Table 3**).[25,48]

Interpretation of results from genetic sequencing platforms should be performed by a certified genetic counselor or gynecologic oncologist, who has experience in making evidence-based recommendations regarding appropriate screening and risk-reduction strategies. This becomes particularly essential to avoid the pitfalls of genetic sequencing, which can include limited mutation assessment with various panels, misinterpretation of somatic and germline mutations and their implications, and VUS.

LIMITATIONS OF COMMERCIAL GENETIC TESTING

Among the commercially available gene sequencing panels mentioned previously, each analyzes a preset list of mutations that are determined most likely to be clinically

Table 3
Review of hereditary cancer syndromes

Syndrome	Mutation	Cancer Site	Cancer Risk (%)
HBOC	BRCA1	Ovary	39–46
	BRCA2	Breast	65–85
		Serous uterine	4
		Ovary	39–46
		Breast	45–85
HOC	BRIP1	Ovary	10–15
	RAD51C		
	RAD51D		
HNPCC	MLH1	Uterine	25–60
	MSH2	Ovary	4–25
	MSH6	Colon	52–82
	PMS2	Uterine	15–26
		Ovary	<5
		Colon	10–22
Peutz-Jeghers	STK11	Ovary (SCTAT)	18–21
		Uterine	9
		Cervical	10
		Breast	45–50
		Colon	39
		Pancreas	11–36
		Gastric	29
Cowden	PTEN	Uterine	19–28
		Breast	25–50
		Colon	9
		Thyroid	3–38
Li-Fraumeni	P53	Breast	Any cancer by age 70 = 90
		Ovary	
		Uterine	
		CNS	
		Sarcoma	
		Leukemia	
PPAP	POLD1	Uterine	—
		Colon	

Abbreviations: CNS, central nervous system; HBOC, hereditary breast and ovarian cancer; HNPCC, hereditary nonpolyposis colon cancer; HOC, hereditary ovarian cancer; PPAP, polymerase proofreading-associated polyposis; SCTAT, sex cord stromal tumor with annular tubules.

relevant. As understanding of clinically relevant mutations expands rapidly, these panels cannot accommodate all possible relevant mutations and thus, it is essential to be aware of the limitations of testing. Additionally, less commonly detected mutations of questionable significance are found with increasing frequency. These are labeled VUS. These variants are not actionable, because the current evidence base does not support application of screening and treatment recommendations to this poorly characterized group.

DIRECT-TO-CONSUMER TESTING

Providers in today's landscape must also face the challenges of direct-to-consumer genetic testing. Specifically, patients have kits mailed to their homes, typically requiring saliva collection, and the results are mailed back detailing any mutations found. Dozens of these companies exist, with specific examples including Color,

Veritas, Helix, or 23andMe. This bypass of traditional health systems allows the benefit of bypassing insurance approvals for patients, but also has many limitations. These include a lack of regulatory oversight, a limitation in the number of genes screened, and often out-of-context reporting of mutations detected.

In 2018, the FDA authorized the first direct-to-consumer testing for *BRCA* genes. This testing reports on three genes most common in people of Ashkenazi Jewish descent. This is in recognition that these three genes are not the most common in the general population and that there are greater than 1000 known *BRCA* mutations that are not evaluable by this testing.[49] The approval clearly advises that these results should not be used to determine treatments or risk-reduction strategies, rather they should guide confirmatory testing and genetic counseling. This approval was offered to 23and Me, Inc.

Unfortunately, these details of the FDA approval are often overlooked and these tests are frequently being used by the general population. In May 2018, the American College of Obstetricians and Gynecologists published a practice advisory regarding direct-to-consumer testing. American College of Obstetricians and Gynecologists discourages direct-to-consumer genetic testing because of the absence of pretest and posttest counseling and the possibility of false-reassurance with a "negative" test result. Furthermore, providers are limited in the ability to counsel patients with a "positive" test result and may subject patients to potential intervention unnecessarily.[50]

GENETIC COUNSELOR REFERRAL GUIDELINES

National Comprehensive Cancer Network guidelines and the Society of Gynecologic Oncology support that all women diagnosed with ovarian and uterine cancer undergo genetic assessment.[51] In those with the high-risk characteristics listed in **Box 1**,

---

Box 1
Review of criteria for genetic counseling assessment

A Personal History of...	A Personal or Family History of...	A Family History of...

• Ovarian cancer
• Breast cancer with 1 criterion:
  ○ Age <50
  ○ Male
  ○ Triple negative age <60
  ○ Ashkenazi Jewish descent
  ○ High-risk family member
• Prostate cancer
	• 3 or more cancers:
	  ○ Breast
	  ○ Pancreas
	  ○ Prostate
	  ○ Melanoma
	  ○ Sarcoma
	  ○ Adrenocortical
	  ○ Brain
	  ○ Leukemia
	  ○ Thyroid
	  ○ Kidney
	  ○ Colon
	  ○ Uterine
	  ○ Gastric
		• First-, second-, third-degree relative with:
		  ○ Ovarian cancer
		  ○ Known cancer mutation
		  ○ >2 breast cancers in 1 person
		  ○ >2 breast cancers on same side of family with 1 person, age <50
		  ○ Male breast cancer
		• First- or second-degree relative with:
		  ○ Breast cancer, age <45 y old

Data from Hampel H, Bennett RL, Buchanan A, et al. A practice guideline from the American College of Medical Genetics and Genomics and the National Society of Genetic Counselors: referral indications for cancer predisposition assessment. Genet Med 2015;17(1):70–87; and Umar A, Boland CR, Terdiman JP, et al. Revised Bethesda guidelines for hereditary nonpolyposis colorectal cancer (Lynch syndrome) and microsatellite instability. J Natl Cancer Inst 2004;96(4):261–8.

referral should be made to a genetic counselor who can guide patients on which, if any, genetic testing should be used. Additionally, the National Comprehensive Cancer Network guidelines on Genetic/Familial High-Risk Assessment: Breast and Ovarian is an excellent resource to guide providers in genetic referral practices.[52]

THE FUTURE OF MOLECULAR MEDICINE

As the fields of genomics and proteomics continue to expand, their applicability to patient screening, tumor interrogation and prognostication, and identification of targetable mutations for novel therapeutic are exciting. For providers, however, this plethora of genetic information can be overwhelming and challenging to navigate. This brief summary of the most applicable technology for an obstetrician/gynecologist or women's physician today should guide surveillance and risk-reduction strategies for the most common syndromes.

REFERENCES

1. Berger AC, Korkut A, Kanchi RS, et al. A comprehensive pan-cancer molecular study of gynecologic and breast cancers. Cancer Cell 2018;33(4):690–705.e9.
2. Cancer Genome Atlas Research Network. Integrated genomic analyses of ovarian carcinoma. Nature 2011;474(7353):609–15.
3. Cancer Genome Atlas Research Network, Albert Einstein College of Medicine, Analytical Biological Services, et al. Integrated genomic and molecular characterization of cervical cancer. Nature 2017;543(7645):378–84.
4. Kandoth C, Schultz N, Cherniack AD, et al. Integrated genomic characterization of endometrial carcinoma. Nature 2013;497(7447):67–73.
5. Berglund EC, Kiialainen A, Syvänen AC. Next-generation sequencing technologies and applications for human genetic history and forensics. Investig Genet 2011;2:23.
6. Jones S, Anagnostou V, Lytle K, et al. Personalized genomic analyses for cancer mutation discovery and interpretation. Sci Transl Med 2015;7(283):283ra53.
7. Carr TH, McEwen R, Dougherty B, et al. Defining actionable mutations for oncology therapeutic development. Nat Rev Cancer 2016;16(5):319–29.
8. Kotelnikova EA, Pyatnitskiy M, Paleeva A, et al. Practical aspects of NGS-based pathways analysis for personalized cancer science and medicine. Oncotarget 2016;7(32):52493–516.
9. Diaz LA Jr, Bardelli A. Liquid biopsies: genotyping circulating tumor DNA. J Clin Oncol 2014;32(6):579–86.
10. Fadare O, DK. Molecular profiling of epithelial ovarian cancer. My cancer genome 2016. Available at: https://www.mycancergenome.org/content/disease/ovarian-cancer/.
11. Meghnani V, Mohammed N, Giauque C, et al. Performance characterization and validation of saliva as an alternative specimen source for detecting hereditary breast cancer mutations by next generation sequencing. Int J Genomics 2016; 2016:2059041.
12. Vnencak-Jones C, Berger M, Pao W. Types of molecular tumor testing. My Cancer Genome 2016. Available at: https://www.mycancergenome.org/content/molecular-medicine/types-of-molecular-tumor-testing/.
13. Siegel RL, Miller KD, Jemal A. Cancer statistics, 2016. CA Cancer J Clin 2016; 66(1):7–30.
14. Ring KL, Garcia C, Thomas MH, et al. Current and future role of genetic screening in gynecologic malignancies. Am J Obstet Gynecol 2017;217(5):512–21.

15. Tanday S. BRCA mutations and risk of uterine cancer. Lancet Oncol 2016;17(8): e324.
16. Loveday C, Turnbull C, Ramsay E, et al. Germline mutations in RAD51D confer susceptibility to ovarian cancer. Nat Genet 2011;43(9):879–82.
17. Loveday C, Turnbull C, Ruark E, et al. Germline RAD51C mutations confer susceptibility to ovarian cancer. Nat Genet 2012;44(5):475–6 [author reply: 476].
18. Lynch HT, Casey MJ, Snyder CL, et al. Hereditary ovarian carcinoma: heterogeneity, molecular genetics, pathology, and management. Mol Oncol 2009;3(2): 97–137.
19. Norquist BM, Harrell MI, Brady MF, et al. Inherited mutations in women with ovarian carcinoma. JAMA Oncol 2016;2(4):482–90.
20. Konstantinopoulos PA, Spentzos D, Karlan BY, et al. Gene expression profile of BRCAness that correlates with responsiveness to chemotherapy and with outcome in patients with epithelial ovarian cancer. J Clin Oncol 2010;28(22): 3555–61.
21. Oncology SoG. SGO clinical practice statement: genetic testing for ovarian cancer. 2014. Available at: https://www.sgo.org/clinical-practice/guidelines/genetic-testing-for-ovarian-cancer/.
22. Randall LM, Pothuri B, Swisher EM, et al. Multi-disciplinary summit on genetics services for women with gynecologic cancers: a Society of Gynecologic Oncology white paper. Gynecol Oncol 2017;146(2):217–24.
23. Huang YW. Association of BRCA1/2 mutations with ovarian cancer prognosis: an updated meta-analysis. Medicine 2018;97(2):e9380.
24. Walsh CS. Two decades beyond BRCA1/2: homologous recombination, hereditary cancer risk and a target for ovarian cancer therapy. Gynecol Oncol 2015; 137(2):343–50.
25. Minion LE, Dolinsky JS, Chase DM, et al. Hereditary predisposition to ovarian cancer, looking beyond BRCA1/BRCA2. Gynecol Oncol 2015;137(1):86–92.
26. Schultz KA, Harris A, Messinger Y, et al. Ovarian tumors related to intronic mutations in DICER1: a report from the international ovarian and testicular stromal tumor registry. Fam Cancer 2016;15(1):105–10.
27. Schultz KA, Pacheco MC, Yang J, et al. Ovarian sex cord-stromal tumors, pleuropulmonary blastoma and DICER1 mutations: a report from the International Pleuropulmonary Blastoma Registry. Gynecol Oncol 2011;122(2):246–50.
28. Conlon N, Silva A, Guerra E, et al. Loss of SMARCA4 expression is both sensitive and specific for the diagnosis of small cell carcinoma of ovary, hypercalcemic type. Am J Surg Pathol 2016;40(3):395–403.
29. Resta N, Pierannunzio D, Lenato GM, et al. Cancer risk associated with STK11/LKB1 germline mutations in Peutz-Jeghers syndrome patients: results of an Italian multicenter study. Dig Liver Dis 2013;45(7):606–11.
30. Richter S, Haroun I, Graham TC, et al. Variants of unknown significance in BRCA testing: impact on risk perception, worry, prevention and counseling. Ann Oncol 2013;24(Suppl 8):viii69–74.
31. Eggington JM, Bowles KR, Moyes K, et al. A comprehensive laboratory-based program for classification of variants of uncertain significance in hereditary cancer genes. Clin Genet 2014;86(3):229–37.
32. Pujade-Lauraine E, Ledermann JA, Penson RT, et al. Treatment with olaparib monotherapy in the maintenance setting significantly improves progression-free survival in patients with platinum-sensitive relapsed ovarian cancer: results from the Phase III SOLO2 Study. Gynecologic Oncology 2017;145(Suppl 1): 219–20.

33. Mirza MR, Monk BJ, Herrstedt J, et al. Niraparib maintenance therapy in platinum-sensitive, recurrent ovarian cancer. N Engl J Med 2016;375(22): 2154–64.

34. Matulonis UA, Harter P, Gourley C, et al. Olaparib maintenance therapy in patients with platinum-sensitive, relapsed serous ovarian cancer and a BRCA mutation: overall survival adjusted for postprogression poly(adenosine diphosphate ribose) polymerase inhibitor therapy. Cancer 2016;122(12):1844–52.

35. Jensen KC, Mariappan MR, Putcha GV, et al. Microsatellite instability and mismatch repair protein defects in ovarian epithelial neoplasms in patients 50 years of age and younger. Am J Surg Pathol 2008;32(7):1029–37.

36. Approved Drugs - FDA grants accelerated approval to pembrolizumab for first tissue/site agnostic indication. Available at: http://www.fda.gov5/2017.

37. Oncology SoG. Clinical practice statement for Lynch syndrome in endometrial cancer. 2014. Available at: https://www.sgo.org/clinical-practice/guidelines/screening-for-lynchsyndrome-in-endometrial-cancer/.

38. Terdiman JP, Gum JR Jr, Conrad PG, et al. Efficient detection of hereditary nonpolyposis colorectal cancer gene carriers by screening for tumor microsatellite instability before germline genetic testing. Gastroenterology 2001;120(1):21–30.

39. Mills AM, Longacre TA. Lynch syndrome screening in the gynecologic tract: current state of the Art. Am J Surg Pathol 2016;40(4):e35–44.

40. Diaz-Padilla I, Romero N, Amir E, et al. Mismatch repair status and clinical outcome in endometrial cancer: a systematic review and meta-analysis. Crit Rev Oncol Hematol 2013;88(1):154–67.

41. Wong YF, Cheung TH, Poon KY, et al. The role of microsatellite instability in cervical intraepithelial neoplasia and squamous cell carcinoma of the cervix. Gynecol Oncol 2003;89(3):434–9.

42. Crafton SM, Salani R. Beyond chemotherapy: an overview and review of targeted therapy in cervical cancer. Clin Ther 2016;38(3):449–58.

43. van Lier MG, Wagner A, Mathus-Vliegen EM, et al. High cancer risk in Peutz-Jeghers syndrome: a systematic review and surveillance recommendations. Am J Gastroenterol 2010;105(6):1258–64 [author reply: 1265].

44. Amadou A, Waddington Achatz MI, Hainaut P. Revisiting tumor patterns and penetrance in germline TP53 mutation carriers: temporal phases of Li-Fraumeni syndrome. Curr Opin Oncol 2018;30(1):23–9.

45. Bellido F, Pineda M, Aiza G, et al. POLE and POLD1 mutations in 529 kindred with familial colorectal cancer and/or polyposis: review of reported cases and recommendations for genetic testing and surveillance. Genet Med 2016;18(4): 325–32.

46. Briggs S, Tomlinson I. Germline and somatic polymerase epsilon and delta mutations define a new class of hypermutated colorectal and endometrial cancers. J Pathol 2013;230(2):148–53.

47. Palles C, Cazier JB, Howarth KM, et al. Germline mutations affecting the proofreading domains of POLE and POLD1 predispose to colorectal adenomas and carcinomas. Nat Genet 2013;45(2):136–44.

48. LaDuca H, Stuenkel AJ, Dolinsky JS, et al. Utilization of multigene panels in hereditary cancer predisposition testing: analysis of more than 2,000 patients. Genet Med 2014;16(11):830–7.

49. FDA authorizes, with special controls, direct-to-consumer test that reports three mutations in the BRCA breast cancer genes. Available at: http://www.fda.gov3/2018.

50. Practice advisory: response to FDA's authorization of BRCA1 and BRCA2 gene mutation direct-to-consumer testing. Available at: https://www.acog.org/Clinical-Guidance-and-Publications/Practice-Advisories/Practice-Advisory-Response-to-FDAs-Authorization-of-BRCA1-and-BRCA2-Genes-Direct-to-Consumer-Testing May 2018.
51. Schorge JO, Modesitt SC, Coleman RL, et al. SGO white paper on ovarian cancer: etiology, screening and surveillance. Gynecol Oncol 2010;119(1):7–17.
52. Daly MB, Axilbund JE, Bryant E, et al. Genetic/familial high-risk assessment: breast and ovarian. J Natl Compr Canc Netw 2006;4(2):156–76.

Less Is More: Minimally Invasive and Quality Surgical Management of Gynecologic Cancer

Evelyn Cantillo, MD, MPH[a],*, Jenna B. Emerson, MD[b],
Cara Mathews, MD[b]

KEYWORDS

• Minimally invasive surgery • ERAS • Gynecologic oncology • Sentinel lymph nodes

KEY POINTS

• The surgical landscape in gynecologic oncology has continued to move toward minimally invasive techniques.
• Sentinel lymph node biopsy in properly selected patients can be performed in lieu of lymphadenectomy.
• Minimally invasive techniques should never come at the expense of oncologic outcomes. Preliminary decreased survival data in early cervical cancer are concerning and need to be further elucidated.
• When properly implemented, Enhanced Recovery After Surgery protocols are appropriate in the gynecologic population.

Since the founding of gynecologic oncology as a specialty in 1969, surgery remains one of its pillars. Although surgical principles remain the same, the ways in which these are performed have changed with time and corresponding advancements in technique. A 2015 survey of the Society of Gynecologic Oncology (SGO) membership found that 83% of respondents performed traditional laparoscopy, whereas 97% performed robotic surgery compared with 91% and 27%, respectively, in 2007.[1] The rapid uptake of the robotic platform, specifically, and minimally invasive surgery (MIS), in general, underscores the need to balance established methods while continuing to push surgical boundaries. In this article, the authors review the evolution of surgical management in cervical, endometrial, and ovarian cancer as well as changes in postoperative management.

[a] Division of Gynecologic Oncology, Department of Obstetrics, Gynecology and Reproductive Sciences, University of Vermont College of Medicine, 111 Colchester Avenue, Smith 408, Burlington, VT 05404, USA; [b] Program in Women' Oncology, Women and Infants Hospital, 101 Dudley Street, Providence, RI 02905, USA
* Corresponding author.
E-mail address: evelyn.cantillo@uvmhealth.org

Obstet Gynecol Clin N Am 46 (2019) 55–66
https://doi.org/10.1016/j.ogc.2018.09.004
0889-8545/19/© 2018 Elsevier Inc. All rights reserved.

obgyn.theclinics.com

CERVICAL CANCER

In 2018, there are estimated to be more than 13,000 new cases of cervical cancer and more than 4000 deaths attributable to the disease in the United States.[2] For early stage cervical cancers, treatment of curative intent is in the form of either radiation therapy (RT) or surgery. Most women deemed to be surgical candidates will undergo hysterectomy with simple or extrafascial hysterectomy being reserved for stage 1A1 lesions without lymphovascular space involvement (LVSI) and radical hysterectomy (RH) with nodal evaluation typically for stage 1A1 with LVSI to 1B1 cancers.

With the advent of MIS, laparoscopic and robotic approaches have become more common and have the benefit of decreased blood loss and shorter hospital stay.[3,4] A systematic review of 12 studies comparing laparoscopic (LRH) versus abdominal radical hysterectomy (ARH) found that oncologic outcome and 5-year survival rates were similar between the 2 groups.[5] A meta-analysis of robotic radical hysterectomy (RRH) compared with laparoscopic and open RH did not find significant differences in survival outcomes.[6] There have been no randomized controlled trials comparing ARH with minimally invasive RH. The phase 3 LACC trial seeks to answer this question and was designed to compare LRH or RRH to ARH in patients with early stage cervical cancer with primary outcome of disease-free survival at 5 years.[7] Preliminary findings have been quite provocative. MIS was found to have more than a 3-fold increase in disease-free survival events (hazard ratio [HR] = 3.74, P = .002) and was also associated with a decrease in overall survival (HR = 6.00, P = .004) compared with ARH.[8] Final analysis is awaited because this may swing the pendulum back to ARH if MIS approaches are found to be inferior.

Table 1			
Sentinel lymph node sensitivity and negative predictive value from select studies			
	n	Sensitivity, %	Negative Predictive Value, %	Identification Technique
Plante et al,[10] 2003	70	93	100	Combined blue dye technique and lymphoscintigraphy
Cormier et al,[11] 2011	122	87.5	97	Blue dye ± technetium-99m sulfur colloid (Tc-99)
Lécuru et al,[12] 2011	145	92	98.2	Combined blue dye technique and lymphoscintigraphy
Salvo et al,[13] 2017	188	96.4	99.3	Combined blue dye technique, Tc-99, and/or indocyanine green (ICG)

Nodal Evaluation

Lymph node metastasis is one of the most important prognostic factors in cervical cancer. Unfortunately, lymphedema, which is a well-known complication among women who have undergone radical surgery with pelvic lymphadenectomy, can be quite debilitating. One prospective, longitudinal study of 227 patients with cervical cancer found that lymphedema and menopausal symptoms were the most disabling treatment-related sequelae.[9] There continues to be an effort to balance adequate nodal evaluation while mitigating complications. The feasibility of sentinel lymph node (SLN) mapping has been explored in several studies (**Table 1**) with findings that suggest that in properly chosen patients, SLN biopsy could be performed in lieu of lymphadenectomy.

The newest version of the National Comprehensive Center Network (NCCN) guidelines include SLN mapping as an option for patients with tumors ≤2 cm with emphasis on adherence to the SLN mapping algorithm (**Fig. 1**).[14]

Besides reducing lymphedema risk, other benefits of SLN biopsy may lie in the ability to detect small volume nodal disease by ultrastaging and identify unusual drainage patterns.[15]

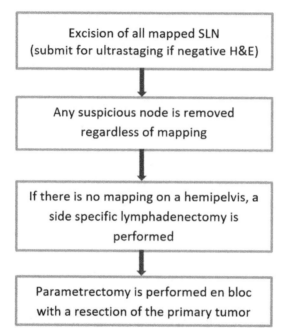

Fig. 1. Surgical algorithm for early cervical cancer. H&E, hematoxylin and eosin staining. (*Adapted from* Cormier B, Diaz JP, Shih K, et al. Establishing a sentinel lymph node mapping algorithm for the treatment of early cervical cancer. Gynecol Oncol 2011;122(2):276; with permission.)

Special Considerations

With a median age at diagnosis of 49, many women are still in their reproductive years. Depending on stage and pathologic factors, the management of cervical cancer may include fertility-sparing options in carefully selected patients, especially those with tumors ≤2 cm (**Table 2**). Nodal metastasis on imaging and the following histologic subtypes: small cell neuroendocrine, gastric type adenocarcinoma, and adenoma malignum, is not suitable for fertility-sparing surgery.

Several studies have found that oncologic outcomes for RH and radical vaginal trachelectomy are similar in tumors ≤2 cm with recurrence rates of less than 5% and overall survival rates of 98%.[16–18] In tumors larger than 2 cm but greater than 4 cm, the recurrence risk is unacceptable with vaginal radical trachelectomy (VRT): 17% compared with 4% in tumors <2 cm.[19] In this population, abdominal radical trachelectomy (ART) may be an option; however, there is a possibility that these patients will require postoperative adjuvant therapy. One systematic review of 485 patients found that ART is a safe treatment option in patients with early stage cervical cancer interested in preserving fertility reporting 4% disease recurrence, 0.4% death rate, 85% fertility rate, and 14% conception rate.[20] This review did not specifically look at tumors greater than 2 cm and less than 4 cm. One retrospective study of 45 women with stage

Table 2
Fertility-sparing treatment in early stage cervical cancer

Stage	Treatment	Imaging
IA1 without LVSI	Cone biopsy with negative margins	
IA1 with LVSI or 1A2	Cone biopsy with negative margins PLND ± PALND OR radical trachelectomy PLND	Consider pelvic MRI to assess extent of local disease
IB1	Radical trachelectomy PLND ± PALND	PET/CT scan or CT chest + abdomen + pelvis

Abbreviations: CT, computed tomography; PALND, para-aortic lymph node dissection; PLND, pelvic lymph node dissection.

IB1-IB2 cancers measuring more than 2 cm found a 5-year survival rate of 93.5% (31% underwent immediate completion of RH due to intraoperative factors), whereas another study of 62 women found zero recurrences at 30-month median follow-up (43% received adjuvant treatment).[21,22] There is not enough evidence to assess the feasibility of a minimally invasive approach. Both RH and trachelectomy are associated with persistent and/or chronic complications, such as urinary issues, sexual dysfunction, and lymphedema.[9,23,24]

In addition, radical trachelectomy has been associated with menstrual disorders and cervical stenosis.[24–26] Given the fertility desires of this population, there has been increased interest in examining the need for a radical approach based on low rates of parametrial involvement in early stage cervical cancer. Several retrospective studies have determined that the risk of parametrial involvement in women with pathologic factors, including tumor ≤2 cm, no LVSI, and negative pelvic lymph nodes on frozen section is ≤1%.[27–30] In a pilot study of 16 patients evaluating the feasibility of simple vaginal trachelectomy and nodal assessment in women with early stage cervical cancer, zero recurrences were documented at 24 months.[31]

The question is how conservative can we be without compromising oncologic outcomes? One phase 2 trial is attempting to establish the safety and feasibility of conservative surgery (cold knife cone or simple hysterectomy) with nodal evaluation in women with low risk cervical cancer.[32]

In addition, the phase 3 SHAPE trial is comparing RH and pelvic node dissection versus simple hysterectomy and pelvic node dissection in patients with previously untreated, low-risk cervical cancer with a primary outcome of pelvic relapse-free survival. Study completion date is September 2020.[33] Last, GOG 278 is currently examining physical function and quality of life before and after nonradical surgery for stage 1A1 with LVSI, 1A2, and 1B1 lesions ≤2 cm.[34]

ENDOMETRIAL CANCER

Endometrial cancer is the most common gynecologic malignancy in US women, and there are estimated to be more than 63,000 newly diagnosed endometrial cancers and 11,350 deaths due to the disease in 2018.[2] From 2006 to 2015, the rates for new uterine cancer cases have risen on average 1.3% each year and death rates have risen on average 1.6% each year; the 5-year overall survival remains stable at greater than

80%.[34] Since the publication of GOG 33 in 1987, which established the inadequacy of clinical staging, endometrial cancer has been surgically staged and traditionally includes extrafascial hysterectomy, bilateral salpingo-oophorectomy, with pelvic and para-aortic lymph node dissection.[35,36] Since that time, there has been an evolution in the approach to surgical route as well as nodal evaluation.

Route of Surgery

A shift from laparotomy to MIS began in the early 1990s as an increase in laparoscopy was seen with concomitant decrease in abdominal procedures.[37] One of the first studies examining laparoscopic staging in clinical stage I endometrial cancers reported an estimated blood loss <200 cc and average hospital stay of 2.9 days, making it an attractive option.[38] Over the years, the oncologic safety of laparoscopy has been examined. In the largest randomized phase 3 trial comparing laparoscopy to laparotomy in the staging of patients with endometrial cancer (GOG-LAP2), overall survival at 5 years was the same in both groups (89.8%) and the 3-year recurrence rate in the laparoscopy arm was 11.4% versus 10.2% in the laparotomy arm.[39] The LAP2 trial also found that laparoscopy resulted in fewer adverse events and shorter hospital stay. Similarly, the LACE trial, which randomly assigned women to total abdominal hysterectomy (n = 353) or total laparoscopic hysterectomy (n = 407), found no difference in overall or recurrence-free survival at 4.5 years.[40] Furthermore, 2 systematic reviews of 17 randomized controlled trials comparing laparoscopy to laparotomy for the treatment of early stage endometrial cancer found similar overall and disease-free survival and no difference in nodal yield between the groups, whereas laparoscopy was associated with reduced operative morbidity and hospital stay.[41,42]

In 2005, the Food and Drug Administration approved the daVinci surgical system (Intuitive Surgical Inc, Sunnyvale, CA, USA) for robotic gynecologic surgery. One of the first series to report the feasibility of and technique for robotic-assisted laparoscopic hysterectomy was published in 2006.[43] The 3-dimensional view, reduction in tremor, and improved ergonomics are some of the reasons the technology was rapidly adopted. Although clinical outcomes appear to be similar between robotic-assisted laparoscopy and traditional laparoscopy, the robotic approach is more expensive.[44] In a 2015 practice bulletin, the SGO in conjunction with the American College of Obstetricians and Gynecologists endorsed MIS as the standard surgical approach for comprehensive surgical staging in women with endometrial cancer.[45]

Nodal Evaluation

Approach to lymphadenectomy in endometrial cancer has undergone a considerable transformation since the publication of GOG 33, which reported a wide range of nodal involvement based on histology and uterine factors. Determining which patients should undergo a lymph node dissection became an important question because patients have different risk profiles. The Mayo Criteria established a cohort of low-risk patients: grade 1 or 2 tumors, ≤2 cm, myometrial invasion ≤50%, and no intraoperative evidence of macroscopic extrauterine spread, in whom lymphadenectomy could be omitted. The 5-year overall cancer-related and recurrence-free survivals in this group were 97% and 96%, respectively.[46] Two randomized controlled trials demonstrated that pelvic lymphadenectomy did not improve disease-free or overall survival.[47,48] It is worth noting that these studies have been criticized for several reasons, including the nonsystemic approach to lymphadenectomy and differences between lymphadenectomy and no lymphadenectomy group to name a few.

Patients with intermediate- or high-risk features still require nodal assessment. A post hoc analysis of GOG LAP2 found that patients with high-risk characteristics on their uterine specimens had 6.3 times the risk of nodal metastasis compared with those with low-risk characteristics.[49] In recent years, there has been a shift toward SLN mapping in lieu of lymphadenectomy. A 2017 meta-analysis of 55 studies and more than 4900 women found the sensitivity of SLN mapping to be 96%. This same study also saw increased bilateral detection rates with ICG compared with blue dye.[50] Similarly, the prospective FIRES trial reported a sensitivity of 97.2% and negative predictive value of 99.6% with SLN mapping.[51] There are also data to suggest that SLN mapping is effective in high-grade histologies, like clear cell and papillary serous.[52,53]

SGO consensus recommendations are for SLN mapping when the NCCN surgical algorithm is closely followed (**Fig. 2**). ICG was also found to be preferable, but radiocolloid Tc-99 combined with dye remains an acceptable alternative.[54]

OVARIAN CANCER

Traditionally, patients with suspected malignant ovarian/fallopian tube/primary peritoneal cancer are staged via laparotomy, which includes extrafascial hysterectomy, bilateral salpingo-oophorectomy, infracolic or infragastric omentectomy, cytoreduction, and possible pelvic and para-aortic lymph node dissection. The importance of cytoreduction is underscored by the improved survival seen in optimally debulked patients: residual tumor <1 cm or no residual tumor (R0), at the end of surgery.[55–57]

The most recent iteration of the NCCN guidelines includes provisions for the use of MIS. The who and why regarding the patient population that might benefit from a laparoscopic approach in ovarian cancer are at the crux of this discussion. There are several studies that show that laparoscopic surgical staging is both feasible and safe with regards to oncologic outcomes in early stage epithelial ovarian cancer.[58,59] One study in particular found that upon 18-month median follow-up, the disease-free survival was 94% and overall survival was 100% in patients who underwent laparoscopy.[60] Oncologic safety was also not affected in women who were laparoscopically staged for their stage I adult granulosa cell tumors.[61] These results suggest that

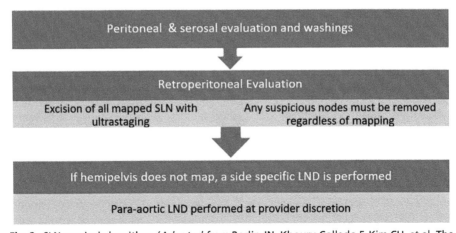

Fig. 2. SLN surgical algorithm. (*Adapted from* Barlin JN, Khoury-Collado F, Kim CH, et al. The importance of applying a sentinel lymph node mapping algorithm in endometrial cancer staging: beyond removal of blue nodes. Gynecol Oncol 2012;125(3):533; with permission.)

patients with early stage ovarian cancer can be laparoscopically staged. This approach is far more controversial for patients requiring primary surgery for advanced ovarian cancer and cannot be recommended at this time.

Laparoscopy in the setting of interval debulking and secondary cytoreduction surgery appears more promising. One study found that patients with ovarian cancer who underwent laparoscopic interval debulking surgery after neoadjuvant chemotherapy had 3-year survival rates similar to women who underwent interval debulking by laparotomy,[62] whereas another study demonstrated that MIS was feasible for secondary cytoreduction in properly selected cases with favorable perioperative outcomes and similar oncologic outcomes.[63] It is clear that more studies need to be performed in this area to determine patient suitability and survival outcomes.

It has also been proposed that laparoscopy can be used to triage patients who can and cannot be optimally debulked. One multicenter, randomized controlled trial in the Netherlands found that diagnostic laparoscopy reduced the number of futile laparotomies in patients with suspected advanced-stage ovarian cancer from 39% to 10%.[64] A more recent prospective validation study found that laparoscopy could avoid 85% of unsuccessful surgeries in patients undergoing interval cytoreduction.[65]

The role of laparoscopy in ovarian cancer continues to be elucidated. It appears that MIS can be performed in select cases and should be performed by an experienced gynecologic oncologist.

ENHANCED RECOVERY AFTER SURGERY

A growing body of literature supports the use of Enhanced Recovery After Surgery (ERAS) protocols for postoperative management in gynecologic surgery patients. Originally developed in colorectal surgery, these protocols are aimed at decreasing postoperative side effects, such as pain, nausea, and vomiting, while also decreasing the length of recovery time to a functional baseline.[66,67] Well-designed clinical trials have demonstrated decreased length of hospital stay, decreased use of postoperative opiate analgesia, and decreased postoperative symptom burden for patients when ERAS is used.[68]

The concept behind ERAS protocols is to maintain and support normal physiology preoperatively and postoperatively, with an objective of improving functional recovery and overall surgical outcome. Initially, ERAS systems were studied as a wide variety of interventions; most now agree that ERAS systems are best implemented as a multimodal bundle of patient care strategies.[69] These strategies are best understood when divided into preoperative, intraoperative, and postoperative interventions. Basic tenets of preoperative care include careful patient preparation preoperatively, including reviewing expectations and postoperative goals, and liberalization of preoperative fasting restrictions. Intraoperatively and postoperatively judicious use of intravenous fluids is prescribed with a goal of euvolemia. Pain control regimens, which minimize opiate use while supplementing with nonopioid adjuncts, are used both during and after surgery. Postoperatively, rapid resumption of a normal diet and normal activities is the goal. A multitude of trials comparing the ERAS approach to more "traditional" postoperative management has consistently demonstrated superiority of ERAS protocols with respect to patient outcomes and hospital length of stay.[70] Although much of the data for patients with gynecologic cancer has been generated out of smaller scale studies, over the past few years the literature has expanded dramatically. A retrospective cohort study of women undergoing gynecologic surgery for gynecologic cancers or pelvic reconstructive surgeries before and after the implementation of ERAS at the Mayo Clinic in Rochester, Minnesota demonstrated significant benefit in the ERAS group.[57]

Within the first 48 hours after surgery, there was a 48% decrease in opiate use, with improvement in pain scores immediately postoperatively in the group using fewer opiates. Although more nausea and vomiting were seen in the ERAS group, the overall amount of antiemetics used to control symptoms was the same between the ERAS and traditional groups. Furthermore, the ERAS group experienced resumption of bowel function 1 day earlier than their counterparts. Importantly, 30-day rates of complications and readmission were no different between the groups.

In addition to these improvements in patient-centered outcomes, ERAS practices are cost saving when compared with traditional postoperative strategies. Reported cost savings are heterogeneous as are the studies from which they are generated; published literature cites savings of $153 to $697 per patient for women undergoing abdominal or vaginal hysterectomy when ERAS is used as compared with traditional postoperative management. Despite this broad range, the cost-saving benefit of ERAS has been consistently demonstrated.[57,71]

Several studies have sought to assess patient acceptability. Many compare data points with historical controls; thus comparable data on patient acceptability are not directly available. However, Ottessen and colleagues[72] surveyed women after enrollment in a "fast-track" vaginal surgery cohort, and 93% of their 41 enrolled patients thought that hospitalization was "as easy" or "easier" than expected. Of their cohort, 85% reported that the hospital length of stay (with a median length of stay of 24 hours) was "convenient." Similarly, Yoong and colleagues[71] surveyed patients undergoing vaginal surgery following implementation of an ERAS protocol and found that 65% of patients reported satisfaction levels of 9 or 10 on a 10-point scale

The success of any ERAS program is contingent on 3 elements: (a) an ERAS protocol, (b) an audit system or database to review protocol compliance and clinical outcomes, and (c) an ERAS team that iterates toward improved compliance and outcomes. Recommendations with how to translate ERAS guidelines into gynecologic oncology practice are available.[60]

SUMMARY

The landscape of gynecologic cancer surgical care continues to evolve. The transition from laparotomy to laparoscopy (both traditional "straight stick" and robotic platforms) has made it possible to perform complicated surgeries with decreased blood loss, less postoperative morbidity, and improved quality of life. In addition, SLN mapping has changed the management of nodal basins maintaining diagnostic accuracy while minimizing toxicity. Although minimally invasive approaches have revolutionized surgical technique, less is only more if improvement in perioperative and postoperative metrics does not compromise oncologic outcomes. Pushing the surgical boundaries with evolving technology must always prioritize patient outcomes as the primary metric of success. The unexpected preliminary decreased survival data in early cervical cancer minimally invasive surgical management have raised a significant concern raising the critical importance of continued scrutiny in the practice changing technologies.

REFERENCES

1. Conrad LB, Ramirez PT, Burke W, et al. Role of minimally invasive surgery in gynecologic oncology: an updated survey of members of the society of gynecologic oncology. Int J Gynecol Cancer 2015;25(6):1121–7.
2. Noone AM, Howlader N, Krapcho M, et al, editors. SEER cancer statistics review, 1975–2015. Bethesda (MD): National Cancer Institute; 2018. Available at: https://seer.cancer.gov/csr/1975_2015.

3. Naik R, Jackson KS, Lopes A, et al. Laparoscopic assisted radical vaginal hysterectomy versus radical abdominal hysterectomy–a randomised phase II trial: perioperative outcomes and surgicopathological measurements. BJOG 2010; 117(6):746.

4. Steed H, Rosen B, Murphy J, et al. A comparison of laparascopic-assisted radical vaginal hysterectomy and radical abdominal hysterectomy in the treatment of cervical cancer. Gynecol Oncol 2004;93(3):588.

5. Wang YZ, Deng L, Xu HC, et al. Laparoscopy versus laparotomy for the management of early stage cervical cancer. BMC Cancer 2015;15:928.

6. Park DA, Yun JE, Kim SW, et al. Surgical and clinical safety and effectiveness of robot-assisted laparoscopic hysterectomycompared to conventional laparoscopy and laparotomy for cervical cancer: a systematic review and meta-analysis. Eur J Surg Oncol 2017;43(6):994–1002.

7. Available at: https://clinicaltrials.gov/ct2/show/NCT00614211. Accessed May 9, 2018.

8. Late breaking abstracts for the 49th Annual Meeting of the Society of Gynecologic Oncology. New Orleans, LA, March 24–28, 2018.

9. Ferrandina G, Mantegna G, Petrillo M, et al. Quality of life and emotional distress in early stage and locally advanced cervical cancer patients: a prospective, longitudinal study. Gynecol Oncol 2012;124(3):389–94.

10. Plante M, Renaud MC, Têtu B, et al. Laparoscopic sentinel node mapping in early-stage cervical cancer. Gynecol Oncol 2003;91(3):494–503.

11. Cormier B, Diaz JP, Shih K, et al. Establishing a sentinel lymph node mapping algorithm for the treatment of early cervical cancer. Gynecol Oncol 2011;122(2): 275–80.

12. Lécuru F, Mathevet P, Querleu D, et al. Bilateral negative sentinel nodes accurately predict absence of lymph node metastasis in early cervical cancer: results of the SENTICOL study. J Clin Oncol 2011;29(13):1686–91.

13. Salvo G, Ramirez P, Levenback C, et al. Sensitivity and negative predictive value for sentinel lymph node biopsy in women with early-stage cervical cancer. Gynecol Oncol 2017;145(1):96–101.

14. NCCN guidelines. Cervical cancer. Version 1.2018.

15. Bats AS, Mathevet P, Buenerd A, et al. The sentinel node technique detects unexpected drainage pathways and allows nodal ultrastaging in early cervical cancer: insights from the multicenter prospective SENTICOL study. Ann Surg Oncol 2013;20(2):413–22.

16. Lanowska M, Mangler M, Spek A, et al. Radical vaginal trachelectomy (RVT) combined with laparoscopic lymphadenectomy: prospective study of 225 patients with early-stage cervical cancer. Int J Gynecol Cancer 2011;21(8):1458.

17. Plante M, Gregoire J, Renaud MC, et al. The vaginal radical trachelectomy: an update of a series of 125 cases and 106 pregnancies. Gynecol Oncol 2011; 121:290–7.

18. Kim CH, Abu-Rustum NR, Chi DS, et al. Reproductive outcomes of patients undergoing radical trachelectomy for early-stage cervical cancer. Gynecol Oncol 2012;125:585.

19. Bentivegna E, Gouy S, Maulard A, et al. Oncological outcomes after fertility-sparing surgery for cervical cancer: a systematic review. Lancet Oncol 2016; 17(6):e240–53.

20. Pareja R, Rendón GJ, Sanz-Lomana CM, et al. Surgical, oncological, and obstetrical outcomes after abdominal radical trachelectomy - a systematic literature review. Gynecol Oncol 2013;131(1):77–82.

21. Lintner B, Saso S, Tarnai L, et al. Use of abdominal radical trachelectomy to treat cervical cancer greater than 2 cm in diameter. Int J Gynecol Cancer 2013;23(6): 1065–70.

22. Li J, Wu X, Li X, et al. Abdominal radical trachelectomy: Is it safe for IB1 cervical cancer with tumors ≥ 2 cm? Gynecol Oncol 2013;131(1):87–92.

23. Carenza L, Nobili F, Giacobini S. Voiding disorders after radical hysterectomy. Gynecol Oncol 1982;13:213.

24. Scotti RJ, Bergman A, Bhatia NN, et al. Urodynamic changes in ureterovesical function after radical hysterectomy. Obstet Gynecol 1986;68:111.

25. Alexander-Sefre F, Chee N, Spencer C, et al. Surgical morbidity associated with radical trachelectomy and radical hysterectomy. Gynecol Oncol 2006;101(3):450.

26. Selo-Ojeme DO, Ind T, Shepherd JH. Isthmic stenosis following radical trachelectomy. Obstet Gynaecol 2002;22(3):327.

27. Gemer O, Eitan R, Gdalevich M, et al. Can parametrectomy be avoided in early cervical cancer? An algorithm for the identification of patients at low risk for parametrial involvement. Eur J Surg Oncol 2013;39:76–80.

28. Frumovitz M, Sun C, Schmeler K, et al. Parametrial involvement in radical hysterectomy specimens for women with early-stage cervical cancer. Obstet Gynecol 2009;114:93–9.

29. Chang S, Bristow R, Ryu H. A model for prediction of parametrial involvement and feasibility of less radical resection of parametrium in patients with FIGO stage IB1 cervical cancer. Gynecol Oncol 2012;126:82–6.

30. Klat J, Sevcik L, Simetka O, et al. What is the risk for parametrial involvement in women with early-stage cervical cancer with tumour <20 mm and with negative sentinel lymph nodes? Aust N Z J Obstet Gynaecol 2012;52(6):540–4.

31. Plante M, Gregoire J, Renaud MC, et al. Simple vaginal trachelectomy in early-stage low-risk cervical cancer: a pilot study of 16 cases and review of the literature. Int J Gynecol Cancer 2013;23(5):916–22.

32. Available at: https://clinicaltrials.gov/ct2/show/study/NCT01048853?show_desc =Y#desc. Accessed May 8, 2018.

33. Available at: https://clinicaltrials.gov/ct2/show/NCT01658930?term=NCT016589 30&rank=1. Accessed May 8, 2018.

34. Available at: https://clinicaltrials.gov/ct2/show/NCT01649089. Accessed May 8, 2018.

35. Creasman WT, Morrow CP, Bundy BN, et al. Surgical pathologic spread patterns of endometrial cancer. A gynecologic oncology group study. Cancer 1987;60(8 Suppl):2035.

36. Pecorelli S. Revised FIGO staging for carcinoma of the vulva, cervix, and endometrium. Int J Gynaecol Obstet 2009;105(2):103–4.

37. Farquhar CM, Steiner CA. Hysterectomy rates in the United States, 1990-1997. Obstet Gynecol 2002;99(2):229–34.

38. Childers JM, Brzechffa PR, Hatch KD, et al. Laparoscopically assisted surgical staging (LASS) of endometrial cancer. Gynecol Oncol 1993;51(1):33–8.

39. Walker JL, Piedmonte MR, Spirtos NM, et al. Recurrence and survival after random assignment to laparoscopy versus laparotomy for comprehensive surgical staging of uterine cancer: Gynecologic Oncology Group LAP2 Study. J Clin Oncol 2012;30(7):695–700.

40. Janda M, Gebski V, Davies LC, et al. Effect of total laparoscopic hysterectomy vs total abdominal hysterectomy on disease-free survival among women with stage I endometrial cancer: a randomized clinical trial. JAMA 2017;317(12):1224–33.

41. Galaal K, Bryant A, Fisher AD, et al. Laparoscopy versus laparotomy for the management of early stage endometrial cancer. Cochrane Database Syst Rev 2012;(9):CD006655.

42. He H, Zeng D, Ou H, et al. Laparoscopic treatment of endometrial cancer: systematic review. J Minim Invasive Gynecol 2013;20(4):413–23.

43. Reynolds RK, Advincula AP. Robot-assisted laparoscopic hysterectomy: technique and initial experience. Am J Surg 2006;191(4):555–60.

44. Smorgick N, As-Sanie S. The benefits and challenges of robotic-assisted hysterectomy. Curr Opin Obstet Gynecol 2014;26(4):290–4.

45. American College of Obstetricians and Gynecologists. Practice Bulletin No. 149: endometrial cancer. Obstet Gynecol 2015;125(4):1006–26.

46. Mariani A, Webb MJ, Keeney GL, et al. Low-risk corpus cancer: is lymphadenectomy or radiotherapy necessary? Am J Obstet Gynecol 2000;182(6):1506–19.

47. Benedetti Panici P, Basile S, Maneschi F, et al. Systematic pelvic lymphadenectomy vs. no lymphadenectomy in early-stage endometrial carcinoma: randomized clinical trial. J Natl Cancer Inst 2008;100(23):1707.

48. ASTEC study group, Kitchener H, Swart AM, Qian Q, et al. Efficacy of systematic pelvic lymphadenectomy in endometrial cancer (MRC ASTEC trial): a randomised study. Lancet 2009;373(9658):125.

49. Milam MR, Java J, Walker JL, et al. Nodal metastasis risk in endometrioid endometrial cancer. Obstet Gynecol 2012;119(2 Pt 1):286–92.

50. Bodurtha Smith AJ, Fader AN, Tanner EJ. Sentinel lymph node assessment in endometrial cancer: a systematic review and meta-analysis. Am J Obstet Gynecol 2017;216(5):459–76.

51. Rossi EC, Kowalski LD, Scalici J, et al. A comparison of sentinel lymph node biopsy to lymphadenectomy for endometrial cancer staging (FIRES trial): a multicentre, prospective, cohort study. Lancet Oncol 2017;18:384–92.

52. Schiavone MB, Zivanovic O, Zhou Q, et al. Survival of patients with uterine carcinosarcoma undergoing sentinel lymph node mapping. Ann Surg Oncol 2016;23: 196–202.

53. Schiavone MB, Scelzo C, Straight CE, et al. Survival of patients with serous uterine carcinoma undergoing sentinel lymph node mapping. Ann Surg Oncol 2017; 24(7):1965–71.

54. Holloway RW, Abu-Rustum NR, Backes FJ, et al. Sentinel lymph node mapping and staging in endometrial cancer: a Society of Gynecologic Oncology literature review with consensus recommendations. Gynecol Oncol 2017;146(2):405–15.

55. Eisenkop SM, Friedman RL, Wang HJ, et al. Complete cytoreductive surgery is feasible and maximizes survival in patients with advanced epithelial ovarian cancer: a prospective study. Gynecol Oncol 1998;69(2):103.

56. Chi DS, Eisenhauer EL, Lang J, et al. What is the optimal goal of primary cytoreductive surgery for bulky stage IIIC epithelial ovarian carcinoma (EOC)? Gynecol Oncol 2006;103(2):559.

57. Bristow RE, Tomacruz RS, Armstrong DK. Survival effect of maximal cytoreductive surgery for advanced ovarian carcinoma during the platinum era: a meta-analysis. J Clin Oncol 2002;20(5):1248–59.

58. Chi DS, Abu-Rustum NR, Sonoda Y, et al. The safety and efficacy of laparoscopic surgical staging of apparent stage I ovarian and fallopian tube cancers. Am J Obstet Gynecol 2005;192(5):1614–9.

59. Park JY, Kim DY, Suh DS, et al. Comparison of laparoscopy and laparotomy in surgical staging of early-stage ovarian and fallopian tubal cancer. Ann Surg Oncol 2008;15(7):2012–9.

60. Brockbank EC, Harry V, Kolomainen D, et al. Laparoscopic staging for apparent early stage ovarian or fallopian tube cancer. First case series from a UK cancer centre and systematic literature review. Eur J Surg Oncol 2013;39(8):912–7.

61. Bergamini A, Ferrandina G, Candiani M, et al. Laparoscopic surgery in the treatment of stage I adult granulosa cells tumors of the ovary: results from the MITO-9 study. Eur J Surg Oncol 2018;44(6):766–70.

62. Melamed A, Nitecki R, Boruta DM 2nd, et al. Laparoscopy compared with laparotomy for debulking ovarian cancer after neoadjuvant chemotherapy. Obstet Gynecol 2017;129(5):861–9.

63. Eriksson AGZ, Graul A, Yu MC, et al. Minimal access surgery compared to laparotomy for secondary surgical cytoreduction in patients with recurrent ovarian carcinoma: perioperative and oncologic outcomes. Gynecol Oncol 2017; 146(2):263–7.

64. Rutten MJ, van Meurs HS, van de Vrie R, et al. Laparoscopy to predict the result of primary cytoreductive surgery in patients with advanced ovarian cancer: a randomized controlled trial. J Clin Oncol 2017;35(6):613–21.

65. Tomar TS, Nair RP, Sambasivan S, et al. Role of laparoscopy in predicting surgical outcomes in patients undergoing interval cytoreduction surgery for advanced ovarian carcinoma: a prospective validation study. Indian J Cancer 2017;54(3): 550–5.

66. Adamina M, Kehlet H, Tomlinson GA, et al. Enhanced recovery pathways optimize health outcomes and resource utilization: a meta-analysis of randomized controlled trials in colorectal surgery. Surgery 2011;149:830–40.

67. Anderson AD, McNaught CE, MacFie J, et al. Randomized clinical trial of multimodal optimization and standard perioperative surgical care. Br J Surg 2003; 90:1497–504.

68. Kalogera E, Bakkum-Gamez J, Jankowski C, et al. Enhanced recovery in gynecologic surgery. Obstet Gynecol 2013;122:319–28.

69. Nelson G, Dowdy S, Lasala J, et al. Enhanced recovery after surgery (ERAS®) in gynecologic oncology – Practical considerations for program development. Gynecol Oncol 2017;147:617–20.

70. Modesitt S, Sarosiek B, Trowbridge E, et al. Enhanced recovery implementation in major gynecologic surgeries. Obstet Gynecol 2016;128:457–66.

71. Yoong W, Sivashanmugarajan V, Relph S, et al. Can enhanced recovery pathways improve outcomes in vaginal hysterectomy? Cohort control study. J Minim Invasive Gynecol 2014;21:83–9.

72. Ottessen M, Sorensen M, Rasmussen Y, et al. Fast track vaginal surgery. Acta Obstet Gynecol Scand 2002;81:138–46.

Ovarian Cancer
Clinical Trial Breakthroughs and Impact on Management

Rebecca Ann Previs, MD, MS*, Angeles Alvarez Secord, MD

KEYWORDS

- Ovarian cancer • Clinical trials • Cytoreduction • PARP inhibitor • Bevacizumab
- Immunotherapy

KEY POINTS

- Clinical trial findings have expanded standard of care treatment options for women with ovarian cancer.
- Women with advanced stage ovarian cancer should be evaluated to determine suitability for primary cytoreduction. Women unlikely to be optimally cytoreduced should receive neoadjuvant chemotherapy.
- Poly-ADP ribose polymerase inhibitors including olaparib, rucaparib, and niraparib, have been approved for maintenance after response to platinum-based chemotherapy.
- Bevacizumab has received approval in the frontline setting followed by maintenance, as well as at the time of recurrence for platinum-sensitive and resistant disease.
- Multiple trials are ongoing to target the immune system with checkpoint inhibitors, vaccine strategies, and adoptive T-cell therapy.

INTRODUCTION

In the past decade, significant advances have been made in the treatment of primary and recurrent epithelial ovarian, tubal, and peritoneal cancer (collectively referred to as epithelial ovarian cancer) in surgical and therapeutic trials. With the addition of anti-angiogenic therapy, poly (adenosine diphosphate-ribose [ADP]) polymerase (PARP) inhibitors, maintenance strategies, and immunotherapy, gynecologic oncologists

Disclosure Statement: R.A. Previs has no conflicts of interest. Dr A.A. Secord discloses that she has received clinical trial grant funding from AbbVie, Amgen, Astellas Pharma, Astex Pharmaceuticals Inc, AstraZeneca, Boerhinger Ingelheim, Bristol-Myers Squibb, Endocyte, Genentech, Incyte, Merck, PharmaMar, and TESARO. She has also received honoraria for Advisory Boards from Alexion, Aravive, AstraZeneca, Clovis, Janssen/Johnson & Johnson, Mesano, Myriad, Roche/Genentech, and TESARO within the past 12 months.
Division of Gynecologic Oncology, Department of Obstetrics and Gynecology, Duke Cancer Institute, Duke University Medical Center, Box 3079, Durham, NC 27710, USA
* Corresponding author.
E-mail address: rebecca.previs@duke.edu

obgyn.theclinics.com

possess a greater armamentarium than ever before to individualize patients' therapies. A better understanding of the heterogeneous nature of ovarian cancer has continued to evolve. Between 2006 and 2015, death rates have declined in almost all racial and ethnic groups owing to improved treatment options.[1] Despite this, 14,070 women will die of their disease in 2018, which emphasizes continued efforts toward treatment advances through clinical trials.

SURGICAL CLINICAL TRIALS: PRIMARY SETTING

In the primary setting for women with suspected ovarian cancer, the standard of care includes surgical cytoreduction followed by platinum-based chemotherapy. Several clinical trials have evaluated outcomes between patients treated with primary surgery or neoadjuvant chemotherapy. This was first evaluated by Vergote and colleagues[2] in a phase III, noninferiority trial, which randomized patients with stage IIIC to stage IV epithelial ovarian cancer. Patients were randomized to undergo primary cytoreductive surgery followed by 6 cycles of chemotherapy or to 3 cycles of neoadjuvant chemotherapy, interval cytoreduction, and 3 more cycles of chemotherapy. This study concluded that primary cytoreduction is the standard of care for patients with advanced stage disease, but that neoadjuvant chemotherapy should be considered a reasonable alternative and the timing of surgery should be tailored to the patient with regard to resectability, age, performance status, and histology. After this development, the CHORUS trial, a phase III, noninferiority, international, randomized, controlled trial evaluated women with stage III or IV ovarian to determine if neoadjuvant chemotherapy represented an effective and safe treatment option. Women with stage III and IV cancer were assigned to undergo primary surgery followed by chemotherapy or 3 cycles of chemotherapy, interval surgery, and 3 additional cycles of chemotherapy. After randomization of 550 women, there were no statistically significant differences between survival outcomes between the 2 groups; however, grades 3 and 4 postoperative adverse events were more frequent in the patients who underwent primary cytoreduction (24% vs 14%; $P = .007$). The authors concluded that, in women with advanced stage disease, neoadjuvant chemotherapy was noninferior to primary surgery and represents an acceptable standard of care. Criticisms of this study include short operative durations (median time was 120 minutes) and optimal debulking rates of 41% and 73% in the primary surgery and neoadjuvant groups, respectively.[3] Subsequently, several other randomized, controlled trials comparing neoadjuvant chemotherapy/interval surgery to primary cytoreduction have been completed and all demonstrated decreased perioperative morbidity and mortality with the administration of neoadjuvant chemotherapy.

The Society of Gynecologic Oncology and the American Society of Clinical Oncology published guidelines on neoadjuvant chemotherapy following this trial and others (**Table 1**).[2–6] These recommendations and studies suggest that women with advanced stage ovarian cancer should be evaluated by a gynecologic oncologist with imaging that includes a computed tomography scan of the abdomen and pelvis with chest imaging (preferably a chest computed tomography scan) to determine if she is a candidate for primary cytoreductive surgery. Women with high perioperative risk factors or who are unlikely to be optimally cytoreduced to less than 1 cm of residual disease should receive neoadjuvant primarily.[6,7] Women who are candidates for surgery can receive either neoadjuvant chemotherapy or surgery first, but primary surgery is recommended over neoadjuvant chemotherapy if there is a high likelihood that surgery would lead to residual disease of less than 1 cm (and ideally, no gross residual disease).

Table 1

Clinical trials evaluating neoadjuvant chemotherapy versus primary cytoreduction in advanced stage ovarian cancer

Reference	Study Type	Enrollment Criteria	Endpoint	Arms (n)	Operative Time (min)	Cytoreduction Rates	Hospital Stay	Time to Start Chemotherapy (d)	Deaths (n)	PFS (mo)	OS (mo)
Fagotti et al,[4] 2016 (SCORPION trial)	Single institution, superiority, randomized phase III trial	Advanced stage EOC s/p staging laparoscopy with predictive indices of ≥8 or ≤12 between 10/2011 and 11/2014	Surgery complications	1. PDS (84) 2. NACT (87)	Median = 451 Median = 275	Optimal = 92.8% Optimal = 100%	Median = 12 d Median = 6 d	Median = 40 Median = 27	2 0	15 14	41 Not reached
Kehoe et al,[3] 2015 (CHORUS trial)	Multiinstitution, noninferiority, randomized phase III trial	Suspected stage III–IV ovarian cancer fit for surgery/ chemotherapy, CA125:CEA >25 (or if less, GI cancer must be excluded) between 3/2004 and 8/2010	OS	1. PDS (276) 2. NACT (274)	Median = 120 Median = 120	R0 = 17% R0 = 39%	<14 d = 80% <14 d = 93%	37% with delays to chemotherapy 28% with delays to chemotherapy	14 1	10.7 12.0	22.6 24.1
Onda et al,[7] (JCOG0602)	Multiinstitution, noninferiority, randomized phase III trial	Stage III–IV ovarian cancers diagnosed clinically with imaging and cytology, CA125 > 200 U/mL, CEA <20 ng/mL between 11/2006 and 10/2011	OS	1. PDS (149) 2. NACT (152)	Median = 240 Median = 302	R0 = 31% R0 = 55%	NR	NR	2 1	15.1 16.4	49.0 44.3

(continued on next page)

Table 1 (*continued*)

Reference	Study Type	Enrollment Criteria	Endpoint	Arms (n)	Operative Time (min)	Cytoreduction Rates	Hospital Stay	Time to Start Chemotherapy (d)	Deaths (n)	PFS (mo)	OS (mo)
Vergote et al (EORTC 55971)	Multiinstitution, randomized phase III trial	Stage IIIC–IV EOC with biopsy-proven disease (FNA acceptable if radiologic criteria also met), CA125:CEA >25 (or if less, GI cancer must be excluded) between 9/1998 and 12/2006	OS	1. PDS (336) 2. NACT (334)	Median = 165 Median-180	R0 = 19.4% R0 = 51.2%	NR	Median = 19 Median = 17	8 2	12 12	29 30
Kumar et al[87]	Randomized trial, phase III trial	Stage IIIC and IV (pleural effusion only) EOC between 10/2001 and 12/2006	OS, DFS, debulking rates	1. PDS (65) 2. NACT (63)	Mean = 110 Mean = 95	Optimal = 23% Optimal = 85%	Mean = 12 Mean = 9.4	NR	6% 1%	NR	42 29

Abbreviations: CEA, carcinoembryonic antigen; DFS, disease free survival; EOC, epithelial ovarian cancer; FNA, fine-needle aspirate; GI, gastrointestinal; NACT, neoadjuvant chemotherapy; NR, not reported; OS, overall survival; PDS, primary debulking surgery; PFS, progression-free survival; R0, no gross residual disease.

Clinical factors associated with suboptimal cytoreductions include age 60 years or older, a CA125 of 500 U/mL or greater, and an American Society of Anesthesiologists physical status classification of 3 or 4.[8] Predictors of suboptimal cytoreduction on pre-operative imaging include suprarenal retroperitoneal lymph nodes greater than 1 cm, diffuse small bowel adhesions/thickening, lesions greater than 1 cm in the small bowel mesentery, root of the superior mesenteria artery, perisplenic area, and the lesser sac.[8]

Diagnostic laparoscopy has also been proposed as a method for diagnosing and assessing disease spread.[9,10] Originally describe by Fagotti and colleagues,[11,12] these studies use a scoring algorithm to predict which patients will have no gross residual disease if cytoreduced in the primary setting. This scoring system includes omental cake with tumor diffusion to the small and large curvature of the stomach, extensive carcinomatosis of the diaphragm, unresectable peritoneal carcinomatosis, mesenteric retraction, bowel infiltration, liver metastases, and stomach infiltration. Surgeons assigned a score of zero or 2 to each criterion, and the likelihood that a patient would have a suboptimal cytoreductive surgery increased to 100% in the cases where a score was equal to or greater than 8.[12] Within the United States, this strategy has been incorporated to improve the proportion of patients with advanced stage ovarian cancer achieving optimal cytoreduction to no gross residual disease (R0). After the implementation of a predictive scoring system, R0 resection rates increased from 44% (before implementation) in 2013 to 84% (after implementation) for patients who were eligible for primary surgery ($P<.01$).[13]

Current surgical guidelines recommend that suspicious and/or enlarged pelvic and paraaortic lymph nodes should be resected in patients with newly diagnosed epithelial ovarian cancer.[14] This has been called into question by a recent prospective, randomized, Lymphadenectomy in Ovarian Neoplasms (LION) study, which included 647 patients with stage IIB to IV disease who were optimally cytoreduced with preoperative and intraoperative assessments of clinically negative lymph nodes were randomized intraoperatively to undergo pelvic and paraaortic lymph node evaluations versus no lymph node evaluation. There was no difference in median overall survival between the 2 groups (69 months in the no lymph node dissection arm and 66 months in the lymph node dissection arm; hazard ratio [HR], 1.06; 95% confidence interval [CI], 0.83–1.34; $P = .65$). There was no difference in the progression-free survival between the groups; however, in the patients who underwent lymph node evaluation, there was a median higher blood loss, more serious complications, and longer surgeries. The authors concluded that resection of clinically negative lymph nodes did not improve survival, despite detecting subclinical involvement in 56% of the patients and should not be routinely performed to avoid additional postoperative morbidity.[15]

In a prospective substudy, LION-PAW (Pleasure Ability of Women), the effect of radical surgery including pelvic and paraaortic lymphadenectomy followed by chemotherapy on women's sexuality was evaluated. A statistically significant difference in the ability of women to achieve an orgasm was observed in sexually active patients after 12 months in women who did not undergo a lymphadenctomy.[16]

SURGICAL CLINICAL TRIALS: RECURRENT SETTING

In patients with recurrent platinum-sensitive ovarian cancer, the role of secondary cytoreductive surgery was evaluated by a randomized controlled phase III study Arbeitsgemeinschaft Gynäkologische Onkologie (AGO) The Descriptive Evaluation of preoperative Selection KriTeria for OPerability in recurrent ovarian cancer (DESKTOP) III/ENGOTOv20. Four hundred seven women were randomized to either second-line chemotherapy or cytoreduction. In the patients who underwent surgery, 67% had a complete resection and median progression-free survival was 19.6 months compared with 14 months in the chemotherapy group (HR, 0.66; 95% CI, 0.52–0.83; $P<.001$). Overall survival data have not reached maturity.[17]

In contrast with these data, GOG-0213, an open-label, randomized phase III trial, evaluated the impact of secondary cytoreductive surgery in 485 women with recurrent ovarian cancer. R0 was achieved in 63% of cases that underwent surgery. Secondary cytoreductive surgery did not improve either progression-free survival (18.2 vs 16.5 months; HR, 0.88; 95% CI, 0.70–1.11) overall survival (53.6 vs 65.7 months; HR, 1.28; 95% CI, 0.92–1.79).[18]

These studies differed based on inclusion criteria. Eligible patients for the DESKTOP study were those that were diagnosed with their first recurrence, had a greater than or equal to 6 month platinum-free interval, had 500 mL of ascites or less, and had a complete resection at the time of their initial cytoreduction. Patients in GOG-0213 were eligible based on the investigator's discretion. A very important difference between these studies may have been the incorporation of bevacizumab into GOG-0213.

CHEMOTHERAPY TRIALS: PRIMARY SETTING

Previous results from Japanese Gynecologic Oncology Group (JGOG) 3016 showed improved overall and progression-free survival in patients with ovarian cancer treated with dose-dense weekly paclitaxel with carboplatin.[19] A randomized, phase III study in Italy and France (MITO-7) compared carboplatin, area under the curve (AUC) 6 plus paclitaxel (175 mg/m^2) every 3 weeks for 6 cycles or carboplatin (AUC 2) plus paclitaxel (60 mg/m^2) every week for 18 weeks. The median progression-free survivals were 17.3 and 18.3 months in the every 3 week and weekly administration groups, respectively.[20] The dose-dense strategy was called further into question after completion of Gynecologic Oncology Group (GOG) 262, which randomized 692 patients with ovarian cancer to carboplatin, AUC 6 with weekly paclitaxel (80 mg/m^2), or carboplatin (AUC 6) with paclitaxel (175 mg/m^2) every 3 weeks. Bevacizumab administration could be added to either group (nonrandomized) and the decision to use bevacizumab had to be made before randomization. There was no difference in median progression-free survival between groups in the intent-to-treat analysis. However, in the subset analysis of the 112 patients who did not receive bevacizumab, there was a 3.9-month improvement in progression-free survival in patients who received dose-dense paclitaxel. Because the use of bevacizumab was not randomized in this study, conclusions about the additional of bevacizumab with dose-dense paclitaxel cannot be firmly drawn.[21] However, most people felt that the subset analysis provided some confirmation of the JGOG 3016 trial, and there was widespread acceptance of dose-dense paclitaxel.

The International Collaborative Ovarian Neoplasm (ICON)-8 trial reaffirmed again the every 3-week dosing schedule for paclitaxel over the dose-dense regimen. In this trial, 1566 women with stage IC grade 3 to stage IV epithelial ovarian cancer were randomized to one of 3 arms: (1) carboplatin (AUC5/6) and paclitaxel (175 mg/m^2) every 3 weeks, (2) carboplatin (AUC5/6) every 3 weeks and weekly paclitaxel (80 mg/m^2), or (3) carboplatin (AUC2) and paclitaxel (80 mg/m^2) weekly. There was no improvement in progression-free survival in weekly administered chemotherapy.[22] Pharmacogenomic differences in drug metabolism in different ethnic groups and different types of epithelial ovarian cancer (with a higher proportion of patients with clear cell carcinomas in the Asian population) could explain the differences seen between the JGOG 3016, MITO-7, and ICON-8 trials.

A randomized, multicenter, phase III study from China evaluated outcomes of nedaplatin with paclitaxel and carboplatin with paclitaxel in women with stages II to IV ovarian cancer with no statistically significant difference between the 2 groups in progression-free or overall survival. The patients receiving nedaplatin has less grade 3 and 4 leukopenia but otherwise, they had similar side effect profiles.[23]

Although the majority of clinical trials have focused on high-grade serous pathology, a phase II study (JGOG3014) evaluated irinotecan plus cisplatin compared with carboplatin plus paclitaxel in ovarian clear cell carcinoma. The progression-free survival was longer in the irinotecan and cisplatin arm, but this difference was not statistically significant.[24] This finding was then evaluated in a phase III randomized clinical trial, which showed no survival differences.[25] Current trials in clear cell cancer are focusing on targeting molecular alterations that are common in this subset of cancers.

INTRAPERITONEAL CHEMOTHERAPY

In 2006, the National Cancer Institute issued an announcement that supported the use of intraperitoneal (IP) chemotherapy based on 8 trials evaluated its use, and together supported a significant improvement in survival. In contrast with GOG 172,[26] GOG 252 evaluated patients with optimally cytoreduced stage II to III ovarian cancer to treatment arms, one of which included a dose-dense intravenous (IV) therapy arm and one included an IV/IP arm (with paclitaxel IV and cisplatin/paclitaxel IP); all arms received bevacizumab. Those who received dose-dense therapy had a similar progression-free survival (27 months) as those who received IV/IP therapy (28 months).[27] The interpretation of this trial is limited by the fact that 28% of patients crossed over from the IV/IP arm to the dose-dense therapy arm, and the effect of bevacizumab added to all arms remains unknown. The uptake of IP chemotherapy at its high was 16.3%[28] owing to challenges with administration and toxicity; physician acceptance has decreased further based on the negative findings of GOG 252.

However, there has been renewed interest in hyperthermic IP chemotherapy (HIPEC) from women with advanced epithelial ovarian cancer. The addition of HIPEC with cisplatin to interval cytoreductive surgery has been evaluated in a multicenter, phase III randomized controlled trial that included 245 patients with stage III ovarian cancer who had at least stable disease after 3 cycles of neoadjuvant chemotherapy. The median recurrence-free survival was 10.7 months in those who underwent surgery alone compared with 14.2 months in the surgery and HIPEC group. The median overall survival was 33.9 months in the surgery group and 45.7 months in the surgery and HIPEC group. There were similar grade 3 and 4 adverse events between the 2 groups.[29]

In a phase I dose escalation trial of HIPEC using carboplatin, 52 women with advanced stage ovarian cancer who underwent a primary or interval cytoreduction to optimal or no gross residual disease were enrolled. Women were treated carboplatin using a closed technique at 41°C for 60 minutes. The posttrial maximum tolerated dose was 1115 mg/m^2.[30]

The future regarding HIPEC remains to be determined and several randomized controlled trials are ongoing.

RECURRENT SETTING

In patients with platinum-sensitive recurrent disease, women are retreated with platinum-based chemotherapy, but the effectiveness of the platinum decreases the longer a patient is from her prior platinum therapy.[31] It has been previously hypothesized that intercalating a nonplatinum treatment between 2 platinum-based treatments may increase the platinum-free interval.[32] The Multicenter Italian Trials in Ovarian Cancer (MITO)-8 tested this hypothesis in an open-label, prospective, randomized, superiority trial. Patients with ovarian cancer who progressed 6 to 12 months after their last platinum-based chemotherapy were randomized to the standard arm (patients received a platinum-based chemotherapy at current relapse followed by a non–platinum-based chemotherapy at subsequent relapse) or the experimental arm (patients received a non–platinum-based chemotherapy at current relapse followed by a platinum-based chemotherapy at subsequent relapse). Non-platinum-based regimens included pegylated liposomal doxorubicin, topotecan, gemcitabine, or other drugs approved in this setting. After enrollment of 215 patients, the trial ended early owing to slow enrollment. No overall survival benefit was seen between the arms. The progression-free survival was shorter in the experimental arm (median, 12.8 months vs 16.4 months, HR, 1.41; 95% CI, 1.04–1.92; $P = .25$). This trial supported the recommendation that platinum-based chemotherapy should be used in women who remain at least partially platinum sensitive.[33]

USE OF POLY (ADENOSINE DIPHOSPHATE-RIBOSE [ADP]) POLYMERASE INHIBITORS FOR MAINTENANCE THERAPY

In women with platinum-sensitive ovarian cancer with a complete or partial response to platinum-based chemotherapy, the US Food and Drug Administration (FDA) has approved 3 PARP inhibitors for maintenance therapy: niraparib, olaparib, and rucaparib (**Table 2**). The efficacy of niraparib in this patient population has been evaluated in all patients, regardless of whether she has a BRCA mutation or homologous recombination deficiency (HRD). In the randomized, double-blind, phase III ENGOT-OV16/NOVA study, women were categorized according to the presence or absence of a germline BRCA mutation. Of the 553 enrolled patients, 203 were in the germline BRCA mutation cohort (138 received niraparib at 300 mg/d vs 65 who received placebo). Patients with a germline BRCA mutation who received niraparib had a significantly longer median progression-free survival versus placebo (21.0 months vs 5.5 months; HR, 0.27; 95% CI, 0.17–0.41). The cohort of patients, who did not have a BRCA germline mutation but had tumors with HRD also derived a survival benefit (12.9 months vs 3.8 months; HR, 0.38; 95% CI, 0.24–0.59). Of note, patients with a somatic BRCA mutation were included in this cohort. Patients without a germline BRCA mutation (including those with an HRD-deficient tumor) also derived an almost

Table 2
Comparison of progression-free survival in patients receiving PARP inhibitors versus placebo for maintenance therapy

PARP Inhibitor	Dose	Progression-Free Survival (mo)						
		BRCA Mutation Status			No Germline Mutation			
		Germline Only	Germline or Somatic	Germline Present or Absent	HRD Positive	HRD Negative	HRD Not Tested	Clinical Trial
Niraparib	300 mg/d	21 vs 5.5	—	—	12.9 vs 3.8	9.3 vs 3.9	—	NOVA
Olaparib	400 mg	—	—	8.4 vs 4.8	—	—	—	Study 19,
	BID	—	11 vs 4	—	—	—	7 vs 5.5	SOLO2
		19.1 vs 5.5	—	—	—	—	—	
Rucaparib	600 mg BID	—	16.6 vs 5.4	—	13.6 vs 5.4	—	—	ARIEL3

Abbreviations: BID, twice daily; HRD, homologous recombination deficiency; PARP, poly (adenosine diphosphate-ribose [ADP]) polymerase.

6-month progression-free survival advantage in the niraparib arm (9.3 mg/d vs 3.9 months; HR, 0.45; 95% CI, 0.34–0.62). Significant side effects were related to bone marrow toxicity and included neutropenia, anemia, and thrombocytopenia.[34] Overall survival results from this study have not been reported.

Study 19, a randomized, double-blind, phase II study, evaluated women with platinum-sensitive recurrent high-grade serous ovarian cancer who had received 2 or more platinum-based regimens and had a complete or partial response to most recent platinum-based regimen. Two hundred sixty-five underwent randomization: 136 received olaparib and 129 received placebo. Progression-free survival was longer in women who received olaparib (8.4 months vs 4.8 months; HR, 0.35; 95% CI, 0.25–0.40). An interim survival analysis at 38% maturity showed no difference (HR, 0.94; 95% CI, 0.63–1.39; $P = .75$); however, 23% of the patients receiving placebo switched to a PARP inhibitor after progression.[35] This was evaluated in a post hoc analysis, which excluded patients from sites where 1 or more patients randomized to placebo received postprogression PARP inhibitor treatment. In this overall survival analysis, the overall HR was 0.52 (95% CI, 0.28–0.97) for the 97 BRCA-mutated patients, suggesting that postprogression PARP treatment did confound the interim overall survival analysis.[36] Common side effects reported in Study 19 included nausea, fatigue, vomiting, and anemia. Other small subanalyses of Study 19 reported maintenance olaparib in patients with either a germline or somatic BRCA mutation, suggesting the benefit was highest in these patients (11-month progression-free survival vs 4-month progression-free survival; HR, 0.18; 95% CI, 0.10–0.31)[37] with a trend toward an improved in overall survival.[38] Women without a BRCA mutation had a small progression survival benefit (2.5 months) with olaparib with no benefit in overall survival.

The phase III SOLO2/ENGOT-Ov21 trial evaluated 295 women with germline BRCA mutations with recurrent, platinum-sensitive, high-grade serous or endometrioid cancer who had received at least 2 lines of prior chemotherapy. Patients who received olaparib had improved progression-free survival (19.1 months vs 5.5 months; HR, 0.30; 95% CI, 0.22–0.41).[39]

Most recently, rucaparib received FDA approval for maintenance therapy with the benefit seen in the phase III ARIEL3 trial. In this trial, 564 patients with platinum-sensitive high-grade serous or endometrioid ovarian cancer who had received 2 or more platinum-based therapies (and who had most recently achieved a complete or partial response to platinum-based treatment) were randomized to receive rucaparib or placebo. Different from other trials, this study permitted enrollment for patients with residual bulky disease.[40,41] Improvement in progression-free survival was seen in women with germline and somatic BRCA mutations, women with HRD, and the intention-to-treat population.

USE OF POLY (ADENOSINE DIPHOSPHATE-RIBOSE [ADP]) POLYMERASE INHIBITORS FOR RECURRENT DISEASE

In women with recurrent ovarian cancer with a known BRCA1 or BRCA2 mutation, treatment with FDA-approved PARP inhibitors remains an option (**Table 3**). Olaparib is approved in women with germline BRCA mutations after at least 3 prior lines of therapy with a companion diagnostic test, BRACAnalysis CDX. The benefit of olaparib was evaluated in a phase II study of patients with germline BRCA 1 or BRCA 2 mutations. Eligibility included ovarian cancer resistant to prior platinum-based therapy, breast cancer with 3 or more chemotherapy regimens, pancreatic cancer with prior gemcitabine treatment, or prostate cancer with progression on hormonal and 1 systemic therapy; 298 patients received treatment. Tumor response rate was 26.2% overall

Table 3
FDA-approved monotherapy PARP inhibitors in patients with recurrent ovarian cancer with BRCA mutations

	BRCA Mutation Status	Platinum Status	Number of Prior Treatments
Olaparib	Germline	Sensitive or resistant	≥ 3
Rucaparib	Germline or somatic	Sensitive or resistant	≥ 2

Abbreviation: PARP, poly (adenosine diphosphate-ribose [ADP]) polymerase.

(95% CI, 21.3–31.6) and 31.1% (95% CI, 24.6–38.1) in patients with ovarian cancer.[42] In a follow-up metaanalysis, which pooled data from 2 phase I trials, and 4 phase II trials, 300 patients with recurrent ovarian cancer with germline BRCA 1 or BRCA2 mutations (205 of which had received ≥ 3 prior therapies) had an objective response rate was 36% (95% CI, 30%–40%).[43]

Rucaparib is also approved for patients with ovarian cancer who have received 2 or more prior chemotherapies and who have a germline or somatic BRCA 1 or BRCA 2 mutations. In a pooled analysis of 2 phase II studies, women who received rucaparib had an objective response rate of 54%.[44] Loss of heterozygosity (LOH) in the tumor may also represent a subset of patients, who are BRCA wild type, but may benefit from rucaparib. Progression-free survival was significantly longer in the BRCA mutants (12.8 months; HR, 0.27; 95% CI, 0.16–0.44) and LOH high subgroups (5.7 months; HR, 0.62; 95% CI, 0.42–0.90) when compared with the LOH low subgroup (5.2 months).[45]

QUADRA, a phase II, single-arm study, evaluated niraparib in 463 patients with recurrent ovarian cancer who had received 3 or more prior chemotherapy regimens. Patients were evaluated for BRCA mutation and HRD status.[46] The median duration of response was 9.2 months (95% CI, 5.9–15.2) and the median overall survival was 19 months.

Another PARP inhibitor, veliparib, is being investigated in a phase II trial, which enrolled 50 patients with germline BRCA1 or BRCA 2 mutations that had received 3 or fewer prior chemotherapy regimens. The overall proportion of patients responding was 26% (90% CI, 16%–38%) with a median progression-free survival of 8.18 months.[47]

ANTIANGIOGENIC THERAPY

The addition of bevacizumab into frontline treatment of women with newly diagnosed ovarian cancer has been evaluated in 2 randomized phase III trials and led to recent FDA approval of bevacizumab in the frontline followed by maintenance bevacizumab (Table 4).[48]

GOG218, a double-blind, placebo-controlled, phase III trial enrolled 1873 patients with incompletely resected stage III or IV epithelial ovarian cancer. All patient received carboplatin and paclitaxel for 6 cycles. The control treatment was chemotherapy with placebo treatment added in during cycles 2 through 22. Arm 2 included bevacizumab in cycles 2 through 6 and placebo added in during cycles 7 through 22. Arm 3 included bevacizumab throughout treatment in cycles 2 through 22. The primary endpoint was progression-free survival. At the final analysis, despite an improvement in progression-free survival seen in patients who received bevacizumab, there was no difference observed in overall survival.[49]

ICON 7, a phase III randomized trial also evaluated the addition of bevacizumab to standard carboplatin and paclitaxel and included 1528 women; 70% had stage IIIC or IV disease. Nine percent of patient were identified as having high-risk early stage disease (defined as stage I or IIA, clear cell, or grade 3 tumors). Compared with standard

Table 4
Clinical trials evaluating bevacizumab in the primary and recurrent treatment of ovarian cancer

	Author, Year, Study	Enrollment Criteria (No. of Enrolled Patients)	Primary Endpoint	Arms	PFS (mo) or [OS (mo)]	Adverse Effects
Primary setting	Burger et al,[49,88] 2011, 2018, GOG 218	Suboptimal stage III or stage IV EOC ovarian cancer s/p debulking (n = 1873)	PFS	1. Carboplatin AUC6, paclitaxel 175 mg/m² (cycles 1–6) + placebo (cycles 2–22)	10.3 [stage III OS = 44.3, stage IV OS = 32.6]	7.2% HTN 1.2% GWD
				2. Carboplatin AUC6, paclitaxel 175 mg/m² (cycles 1–6) + bevacizumab (cycles 2–6) and placebo (cycles 7–22)	11.2 [stage III OS = 42.9, stage IV OS = 34.5]	16.5% HTN 2.8% GWD
				3. Carboplatin AUC6, paclitaxel 175 mg/m² (cycles 1–6) + bevacizumab (cycles 2–22)	14.1 [stage III OS = 44.2, stage IV OS = 42.8]	22.9% HTN 2.6% GWD
	Perren et al,[50] 2011, ICON7	Stage I–IIa, grade 3 or clear histology; stage IIb–IV ovarian cancer s/p debulking (n = 1528)	PFS	1. Carboplatin (AUC 5 or 6), Paclitaxel 175 mg/m²	17.3 (22 at 42 mo)	2% HTN
				2. Carboplatin (AUC 5 or 6), paclitaxel 175 mg/m² plus bevacizumab (7.5 mg/kg) (6 cycles), then bevacizumab (continued for up to 12 further cycles)	19.0 (24 at 42 mo)	18% HTN

(continued on next page)

Table 4 (continued)					
	Author, Year, Study	Enrollment Criteria (No. of Enrolled Patients)	Primary Endpoint	Arms	PFS (mo) or [OS (mo)]	Adverse Effects
Platinum-sensitive recurrent disease	Aghajanian et al,[52] 2012, OCEANS	Recurrent platinum-sensitive ovarian cancer, ≥6 mo after first-line platinum-based therapy, measurable disease (n = 484)	PFS	1. Gemcitabine (1000 mg/m^2 on days 1 and 8), carboplatin (AUC 4 on day 1), placebo (6–10 cycles), placebo was continue until progression	8.4	<1% HTN <1% proteinuria 1% bleeding
				2. Gemcitabine, carboplatin, bevacizumab (15 mg/kg on day 1 for 6–10 cycles), bevacizumab was continued until progression	12.4	17.4% HTN 8.5% proteinuria 6% bleeding
	Coleman et al,[18] 2015; Coleman et al,[47] 2018, GOG 213	Recurrent, platinum-sensitive ovarian cancer, ≥6 mo after first-line platinum-based chemotherapy, measurable disease, and surgical candidates (n = 674)	If secondary cytoreduction + adjuvant chemotherapy increases OS. If the addition of bevacizumab improves OS.	1. Carboplatin (AUC5), paclitaxel (175 m/gm^2) (day 1, 6 cycles)	10 [37.3]	1% HTN, 2% fatigue
				2. Carboplatin, paclitaxel, bevacizumab (15 mg/kg) (day 1, 6 cycles, and bevacizumab continued for maintenance)	14 [42.2]	0% proteinuria, 1% death
				3. Secondary cytoreductive surgery followed by platinum-based chemotherapy	18.2 [53.6]	12% HTN, 8% fatigue
				4. Platinum-based chemotherapy	16.5 [65.7]	8% proteinuria, 3% death

Platinum-resistant recurrent disease	Burger et al,[57] 2007, GOG 170D	Platinum-resistant, persistent or recurrent ovarian cancer, 1–2 prior regimens, measurable disease (n = 62)	PFS at 6 mo and clinical response	Bevacizumab (15 mg/kg, day 1)	4.7 [17]	
	Cannistra et al,[58] 2007	Platinum-resistant, progressive ovarian cancer within 3 mo of topotecan or liposomal doxorubicin discontinuation (n = 44)	PFS	Bevacizumab (15 mg/kg)	4.4	9.1% HTN 15.9% proteinuria, 2.3% bleeding, 11.4% GWD
	Pujade-Lauraine et al,[59] 2014, AURELIA	Platinum-resistant ovarian cancer with measurable disease (n = 361)	PFS	1. Single-agent chemotherapy (pegylated doxorubicin, weekly paclitaxel, or topotecan)	3.4 [13.3]	1% HTN, 0% proteinuria, GWD 0%
				2. Chemotherapy (above regimens) with bevacizumab (10 mg/kg every 2 wk or 15 mg/kg every 3 wk)	6.7 [16.6]	7% HTN, 2% proteinuria, GWD 2%

Abbreviations: EOC, epithelial ovarian cancer; GWD, gastrointestinal wall disruption; HTN, hypertension; OS, overall survival; PARP, poly (adenosine diphosphate-ribose [ADP]) polymerase inhibitor; PFS, progression-free survival.

chemotherapy, the addition of bevacizumab increased overall response rate, longer progression-free survival, and more serious adverse events. There were no differences in overall survival or the quality of life of patients.[50,51] For patients who were determined to be at a high risk for progression (defined as stage III with >1 cm of residual disease after surgery, inoperable stage III or IV disease) the addition of bevacizumab was associated with improved progression-free survival and overall survival; however, this was a post hoc subgroup analysis.[51]

In the recurrent, platinum-sensitive setting, bevacizumab has been evaluated in the OCEANS and GOG 2013 trials. OCEANS, a phase III study, randomized 484 patients to receive carboplatin and gemcitabine with or without bevacizumab every 21 days for up to 10 cycles, followed by maintenance bevacizumab. This resulted in improved progression-free survival in the patients who received bevacizumab (12 months vs 8 months; HR, 0.48; 95% CI, 0.39–0.61), high objective response rate, and a higher rate of adverse events.[52,53] There was no difference in overall survival (58.2 months in bevacizumab arm and 56.4 months in the control arm).[54]

GOG 213, a randomized phase III clinical trial, enrolled 674 women with platinum-sensitive ovarian cancer. Patient were randomized to standard chemotherapy with or without the addition of bevacizumab followed by bevacizumab maintenance. The primary endpoint was median overall survival and, based on pretreatment stratification data, was prolonged in those patients who received bevacizumab: 42.2 months versus 37.3 months (HR, 0.829; 95% CI, 0.2683–10.0050; $P = .056$). Incorrect treatment-free intervals were identified in 7% of patients and a sensitivity analysis based on audited results gave an adjusted HR of 0.823 (95% CI, 0.680–0.996; $P = .0447$).[55]

For platinum-sensitive patients, the randomized phase III MITO16B-MaNGO OV2B-ENGOT OV17 trial evaluated whether the additional of bevacizumab to platinum-based chemotherapy improved progression-free survival in patients who received bevacizumab during front-line therapy. A significantly longer median progression-free survival was reported in women who received bevacizumab retreatment (11.8 months vs 8.8 months; HR, 0.51; 95% CI, 0.41–0.64; $P<.001$), although there was no difference in overall survival.[56]

The platinum-resistant patient population remains one of the most challenging clinical situations faced by gynecologic oncologists. Single agent bevacizumab has been evaluated in this situation in GOG 170D, a phase II clinical trial of 36 platinum-resistant patients; 21% of patients had clinical responses (2 complete and 11 partial responses).[57] Another phase II study evaluating single-agent bevacizumab showed a median progression-free survival of 4.4 months (95% CI, 3.1–5.5 months).[58] AURELIA, a phase III trial evaluated platinum-resistant patients who were randomly assigned to single-agent chemotherapy (pegylated liposomal doxorubicin, weekly paclitaxel, or topotecan) with bevacizumab until progression. The median progression-free survival was 3.4 months with chemotherapy alone versus 6.7 months with chemotherapy plus bevacizumab; there was no difference is overall survival.[59]

ICON6, a phase III randomized controlled trial, evaluated cediranib, a vascular endothelial growth factor receptor (VEGFR)-1-3 oral inhibitor in patients with platinum-sensitive ovarian cancer. Patients who received cediranib in combination with platinum-based chemotherapy followed by maintenance cediranib had improved progression-free survival, but with more side effects including diarrhea, neutropenia, hypertension, voice changes, and hypothyroidism.[60] A recently reported phase II study evaluated the activity of cediranib in combination with olaparib in both a platinum-resistant and platinum-sensitive setting. The overall response rate was 77% among platinum-sensitive patients and the presence of a germline BRCA mutation was correlated with an increased likelihood of response.[61] Cediranib is being evaluated in combination with olaparib in the platinum-sensitive (NCT02446600) and platinum-resistant (NCT02502266) settings.

Nintedanib, a VEGFR-1-3, platelet-derived growth factor receptor (PDGFR), and fibroblast growth factor receptor kinase inhibitor was evaluated in combination with carboplatin and paclitaxel in patients with newly diagnosed ovarian cancer in a phase III randomized, controlled trial. After an upfront debulking, 1366 patients were randomized and treated. The median progression-free survival was longer in the nintedanib group (17.2 months vs 16.6 months; HR, 0.84; 95% CI, 0.72–0.98; $P = .024$), but patients who received nintedanib experienced more gastrointestinal-related side effects.[62]

Other agents such as apatinib, an oral tyrosine kinase inhibitors, which selectively inhibits VEGFR-2, have been assessed in combination with oral etoposide in platinum-resistant patients. A phase II, single-arm study enrolled 35 patients with a 54.3% objective response rate and median progression-free survival of 8.1 months (95% CI, 2.8–13.4).[63]

AGO-OVAR16, a phase III randomized trial, evaluated pazopanib, an oral multikinase inhibitor of VEGFR-1, -2, -3, PDGFR-α, PDGFR-β, and c-Kit, versus placebo as a maintenance therapy after patients with advanced ovarian cancer received frontline therapy. In an updated analysis of this trial, there was no observed difference in overall survival between women who received pazopanib (59.1 months) and placebo (64.0 months).[64]

IMMUNOTHERAPY

A cancer cells' ability to evade the immune system is made possible by immunosuppressive cosignals such as programmed cell death 1 (PD-1) and its corresponding ligand.[65] T cells express PD-1, and PD-1 ligand (PD-L1) is expressed on tumor infiltrating immune cells, ovarian cancer cells, and other cells within the tumor microenvironment. The presence of tumor-infiltrating T cells correlates with improved outcomes in ovarian cancer.[66] The success of checkpoint inhibitors in other solid malignancies, such as lung cancer[67,68] and melanoma,[69–71] has increased interest of immunotherapy in ovarian cancer. PD-L1 expression has been associated with poor prognosis in ovarian cancer[66] and induces an immunosuppressive tumoral microenvironment through dysfunction of T cells. These findings have led to multiple clinical trials evaluating agents that target immune checkpoints.[72]

Nivolumab is an anti–PD-1 antibody that was evaluated in a phase II clinical trial of 20 patients with platinum-resistant ovarian cancer with the primary endpoint as best overall response. Patients were treated with an infusion of nivolumab every 2 weeks at doses of either 1 or 3 mg/kg. The best overall response was 15%, which included 2 patients with a complete response. The overall disease control rate was 45%; median progress-free survival was 3.5 months (95% CI, 1.7–3.9 months). Grade 3 or 4 adverse events related to treatment occurred in 40% of all patients.[73]

Avelumab is an anti–PD-L1 antibody that was evaluated in a phase Ib study of recurrent or refractory ovarian cancer. Seventy-five patients were treated with avelumab at 10 mg/kg every 2 weeks. For the 23 patients with a follow-up of greater than or equal to 2 months, 17.4% of patients achieved a partial response and 47.8% had stable disease; the median progression-free survival was 11.9 weeks. Emergent treatment-related adverse events were reported in 78.3% of patients.[74]

Pembrolizumab, an anti–PD-1 antibody, has been evaluated in KEYNOTE-028, a nonrandomized, multicohort phase Ib trial. Patients in the cohort with ovarian cancer had recurrent disease, failure of prior therapy, PD-L1 expression of 1% of cells or greater in tumor nests, or PD-L1[+] bands in stroma. Pembrolizumab 10 mg/kg was administered every 2 weeks; 26 patients were enrolled. One patient achieved a complete response, 2 patients experienced a partial response, and 6 patients had stable disease. The best overall response was 11.5% (95% CI, 2.4–30.2). Drug-related adverse events occurred in 69.2% of patients.[75] In an update of a phase I/II study (TOPACIO/Keynote-162) evaluating niraparib in combination with pembrolizumab in a platinum-resistant population of 60 patients, objective response rates were 45% in patients with tumor associated BRCA mutations and 25% in patients with platinum-resistant disease.[76]

Multiple phase III trials are ongoing that include checkpoint inhibitors, including JAVELIN OVARIAN 100 (NCT02718417), JAVELIN Ovarian 200 (NCT02580058),[77] ATALANTE (NCT02891824), IMagyn050 (NCT03038100), and NRG-GY009 (NCT02839707).

Aside from checkpoint inhibition, other immune interventions include cancer vaccines and adoptive cell therapy. Cancer vaccines may be administered prophylactically (to mount an immune response to prevent disease progression) or therapeutically (to activate the antitumor response of the immune system). For example, cancer testis antigens that have been identified as targetable include NY-ESO-1[78] and MAGE. Multiple trials have demonstrated efficacy and larger studies are ongoing.[79–81] Galinpepimut is a WT-1 targeting vaccine and has shown efficacy in other solid and hematologic malignancies and has been evaluated in combination with nivolumab. In a phase I study of 11 patients with ovarian cancer whose tumors expressed WT-1, a 1-year progression-free survival rate was 64% in the intention-to-treat analysis with favorable T-cell and B-cell immune responses.[82]

In an effort to elicit a durable immune response, a phase II, randomized trial evaluated an autologous dendritic cell vaccine added to chemotherapy in patients with newly diagnosed ovarian cancer who had undergone an optimal cytoreduction. In a planned interim analysis, the median progression-free survival was 18.3 months in patients who received the vaccine concomitantly with chemotherapy. This outcome was compared with 24.3 months for patients who received the vaccine sequentially after chemotherapy and 18.6 months for patients who just received chemotherapy. The median overall survival has not been reached.[83] Similar results in response rates and improved outcomes have been reported in the recurrent setting with dendritic cell vaccines.[83]

Adoptive cell therapy requires T cells from individual patients, which can come from peripheral blood or tumor. Antigen-specific T cells are selected within a laboratory, expanded, and then infused into the patient after she receives chemotherapy, which depletes lymphocyte populations. Current strategies focus on genetically modifying T-cell receptors or chimeric antigen receptors, and clinical trials are going[84–86] (NCT02498912, NCT02482090, NCT01883297, NCT01583686, NCT01567891, and NCT02457650).

SUMMARY

Clinical trials over the past decade have made significant progression in the standard of care for patients with ovarian cancer. A better understanding of disease biology has informed surgical decision making. PARP inhibitors and antiangiogenic therapy represent newer options for patients who develop recurrent disease. In the next decade, further progress will be made in leveraging a woman's own immune system to target disease. The patients who choose to enroll on clinical trials will pioneer our future efforts moving forward to further individualize therapy.

REFERENCES

1. Cancer facts & figures 2018: special section: ovarian cancer. 2018. Available at: https://www.cancer.org/research/cancer-facts-statistics/all-cancer-facts-figures/cancer-facts-figures-2018.html.
2. Vergote I, Trope CG, Amant F, et al. Neoadjuvant chemotherapy or primary surgery in stage IIIC or IV ovarian cancer. N Engl J Med 2010;363(10):943–53.
3. Kehoe S, Hook J, Nankivell M, et al. Primary chemotherapy versus primary surgery for newly diagnosed advanced ovarian cancer (CHORUS): an open-label, randomised, controlled, non-inferiority trial. Lancet 2015;386(9990):249–57.
4. Fagotti A, Ferrandina G, Vizzielli G, et al. Phase III randomised clinical trial comparing primary surgery versus neoadjuvant chemotherapy in advanced epithelial ovarian cancer with high tumour load (SCORPION trial): final analysis of peri-operative outcome. Eur J Cancer 2016;59:22–33.
5. Onda T, Satoh T, Saito T, et al. Comparison of treatment invasiveness between up-front debulking surgery versus interval debulking surgery following neoadjuvant chemotherapy for stage III/IV ovarian, tubal, and peritoneal cancers in a phase III randomised trial: Japan Clinical Oncology Group Study JCOG0602. Eur J Cancer 2016;64:22–31.
6. Wright AA, Bohlke K, Armstrong DK, et al. Neoadjuvant chemotherapy for newly diagnosed, advanced ovarian cancer: Society of Gynecologic Oncology and American Society of Clinical Oncology Clinical practice guideline. Gynecol Oncol 2016;143(1):3–15.
7. Onda T, Satoh T, Saito T, et al. Comparison of survival between upfront primary debulking surgery versus neoadjuvant chemotherapy for stage III/IV ovarian, tubal and peritoneal cancers in phase III randomized trial: JCOG0602. J Clin Oncol 2018;36(suppl) [abstract: 5500].
8. Suidan RS, Ramirez PT, Sarasohn DM, et al. A multicenter prospective trial evaluating the ability of preoperative computed tomography scan and serum CA-125 to predict suboptimal cytoreduction at primary debulking surgery for advanced ovarian, fallopian tube, and peritoneal cancer. Gynecol Oncol 2014;134(3):455–61.
9. Fagotti A, Vizzielli G, De Iaco P, et al. A multicentric trial (Olympia-MITO 13) on the accuracy of laparoscopy to assess peritoneal spread in ovarian cancer. Am J Obstet Gynecol 2013;209(5):462.e1–11.
10. Fagotti A, Vizzielli G, Fanfani F, et al. Introduction of staging laparoscopy in the management of advanced epithelial ovarian, tubal and peritoneal cancer: impact on prognosis in a single institution experience. Gynecol Oncol 2013;131(2):341–6.
11. Fagotti A, Fanfani F, Ludovisi M, et al. Role of laparoscopy to assess the chance of optimal cytoreductive surgery in advanced ovarian cancer: a pilot study. Gynecol Oncol 2005;96(3):729–35.
12. Fagotti A, Ferrandina G, Fanfani F, et al. Prospective validation of a laparoscopic predictive model for optimal cytoreduction in advanced ovarian carcinoma. Am J Obstet Gynecol 2008;199(6):642.e1–6.
13. Gomez-Hidalgo NR, Martinez-Cannon BA, Nick AM, et al. Predictors of optimal cytoreduction in patients with newly diagnosed advanced-stage epithelial ovarian cancer: time to incorporate laparoscopic assessment into the standard of care. Gynecol Oncol 2015;137(3):553–8.
14. National Comprehensive Cancer Network (US). NCCN Clinical Practice Guidelines in Oncology. Ovarian cancer including fallopian tube cancer and primary peritoneal cancer. version 2.2018. Available at: https://www.nccn.org/professionals/physician_gls/pdf/ovarian.pdf.

15. Harter P, Sehouli J, Lorusso D, et al. LION: Lymphadenectomy In Ovarian Neoplasms—A prospective randomized AGO study group led gynecologic cancer intergroup trial. J Clin Oncol 2017;35(15_suppl):5500.

16. Hasenburg A, Sehouli J, Lampe B, et al. LION-PAW: Lymphadenectomy In Ovarian Neoplasm–Pleasure Ability of Women—Prospective substudy of the randomized multicenter LION study. J Clin Oncol 2018;36(suppl) [abstract: 5575].

17. Bois AD, Vergote I, Ferron G, et al. Randomized controlled phase III study evaluating the impact of secondary cytoreductive surgery in recurrent ovarian cancer: AGO DESKTOP III/ENGOT ov20. J Clin Oncol 2017;35(15_suppl):5501.

18. Robert L, Coleman DE, Spirtos N, et al. A phase III randomized controlled trial of secondary surgical cytoreduction (SSC) followed by platinum-based combination chemotherapy (PBC), with or without bevacizumab (B) in platinum-sensitive, recurrent ovarian cancer (PSOC): a NRG Oncology/Gynecologic Oncology Group (GOG) study. J Clin Oncol 2018;36(suppl) [abstract: 5501].

19. Katsumata N, Yasuda M, Isonishi S, et al. Long-term results of dose-dense paclitaxel and carboplatin versus conventional paclitaxel and carboplatin for treatment of advanced epithelial ovarian, fallopian tube, or primary peritoneal cancer (JGOG 3016): a randomised, controlled, open-label trial. Lancet Oncol 2013;14(10):1020–6.

20. Pignata S, Scambia G, Katsaros D, et al. Carboplatin plus paclitaxel once a week versus every 3 weeks in patients with advanced ovarian cancer (MITO-7): a randomised, multicentre, open-label, phase 3 trial. Lancet Oncol 2014;15(4):396–405.

21. Chan JK, Brady MF, Penson RT, et al. Weekly vs. every-3-week paclitaxel and carboplatin for ovarian cancer. N Engl J Med 2016;374(8):738–48.

22. Clamp AR, McNeish I, Dean A, et al. 929O_PRICON8: a GCIG phase III randomised trial evaluating weekly dose- dense chemotherapy integration in first-line epithelial ovarian/fallopian tube/primary peritoneal carcinoma (EOC) treatment: results of primary progression- free survival (PFS) analysis. Ann Oncol 2017; 28(suppl_5):v605–49.

23. Li L, Zhuang Q, Cao Z, et al. Paclitaxel plus nedaplatin vs. paclitaxel plus carboplatin in women with epithelial ovarian cancer: a multi-center, randomized, open-label, phase III trial. J Clin Oncol 2018;36(suppl) [abstract: e17519].

24. Takakura S, Takano M, Takahashi F, et al. Randomized phase II trial of paclitaxel plus carboplatin therapy versus irinotecan plus cisplatin therapy as first-line chemotherapy for clear cell adenocarcinoma of the ovary: a JGOG study. Int J Gynecol Cancer 2010;20(2):240–7.

25. Sugiyama T, Okamoto A, Enomoto T, et al. Randomized phase III trial of irinotecan plus cisplatin compared with paclitaxel plus carboplatin as first-line chemotherapy for ovarian clear cell carcinoma: JGOG3017/GCIG trial. J Clin Oncol 2016;34(24):2881–7.

26. Armstrong DK, Bundy B, Wenzel L, et al. Intraperitoneal cisplatin and paclitaxel in ovarian cancer. N Engl J Med 2006;354(1):34–43.

27. Walker JL, BM, DiSilvestro PA, et al. A phase III trial of bevacizumab with IV versus IP chemotherapy in ovarian, fallopian tube, and peritoneal carcinoma NCI-supplied agent(s): a GOG/NRG trial (GOG 252). Society of Gynecologic Oncology Annual Meeting Late-breaking abstract 6 Presented San Diego, CA, March 21, 2016. 2016.

28. Wright JD, Hou JY, Burke WM, et al. Utilization and toxicity of alternative delivery methods of adjuvant chemotherapy for ovarian cancer. Obstet Gynecol 2016; 127(6):985–91.

29. van Driel WJ, Koole SN, Sikorska K, et al. Hyperthermic intraperitoneal chemotherapy in ovarian cancer. N Engl J Med 2018;378(3):230–40.

30. Leslie M, Randall DG, Krill LS, et al. A phase I dose-escalation of hyperthermic intraoperative intraperitoneal chemotherapy (HIPEC) carboplatin for the frontline treatment of advanced ovarian cancer. J Clin Oncol 2018;36(suppl) [abstract: 5554].

31. Markman M, Rothman R, Hakes T, et al. Second-line platinum therapy in patients with ovarian cancer previously treated with cisplatin. J Clin Oncol 1991;9(3): 389–93.

32. Bookman MA. Extending the platinum-free interval in recurrent ovarian cancer: the role of topotecan in second-line chemotherapy. Oncologist 1999;4(2):87–94.

33. Pignata S, Scambia G, Bologna A, et al. Randomized controlled trial testing the efficacy of platinum-free interval prolongation in advanced ovarian cancer: the MITO-8, MaNGO, BGOG-Ov1, AGO-Ovar2.16, ENGOT-Ov1, GCIG Study. J Clin Oncol 2017;35(29):3347–53.

34. Mirza MR, Monk BJ, Herrstedt J, et al. Niraparib maintenance therapy in platinum-sensitive, recurrent ovarian cancer. N Engl J Med 2016;375(22): 2154–64.

35. Ledermann J, Harter P, Gourley C, et al. Olaparib maintenance therapy in platinum-sensitive relapsed ovarian cancer. N Engl J Med 2012;366(15):1382–92.

36. Matulonis UA, Harter P, Gourley C, et al. Olaparib maintenance therapy in patients with platinum-sensitive, relapsed serous ovarian cancer and a BRCA mutation: overall survival adjusted for postprogression poly(adenosine diphosphate ribose) polymerase inhibitor therapy. Cancer 2016;122(12):1844–52.

37. Ledermann J, Harter P, Gourley C, et al. Olaparib maintenance therapy in patients with platinum-sensitive relapsed serous ovarian cancer: a preplanned retrospective analysis of outcomes by BRCA status in a randomised phase 2 trial. Lancet Oncol 2014;15(8):852–61.

38. Ledermann JA, Harter P, Gourley C, et al. Overall survival in patients with platinum-sensitive recurrent serous ovarian cancer receiving olaparib maintenance monotherapy: an updated analysis from a randomised, placebo-controlled, double-blind, phase 2 trial. Lancet Oncol 2016;17(11):1579–89.

39. Pujade-Lauraine E, Ledermann JA, Selle F, et al. Olaparib tablets as maintenance therapy in patients with platinum-sensitive, relapsed ovarian cancer and a BRCA1/2 mutation (SOLO2/ENGOT-Ov21): a double-blind, randomised, placebo-controlled, phase 3 trial. Lancet Oncol 2017;18(9):1274–84.

40. Coleman RL, Oza AM, Lorusso D, et al. Rucaparib maintenance treatment for recurrent ovarian carcinoma after response to platinum therapy (ARIEL3): a randomised, double-blind, placebo-controlled, phase 3 trial. Lancet 2017; 390(10106):1949–61.

41. Aghajanian C, Coleman RL, Oza AM, et al. Evaluation of rucaparib in platinum-sensitive recurrent ovarian carcinoma (rOC) in patients (pts) with or without residual bulky disease at baseline in the ARIEL3 study. J Clin Oncol 2018;36(suppl) [abstract: 5537].

42. Kaufman B, Shapira-Frommer R, Schmutzler RK, et al. Olaparib monotherapy in patients with advanced cancer and a germline BRCA1/2 mutation. J Clin Oncol 2015;33(3):244–50.

43. Matulonis UA, Penson RT, Domchek SM, et al. Olaparib monotherapy in patients with advanced relapsed ovarian cancer and a germline BRCA1/2 mutation: a multistudy analysis of response rates and safety. Ann Oncol 2016;27(6):1013–9.

44. Kristeleit RS, Shapira-Frommer R, Oaknin A, et al. Clinical activity of the poly(ADP-ribose) polymerase (PARP) inhibitor rucaparib in patients (pts) with high-grade ovarian carcinoma (HGOC) and a BRCA mutation (BRCAmut): analysis of pooled data from Study 10 (parts 1, 2a, and 3) and ARIEL2 (parts 1 and 2). Ann Oncol 2016;27(suppl_6):856O.

45. Swisher EM, Lin KK, Oza AM, et al. Rucaparib in relapsed, platinum-sensitive high-grade ovarian carcinoma (ARIEL2 Part 1): an international, multicentre, open-label, phase 2 trial. Lancet Oncol 2017;18(1):75–87.

46. Kathleen N, Moore AAS, Geller MA, et al. QUADRA: a phase 2, open-label, single-arm study to evaluate niraparib in patients (pts) with relapsed ovarian cancer (ROC) who have received ≥3 prior chemotherapy regimens. J Clin Oncol 2018; 36(suppl) [abstract: 5514].

47. Coleman RL, Sill MW, Bell-McGuinn K, et al. A phase II evaluation of the potent, highly selective PARP inhibitor veliparib in the treatment of persistent or recurrent epithelial ovarian, fallopian tube, or primary peritoneal cancer in patients who carry a germline BRCA1 or BRCA2 mutation - an NRG Oncology/Gynecologic Oncology Group study. Gynecol Oncol 2015;137(3):386–91.

48. Administration USFD. FDA approves bevacizumab in combination with chemotherapy for ovarian cancer. Available at: https://www.fda.gov/drugs/informationondrugs/approveddrugs/ucm610664.htm.

49. Burger RA, Enserro D, Tewari KS, et al. Final overall survival (OS) analysis of an international randomized trial evaluating bevacizumab (BEV) in the primary treatment of advanced ovarian cancer: a NRG oncology/Gynecologic Oncology Group (GOG) study. J Clin Oncol 2018;36(suppl) [abstract: 5517].

50. Perren TJ, Swart AM, Pfisterer J, et al. A phase 3 trial of bevacizumab in ovarian cancer. N Engl J Med 2011;365(26):2484–96.

51. Oza AM, Cook AD, Pfisterer J, et al. Standard chemotherapy with or without bevacizumab for women with newly diagnosed ovarian cancer (ICON7): overall survival results of a phase 3 randomised trial. Lancet Oncol 2015;16(8):928–36.

52. Aghajanian C, Blank SV, Goff BA, et al. OCEANS: a randomized, double-blind, placebo-controlled phase III trial of chemotherapy with or without bevacizumab in patients with platinum-sensitive recurrent epithelial ovarian, primary peritoneal, or fallopian tube cancer. J Clin Oncol 2012;30(17):2039–45.

53. Aghajanian C, Goff B, Nycum LR, et al. Independent radiologic review: bevacizumab in combination with gemcitabine and carboplatin in recurrent ovarian cancer. Gynecol Oncol 2014;133(1):105–10.

54. Aghajanian C, Goff B, Nycum LR, et al. Final overall survival and safety analysis of OCEANS, a phase 3 trial of chemotherapy with or without bevacizumab in patients with platinum-sensitive recurrent ovarian cancer. Gynecol Oncol 2015;139(1):10–6.

55. Coleman RL, Brady MF, Herzog TJ, et al. Bevacizumab and paclitaxel-carboplatin chemotherapy and secondary cytoreduction in recurrent, platinum-sensitive ovarian cancer (NRG Oncology/Gynecologic Oncology Group study GOG-0213): a multicentre, open-label, randomised, phase 3 trial. Lancet Oncol 2017;18(6):779–91.

56. Pignata S, Lorusso D, Joly F, et al. Chemotherapy plus or minus bevacizumab for platinum-sensitive ovarian cancer patients recurring after a bevacizumab containing first line treatment: the randomized phase 3 trial MITO16B-MaNGO OV2B-ENGOT OV17. J Clin Oncol 2018;36(suppl) [abstract: 5506].

57. Burger RA, Sill MW, Monk BJ, et al. Phase II trial of bevacizumab in persistent or recurrent epithelial ovarian cancer or primary peritoneal cancer: a Gynecologic Oncology Group Study. J Clin Oncol 2007;25(33):5165–71.

58. Cannistra SA, Matulonis UA, Penson RT, et al. Phase II study of bevacizumab in patients with platinum-resistant ovarian cancer or peritoneal serous cancer. J Clin Oncol 2007;25(33):5180–6.

59. Pujade-Lauraine E, Hilpert F, Weber B, et al. Bevacizumab combined with chemotherapy for platinum-resistant recurrent ovarian cancer: the AURELIA open-label randomized phase III trial. J Clin Oncol 2014;32(13):1302–8.

60. Ledermann JA, Embleton AC, Raja F, et al. Cediranib in patients with relapsed platinum-sensitive ovarian cancer (ICON6): a randomised, double-blind, placebo-controlled phase 3 trial. Lancet 2016;387(10023):1066–74.

61. Liu JF, Barry WT, Wenham RM, et al. A phase 2 biomarker trial of combination cediranib and olaparib in relapsed platinum (plat) sensitive and plat resistant ovarian cancer (ovca). J Clin Oncol 2018;36(suppl) [abstract: 5519].

62. du Bois A, Kristensen G, Ray-Coquard I, et al. Standard first-line chemotherapy with or without nintedanib for advanced ovarian cancer (AGO-OVAR 12): a randomised, double-blind, placebo-controlled phase 3 trial. Lancet Oncol 2016;17(1): 78–89.

63. Lan C, Wang Y, Xiong Y, et al. Apatinib, a novel VEGFR inhibitor, combined with oral etoposide in patients with platinum-resistant or platinum-refractory ovarian cancer: a single-arm, open-label, phase 2 study. J Clin Oncol 2018;36(suppl) [abstract: 5515].

64. Vergote I, Hanker LC, Floquet A, et al. AGO-OVAR 16: a phase III study to evaluate the efficacy and safety of pazopanib (PZ) monotherapy versus placebo in women who have not progressed after first line chemotherapy for epithelial ovarian, fallopian tube, or primary peritoneal cancer—Overall survival (OS) results. J Clin Oncol 2018;36(suppl) [abstract: 5518].

65. Hamanishi J, Mandai M, Matsumura N, et al. PD-1/PD-L1 blockade in cancer treatment: perspectives and issues. Int J Clin Oncol 2016;21(3):462–73.

66. Zhang L, Conejo-Garcia JR, Katsaros D, et al. Intratumoral T cells, recurrence, and survival in epithelial ovarian cancer. N Engl J Med 2003;348(3):203–13.

67. Brahmer J, Reckamp KL, Baas P, et al. Nivolumab versus docetaxel in advanced squamous-cell non-small-cell lung cancer. N Engl J Med 2015;373(2):123–35.

68. Borghaei H, Paz-Ares L, Horn L, et al. Nivolumab versus docetaxel in advanced nonsquamous non-small-cell lung cancer. N Engl J Med 2015;373(17):1627–39.

69. Robert C, Long GV, Brady B, et al. Nivolumab in previously untreated melanoma without BRAF mutation. N Engl J Med 2015;372(4):320–30.

70. Robert C, Schachter J, Long GV, et al. Pembrolizumab versus ipilimumab in advanced melanoma. N Engl J Med 2015;372(26):2521–32.

71. Weber JS, D'Angelo SP, Minor D, et al. Nivolumab versus chemotherapy in patients with advanced melanoma who progressed after anti-CTLA-4 treatment (CheckMate 037): a randomised, controlled, open-label, phase 3 trial. Lancet Oncol 2015;16(4):375–84.

72. Abiko K, Mandai M, Hamanishi J, et al. PD-L1 on tumor cells is induced in ascites and promotes peritoneal dissemination of ovarian cancer through CTL dysfunction. Clin Cancer Res 2013;19(6):1363–74.

73. Hamanishi J, Mandai M, Ikeda T, et al. Safety and antitumor activity of anti-PD-1 antibody, nivolumab, in patients with platinum-resistant ovarian cancer. J Clin Oncol 2015;33(34):4015–22.

74. Disis ML, Patel MR, Pant S, et al. Avelumab (MSB0010718C), an anti-PD-L1 antibody, in patients with previously treated, recurrent or refractory ovarian cancer: a phase Ib, open-label expansion trial. J Clin Oncol 2015;33(15_suppl):5509.

75. Varga A, Piha-Paul SA, Ott PA, et al. Antitumor activity and safety of pembrolizumab in patients (pts) with PD-L1 positive advanced ovarian cancer: interim results from a phase Ib study. J Clin Oncol 2015;33(15_suppl):5510.
76. Konstantinopoulos PA, Waggoner SE, Vidal GA, et al. TOPACIO/Keynote-162 (NCT02657889): a phase 1/2 study of niraparib + pembrolizumab in patients (pts) with advanced triple-negative breast cancer or recurrent ovarian cancer (ROC)—Results from ROC cohort. J Clin Oncol 2018;36(suppl) [abstract: 106].
77. Pujade-Lauraine E, Fujiwara K, Dychter SS, et al. Avelumab (anti-PD-L1) in platinum-resistant/refractory ovarian cancer: JAVELIN ovarian 200 phase III study design. Future Oncol 2018;14(21):2103–13.
78. Szender JB, Papanicolau-Sengos A, Eng KH, et al. NY-ESO-1 expression predicts an aggressive phenotype of ovarian cancer. Gynecol Oncol 2017;145(3):420–5.
79. Tsuji T, Sabbatini P, Jungbluth AA, et al. Effect of Montanide and poly-ICLC adjuvant on human self/tumor antigen-specific CD4+ T cells in phase I overlapping long peptide vaccine trial. Cancer Immunol Res 2013;1(5):340–50.
80. Odunsi K, Matsuzaki J, Karbach J, et al. Efficacy of vaccination with recombinant vaccinia and fowlpox vectors expressing NY-ESO-1 antigen in ovarian cancer and melanoma patients. Proc Natl Acad Sci U S A 2012;109(15):5797–802.
81. Odunsi K, Matsuzaki J, James SR, et al. Epigenetic potentiation of NY-ESO-1 vaccine therapy in human ovarian cancer. Cancer Immunol Res 2014;2(1):37–49.
82. O'Cearbhaill RE, Gnjatic S, Aghajanian C, et al. A phase I study of concomitant galinpepimut-s (GPS) in combination with nivolumab (nivo) in patients (pts) with WT1+ ovarian cancer (OC) in second or third remission. J Clin Oncol 2018;36(suppl) [abstract: 5553].
83. Rob L, Mallmann P, Knapp P, et al, SOV01 Investigators. Dendritic cell vaccine (DCVAC) with chemotherapy (ct) in patients (pts) with epithelial ovarian carcinoma (EOC) after primary debulking surgery (PDS): interim analysis of a phase 2, open-label, randomized, multicenter trial. J Clin Oncol 2018;36(suppl) [abstract: 5509].
84. Odunsi K. Immunotherapy in ovarian cancer. Ann Oncol 2017;28(suppl_8):viii1–7.
85. Zhu X, Cai H, Zhao L, et al. CAR-T cell therapy in ovarian cancer: from the bench to the bedside. Oncotarget 2017;8(38):64607–21.
86. Koneru M, O'Cearbhaill R, Pendharkar S, et al. A phase I clinical trial of adoptive T cell therapy using IL-12 secreting MUC-16(ecto) directed chimeric antigen receptors for recurrent ovarian cancer. J Transl Med 2015;13:102.
87. Kumar L, Hariprasad R, Kumar S, et al. Neoadjuvant chemotherapy in advanced epithelial ovarian oancer (EOC): A phase III randomized study. Journal of Clinical Oncology 2006;24(June 20 Supplement):18S.
88. Burger RA, Brady MF, Bookman MA, et al. Incorporation of bevacizumab in the primary treatment of ovarian cancer. N Engl J Med 2011;365(26):2473–83.

Endometrial Cancer
Obesity, Genetics, and Targeted Agents

Megan E. McDonald, MD, David P. Bender, MD*

KEYWORDS

- Endometrial cancer • Obesity • Genetics • Targeted therapeutics

KEY POINTS

- Endometrial cancer incidence and mortality in the United States is increasing. Although most women are diagnosed with early stage disease and have a good prognosis, up to 30% present with advanced-stage disease and suffer lower 5-year survival rates.
- Obesity is a known risk factor for endometrial cancer. Estrogens and proinflammatory adipokines stimulate cell proliferation as seen in endometrial hyperplasia and carcinoma.
- Newly characterized genomic events in endometrial cancer compliment the histologic classification of this disease and broaden our understanding of endometrial carcinogenesis.
- Agents targeting hormonal activity, cell surface receptors, cell proliferation pathways, and DNA repair mechanisms have had limited durable responses to date.
- Further understanding of actionable molecular and genomic targets is critical to selecting optimal therapeutic regimens and improving the treatment of advanced endometrial cancer.

INTRODUCTION

As the most common gynecologic malignancy in the United States, endometrial cancer incidence and mortality are increasing with 63,230 new cases projected in 2018 and 11,350 deaths.[1] Most women are diagnosed with early stage disease and have a good prognosis with 5-year overall survival (OS) rates of nearly 90%. Unfortunately, roughly 30% of women present with stage III or IV disease, with significantly worse 5-year survival rates of 60% and 20%, respectively.[2] Although the prognosis for endometrial cancer is favorable for early stages, incidence and recurrence remain on the increase. A recent estimate projects a 55% increase in incidence by 2030.[3] Thus, it is imperative to understand the underlying mechanisms

Disclosures: The authors have no conflicts of interest to disclose.
Division of Gynecologic Oncology, Department of Obstetrics and Gynecology, University of Iowa, University of Iowa Hospitals and Clinics, 200 Hawkins Drive, Iowa City, IA 52242, USA
* Corresponding author.
E-mail address: david-bender@uiowa.edu

Obstet Gynecol Clin N Am 46 (2019) 89–105
https://doi.org/10.1016/j.ogc.2018.09.006
obgyn.theclinics.com

of endometrial carcinogenesis and recurrence to develop more effective prevention strategies and treatment. This article reviews available genomic data, the interplay between endometrial carcinogenesis with obesity and genetics, as well as current targeted therapies.

OVERVIEW OF TYPE I AND II ENDOMETRIAL CANCER
Type I and Type II Tumors

Classically, endometrial cancer has been divided into type I and type II tumors, as first described by Bokhman in 1983 (**Table 1**).[4] Pathogenically, type I tumors are thought to be related to hyperestrogenism. Patients with these tumors are phenotypically characterized by anovulatory bleeding and infertility in the premenopausal state, obesity, and associated metabolic disturbances. These tumors are histologically endometrioid, low-grade, early stage with superficial myometrial invasion, slow growing, and highly sensitive to progestins. For these reasons, the prognosis for type I tumors is favorable. Conversely, type II tumors seem unrelated to hyperestrogenism. Unlike type I tumors, the endometrium in these women often seems atrophic. Type II tumors portend a worse prognosis because they are often poorly differentiated, of nonendometrioid histology, deeply invasive at diagnosis, and carry a high potential for lymphovascular spread.

Integrated Genomic Characterization of Endometrial Cancer

In 2013, a comprehensive genomic characterization of endometrial carcinomas within The Cancer Genome Atlas (TCGA) was published and introduced a new classification schema for these tumors.[5] Unlike the Bokhman characterization, TCGA classified endometrial cancers into 4 categories: POLE ultramutated, microsatellite instability (MSI) hypermutated, copy-number low, and copy-number high (**Table 2**). The POLE ultramutated group accounted for 7% of tumors within TCGA and was characterized by low numbers of somatic copy number alterations (SCNAs). Most importantly, these tumors were characterized by a markedly increased somatic mutational burden (232×10^{-6}) and an improved progression-free survival (PFS) compared with the other 3 groups (log-rank $P = .0004$). The second group, MSI hypermutated, was characterized by a mix of low- (28.6%) and high-grade (54.3%) endometrioid endometrial

Table 1 Classification of endometrial cancer		
	Type I	**Type II**
Phenotype	Younger age Obese Associated lipid and metabolic disturbances Thickened endometrium	Older age Nonobese Lack of associated lipid and metabolic disturbances Atrophic/transitional endometrium
Pathogenesis	Estrogen dependent	Estrogen independent
Histology	Endometrioid	Nonendometrioid
Differentiation	Well/moderately differentiated	Poorly differentiated
Prognosis	Good	Poor
Molecular Aberrations	PTEN, MSI, PI3K/AKT, KRAS	p53, Her2, PI3K/AKT, KRAS

From Bokhman JV. Two pathogenetic types of endometrial carcinoma. Gynecol Oncol 1983;15(1):10–7; with permission.

Table 2
TCGA genomic characterization of endometrial cancer

	POLE Ultramutated	MSI Hypermutated	Copy-Number Low	Copy-Number High
Copy-Number Alterations	Low	Low	Low	High
Histologic Subtype	Endometrioid	Endometrioid	Endometrioid	Serous, mixed histology, grade 3 endometrioid
Microsatellite Stability	Mixed	Instable (MLH1 promoter methylation common)	Stable	Stable
Mutation Rate	232×10^{-6}	18×10^{-6}	2.9×10^{-6}	2.3×10^{-6}
Frequent Molecular Aberrations	POLE, PTEN, PI3K/ AKT/mTOR, ARID1A	PTEN, KRAS, PI3K/AKT, ARID1A	PTEN, CTNNB1, PI3K/AKT, FGFR	TP53, FGFR, ERBB2/ Her2
Prognosis	Good	Intermediate	Intermediate	Poor

Data from Cancer Genome Atlas Research Network, Kandoth C, Schultz N, Cherniack AD, et al. Integrated genomic characterization of endometrial carcinoma. Nature 2013;497(7447):67–73.

cancers, a 10-fold greater mutation frequency than the microsatellite stable tumors, few SCNAs, frequent KRAS mutations, and infrequent TP53 mutations. The copy-number low group had a worse PFS than the MSI hypermutated group (log-rank $P = .003$) and contained frequent CTNNB1 mutations. Most of the serous and mixed histology tumors clustered into the fourth group, copy-number high, a group with frequent SCNAs and TP53 mutations, few PTEN mutations, and little MSI. Tumors within this cluster were associated with worse PFS than tumors within all other clusters. Approximately 25% of tumors, classified as high-grade endometrioid, clustered into group 4 based on their molecular phenotype that warrants consideration of treating these patients similar to other copy-number high tumors rather than the conventional type I tumors.

OBESITY

The association between obesity and increased risk of malignancy is well established within the literature, with the risk of endometrial cancer demonstrating the strongest association (risk ratio of 1.52).[6] Furthermore, obesity is associated with an increased risk of recurrence and death from cancer.[6] Adipose tissue functions as an endocrine organ contributing to hormone production, inflammatory responses, and stimulation of cellular proliferation pathways. Classically, aromatization of androstenedione to estrone within adipose tissue was felt to drive the development of type 1 endometrial cancers (**Fig. 1**).[7] Excess endogenous estrogens directly stimulate endometrial growth through activation of the estrogen receptor, ERα. The most potent of the endogenous female sex hormones, estradiol, is also thought to play a role in carcinogenesis through activation of insulin-like growth factor I receptor and epidermal growth factor receptor (EGFR), thereby activating the downstream phosphatidylinositol 3-kinase–AKT–mammalian target of rapamycin (PI3K-AKT-mTOR) pathway.[8]

In addition to hyperestrogenism, obesity promotes carcinogenesis through production of adipokines and maintenance of a proinflammatory state. Secreted adipokines

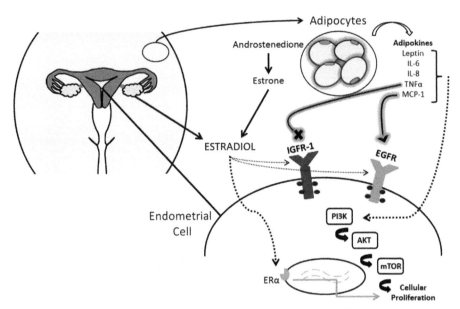

Fig. 1. Obesity and carcinogenesis. Hyperestrogenism leads to direct ERα stimulation, resulting in endometrial cell proliferation. Adipose tissue produces proinflammatory adipokines, leading to insulin resistance and stimulation of the PI3K-AKT-mTOR pathway subsequently resulting in cell proliferation.

include leptin, tumor necrosis factor alpha (TNF-α), interleukin 6 (IL-6), IL-8, and monocyte chemoattractant protein-1 (MCP-1).[9–12] Elevated levels of adipokines (leptin) have been connected with an increased risk of endometrial cancer. In turn, insulin resistance has been shown to be an independent risk factor for the development of endometrial cancer.[13]

Inflammation-mediated hyperactivation of the PI3K-AKT-mTOR pathway has also been shown, most commonly in type 1 tumors.[14] In addition to downstream regulation of mTOR, activation of PI3K-AKT leads to production of COX-2 and PGE2. Overexpression of COX-2 and PGE2 has been linked with carcinogenesis, because they are antiapoptotic, proangiogenic, and can induce invasion.[15–17] The antiinflammatory effect of aspirin via suppression of the COX-2/PGE2 pathway has become an attractive therapeutic option to mitigate cancer risk.

Hormonal Therapy

Progestin-based hormonal therapy has long been used to counter the hyperestrogenism associated with endometrial hyperplasia and carcinoma. A Gynecologic Oncology Group (GOG) study of high-dose megestrol acetate in advanced and recurrent endometrial cancer showed a 24% clinical RR,[18] but response was not sustained. Shortened response duration to progestins has been attributed to down-regulation of progesterone receptors (PR). Alternatively, estrogenic stimulation of the endometrium, via ERα binding by tamoxifen, is known to increase PR expression through activation of gene transcription. The combination of progesterone and tamoxifen, evaluated in phase II trials, resulted in RRs of 27% to 33%.[19,20] Among those who responded favorably to this regimen, 53% of the responses exceeded 20 months.[20]

Decreased hormone efficacy is thought to be due to decreased PR expression in response to progesterone exposure. PR was also found to be downregulated through epigenetic silencing mechanisms such as promoter methylation and histone modification.[21,22] In vitro studies demonstrated that treatment of endometrial cancer cells with a DNA methyltransferase inhibitor or histone deacetylase (HDAC) inhibitor counters these epigenetic modifications, thereby increasing PR expression.[21,22] Trials incorporating HDAC inhibitors as sensitizing agents in combination with hormonal therapy are ongoing.

As noted earlier, hyperestrogenism leads to stimulation of the PI3K-AKT-mTOR pathway via ER activation.[8] Hence, endocrine therapy, in combination with mTOR inhibitors, was explored in endometrial cancer. A phase II trial of letrozole with everolimus resulted in an objective response rate (RR) of 32% and median PFS of 3 months,[23] whereas another phase II trial of letrozole, everolimus, and metformin demonstrated an overall RR of 29%.[24] Temsirolimus administered with alternating megestrol acetate and tamoxifen led to a modest RR of 14%, but the complication rate of venous thromboembolism was unacceptably high.[25]

Aspirin

Aspirin blockade of COX-2 activity and PGE2 production is a targetable pathway in endometrial cancer. Proinflammatory cytokines, such as leptin, TNF-α, IL-6, IL-8, and MCP-1, often elevated in obesity, induce COX-2 expression and PGE2 production. Higher COX-2 expression in endometrial cancers has been associated with deeper myometrial invasion and shorter disease-free survival.[26] Daily aspirin of greater than or equal to 3 years was associated with a decreased incidence of uterine cancers ($P = .003$).[27] A case-control study demonstrated a lower risk of endometrial cancer among women who had ever used aspirin within the last 5 years, particularly among obese patients. Furthermore, this finding seemed to be dose dependent where use greater than or equal to 2x per week proved the most beneficial (odds ratio 0.54).[28]

In addition to decreased incidence, survival benefit was observed with aspirin use. Matsuo and colleagues[29] found low-dose aspirin was associated with an improved 5 year PFS (hazard ratio [HR] 0.46, $P = .014$), as well as OS (HR 0.23, $P = .005$). The protective effects of aspirin were most pronounced in obese patients, patients with type 1 tumors, and women younger than 60 years. Conversely, GOG 210 evaluated nonsteroidal antiinflammatory drug use with cancer-specific recurrence and mortality in patients with endometrial cancer and showed an increased risk of mortality in patients with type 1 tumors (HR 1.66).[30] Investigations are ongoing to further delineate the relationship between aspirin and endometrial cancer.

Metformin

Epidemiologic studies have shown metformin to decrease cancer-related deaths among diabetic patients.[31,32] In addition to insulin sensitization and inhibition of hepatic gluconeogenesis, metformin inhibits the mTOR pathway through activation of adenosine monophosphate–activated protein kinase.[33] In vitro studies demonstrated cellular growth inhibition in endometrial cancer cells treated with metformin.[33] Furthermore, as with mTOR inhibitors, efficacy improved when used in combination with other agents. Hanna and colleagues[34] demonstrated a synergistic effect between metformin and paclitaxel in endometrial cancer cells. Given promising preclinical data, a phase III randomized trial comparing combination therapy of carboplatin and paclitaxel with that of carboplatin, paclitaxel, and metformin in patients with advanced or recurrent endometrial cancer was completed through the GOG. Mature data regarding tolerability and efficacy are currently pending.

GENETICS

Lynch Syndrome

A small number of endometrial cancer cases are related to hereditary genetic syndromes, such as Lynch syndrome. It is estimated that Lynch syndrome accounts for up to 5% of endometrial cancers.[35] Lynch syndrome is an autosomal dominantly inherited germline mutation in one of the DNA mismatch repair genes. Mutations in MLH1, MSH2, MSH6, and PMS2 are the most commonly mutated genes and found in 37%, 41%, 13%, and 9% of affected individuals, respectively.[36] The lifetime risk of developing endometrial cancer with Lynch syndrome is up to 60% but largely depends on the mutated genes. The National Comprehensive Cancer Network recommends an endometrial biopsy every 1 to 2 years for endometrial cancer screening and risk-reducing hysterectomy when childbearing is complete. Given the increased lifetime risk of ovarian cancer (10%), risk-reducing salpingo-oophorectomy should also be considered at the time of hysterectomy.[37]

Defects in mismatch repair (MMR) genes lead to microsatellite instability (MSI). However, MSI is not unique to Lynch syndrome. MSI can also occur due to alternate causes of MMR gene defects, most commonly sporadic methylation of the MLH-1 promotor. One study suggests that nearly 15% of sporadic tumors are MSI[38] and that greater than 90% of MSI endometrial tumors are due to MLH-1 promoter methylation.[39]

Identifying MMR-deficient or MSI tumors through immunohistochemical staining may have treatment implications and as such is an integral part of the workup of newly diagnosed endometrial cancer. Not only will this dictate management and surveillance of patients found to have Lynch syndrome, which are at risk for other cancers, but also may direct the use of novel therapeutic agents. The immune checkpoint inhibitor pembrolizumab has recently been approved by the Food and Drug Administration for the treatment of solid tumors with MSI or MMR deficiency, including endometrial cancer.[40] Use of pembrolizumab is generally reserved for patients who are refractory to other treatment options, such as cytotoxic chemotherapy or hormonal therapy.

Homologous Recombination Deficiency

Genomic events in endometrial cancer may result in homologous recombination deficiency (HRD), altering the cells' ability to repair DNA. Mutations described in classic homologous recombination pathways include BRCA1, BRCA2, ATR, ATM, RAD51, PALB2, and MRE11A. More frequent mutations reported in endometrial cancers such as PTEN (~50%)[41,42] and ARID1A complexes (46%–60%) also contribute to HRD.[43] The identification of HRD within endometrial cancers has led to the intense pursuit for therapeutic agents inhibiting DNA repair.

Literature regarding the risk of endometrial cancer in patients with BRCA mutations is contradictory and often confounded by tamoxifen use in patient cohorts. Recently, evidence suggests there may be a slight increased risk of serous endometrial cancers, particularly in BRCA1 mutant patients. Within a prospective cohort study of 1083 BRCA patients, 5 developed a serous or serouslike endometrial cancer with an observed/expected ratio of 22.2 in BRCA1 and 6.4 in BRCA2 patients.[44] However, it must be noted that the overall risk of serous carcinoma in this patient population was 0.4% and not increased over baseline. As such, the decision to proceed with risk-reducing hysterectomy at the time of salpingo-oophorectomy should not be automatic and should include consideration of patient and surgical morbidity.

Polymerase ε

As described by TCGA, there exists a subgroup of tumors distinguished by mutations in the DNA polymerase ε (POLE) exonuclease domain with a markedly increased somatic mutation burden. Within the TCGA report, this group had an improved PFS compared with the other 3 subgroups of endometrial cancer, MSI, copy-number low, and copy number high,[5] although this finding is likely confounded by the large proportion of low-grade tumors comprising the POLE subgroup relative to the higher proportion of aggressive histologies found in other subgroups. Moreover, follow-up studies failed to conclusively demonstrate an improved survival within this POLE group.[45]

In an attempt to develop a more clinically applicable molecular classification system for endometrial cancers, the NRG oncology/GOG study group classified 1040 endometrioid endometrial cancers into 4 classes; copy-number stable, MMR deficient, copy-number altered, or POLE.[46] Although the POLE group trended toward improved survival, this did not reach statistical significance. The POLE group also received the highest rate of adjuvant treatment of all 4 classes. Few studies to date have looked specifically at grade 3 endometrioid endometrial cancers. Within this particular group, the POLE mutant tumors did demonstrate improved PFS.[47] As of now, the prognostic significance of POLE mutations remains unclear.

Consistently throughout the literature, POLE mutant tumors were found to occur in younger women.[45–47] Furthermore, the same studies demonstrated equal distribution of POLE mutant tumors between microsatellite stable and instable tumors. The MSI POLE group, however, was more common in somatic or germline mutant tumors than in those characterized by MLH1 promoter methylation. This has clinical implications in that MSI/POLE mutant endometrioid endometrial cancers should be tested for germline or somatic MMR mutations.

POLE mutant tumors were also found to harbor large numbers of tumor-infiltrating lymphocytes and showed high levels of PD-1 and PD-L1expression.[48,49] A recent case report demonstrated excellent activity of the anti-PD-1 antibody, pembrolizumab, in a patient with POLE mutant endometrial cancer.[50] Identification of POLE mutant tumors may define a population that could benefit from immunotherapy.

TARGETING ABERRANT PATHWAYS
Angiogenesis

In endometrial tumors, VEGF overexpression has been associated with deep myometrial invasion and lymph node metastasis.[51] Given these findings, the use of antiangiogenic agents in the treatment of endometrial cancer has been explored. Most notably, within the GOG 229 series, bevacizumab, a monoclonal antibody targeting VEGF-A, showed activity with an RR of 13.5%.[52] The multifunctional tyrosine kinase inhibitor, cediranib, targeting vascular EGFR (VEGFRs), platelet-derived growth factor (PDGF) alpha and beta receptors, and fibroblast growth factor (FGF) receptor was deemed active as well, with an RR of 12.5% and 29% 6-month event-free survival.[53] Among recurrent endometrial cancers, median PFS with bevacizumab or cediranib alone was limited to 4.3 and 3.6 months, respectively.[52,53] Additional studies, evaluating similar agents as monotherapy in the GOG 229 queue showed minimal benefit.[54–57]

In light of the limited response to antiangiogenic monotherapy, combinations with cytotoxic agents were evaluated. Bevacizumab was added to carboplatin and paclitaxel in a randomized phase II trial as initial therapy for advanced or recurrent endometrial cancer (GOG 86P). Although PFS was not improved with the addition of bevacizumab, OS was longer when compared with historical controls.[58] Among a similar patient population, combination therapy (bevacizumab, carboplatin, paclitaxel) followed by bevacizumab maintenance led to improved PFS compared with chemotherapy alone (PFS 12 vs 8.7 months, $P<.039$).[59] Bevacizumab was also studied in combination with the mTOR inhibitor, temsirolimus, in patients with recurrent or persistent disease. Although a 24.5% RR and a 46.9% 6-month event-free survival were impressive, this combination was associated with significant toxicity.[60] The definitive role of antiangiogenic agents in endometrial cancer has yet to be determined. Potential combinations with other therapies warrant further investigation.

Phosphatidylinositol 3-Kinase-AKT-Mammalian Target of Rapamycin Pathway

In addition to phenotypic and histologic differences, recent DNA sequencing of type I and II tumors have elucidated differences in aberrant molecular pathways as well. The PI3K-AKT-mTOR pathway is the most commonly aberrant pathway within type I tumors, because 30% to 80% of sporadic endometrioid endometrial cancers harbor a PTEN mutation.[42,61,62] It is through the loss of PTEN tumor suppressor function that the PI3K-AKT-mTOR pathway is constitutively activated. In addition, activation of the PI3K-AKT-mTOR pathway is seen in the presence of AKT[63,64] and PIK3CA mutations,[65,66] also common within type I tumors. The activation of the PI3K-AKT-mTOR pathway leads to upregulation of mTOR, a serine/threonine kinase involved in regulation of protein translation. Although present, mutations within this pathway are less frequent in type II tumors (60%).

The relatively high frequency of mutations in both type I and type II tumors has made the PI3K-AKT-mTOR pathway appealing for targeted therapy. Single-agent mTOR inhibitors, ridaforolimus and everolimus, have been tested in advanced endometrial cancers. Twenty-nine percent of patients receiving ridaforolimus achieved clinical benefit (objective response or stable disease) in one study,[67] whereas 35% had stable disease in another phase II trial.[68] Patients treated with single-agent everolimus as second- or third-line therapy demonstrated a 36% stable disease rate at 3 months.[69]

RAS/RAF/MEK Pathway

Alterations with the RAS/RAF/MEK pathway are seen within type I endometrial cancers at an estimated rate of 10% to 36% and less frequently in type II tumors.[70–72] Constitutive activation of the MEK pathway occurs through various mechanisms including somatic mutations within RAS (most commonly KRAS), BRAF, and/or MEK. Dysregulated activation of this cascade leads to uncontrolled cellular growth. The oral MEK inhibitor selumetinib was used in the treatment of recurrent endometrial cancer in a phase II trial.[73] Although selumetinib was well tolerated, it did not meet pretrial specifications for efficacy. There are a large proportion of tumors with mutations in both PI3K-AKT-mTOR and RAS/RAF/MEK pathways, and an intricate relationship of coregulation between these pathways exists, where downregulation of one pathway may induce upregulation of the other.[74] This highlights the importance of dual inhibition of both pathways to achieve maximum therapeutic benefit and may explain the limited activity of MEK inhibitor monotherapy. With this in mind, investigators randomized patients with recurrent or persistent endometrial cancer to an MEK inhibitor (trametinib) versus an MEK inhibitor plus an AKT inhibitor (trametinib + GSK2141795). Unfortunately, the study was closed after a safety lead-in because the combination therapy was associated with unacceptable toxicity. Improved toxicity was seen at reduced dosing but efficacy at this dosing was insufficient to warrant further investigation.[75]

Table 3
Summary of clinical trials of targeted therapies for endometrial cancer

	Cohort	Regimen	No. Pts	RR No (%)	PFS (mo)	OS (mo)
Hormonal Therapy[Ref]						
Megestrol Acetate (MA)[18]	Advanced/Recurrent EC No prior hormonal or cytotoxic therapy	MA 800 mg/d PO	58	CR: 6 (11) PR: 7 (13)	2.5	7.6
Medroxyprogesterone Acetate (MPA) + Tamoxifen[19]	Advanced/Recurrent EC No prior hormonal or cytotoxic therapy	Tamoxifen 40 mo qday PO + MPA 200 mg qday PO on even numbered weeks	58	CR: 6 (10) PR: 13 (22)	3.0	13.0
Megestrol Acetate (MA) + Tamoxifen[20]	Advanced/Recurrent EC No prior hormonal or cytotoxic therapy	MA 80 mg BID PO x3 wks alternating with Tamoxifen 20 mg BID PO x3 wks	56	CR: 12 (21) PR: 3 (5)	2.7	14.0
Antiangiogenics						
Bevacizumab[52]	Persistent/Recurrent 1–2 prior cytotoxic regimens allowed	Bevacizumab 15 mg/kg IV q3 wks	52	CR: 1 (2) PR: 6 (12)	4.2	10.5
Cediranib[53]	Persistent/Recurrent 1–2 prior cytotoxic regimens allowed	Cediranib 30 mg qday PO	48	CR: 0 (0) PR: 6 (13)	3.7	12.5
Carboplatin/Paclitaxel + Bevacizumab[a,58]	Advanced/Recurrent EC No prior cytotoxic therapy	Carboplatin AUC 6 + Paclitaxel 175 mg/m² + Bevacizumab 15 mg/m² Day 1 q21 d	116	ORR: 70 (60)	N/A	34.0

(continued on next page)

Table 3
(continued)

Cohort	Regimen	No. Pts	RR No (%)	PFS (mo)	OS (mo)
	Maintenance Bevacizumab 15 mg/m² q21 d				
Carboplatin/Paclitaxel + Bevacizumab[a,59]	Advanced/Recurrent EC 1 prior cytotoxic regimens allowed	Carboplatin AUC 6 + Paclitaxel 175 mg/m² + Bevacizumab 15 mg/m² Day 1 q21 d Maintenance Bevacizumab 15 mg/m² q21 d	54	ORR: 39 (73)	13.0	N/A
Bevacizumab + Temsirolimus[60]	Persistent/Recurrent EC 1–2 prior cytotoxic regimens allowed	Bevacizumab 10 mg/kg IV qo wk + Temsirolimus 25 mg IV qweek	49	CR: 1 (2) PR: 11 (22)	5.6	16.9
PI3K-Akt-mTOR					
Ridaforolimus[67]	Recurrent/Persistent EC	Ridaforolimus 12.5 mg IV qday x5 days q2 weeks	45	PR: 5 (11) SD: 8 (18)	3.3 – prior chemo 7.3 – chemo naïve	N/A
Ridaforolimus[68]	Advanced/Recurrent EC	40 mg PO qday x5 days weekly	64	ORR: 0 (0) SD: 22 (35)	3.6	N/A
Everolimus[69]	Advanced/Recurrent 1–2 prior cytotoxic regimens allowed	Everolimus 10 mg qday	44	PR: 4 (10)	2.8	8.1
Letrozole + Everolimus[23]	Recurrent EC 1–2 prior cytotoxic regimens allowed	Everolimus 10 mg qday + Letrozole 2.5 mg qday	35	CR: 9 (26) PR: 2 (6)	3.0	14.0

			N			
Letrozole + Everolimus + Metformin[a,24]	Advanced/Recurrent endometrioid EC 1–2 prior cytotoxic regimens allowed	Everolimus 10 mg qday + Letrozole 2.5 mg PO qday + Metformin 500 mg POD BID	48	CR: 0 (0) PR: 14 (29) SD: 18 (38)	N/A	N/A
Temsirolimus + Megestrol Acetate (MA) + Tamoxifen[25]	Advanced/Recurrent EC	Temsirolimus 25 mg IV qweek + MA 80 mg BID + Tamoxifen 20 mg BID	71	CR: 0 (0) PR: 3 (14)	4.9 – prior chemo 8.2 –chemo naive	10.8 – prior chemo 20.7 – chemo naive
RAS/RAF/MEK						
Selumetinib[73]	Persistent/Recurrent EC 1–2 prior cytotoxic regimens allowed	Selumetinib 75 mg PO BID qday	52	CR: 1 (2) PR: 2 (4) SD: 13 (25)	2.3	8.5
Cell Surface Receptors						
Gefitinib[55]	Persistent/Recurrent EC	Gefitinib 500 mg PO qday	26	CR: 1 (8) SD: 7 (30)	1.8	7.1
Erlotinib[78]	Advanced/Recurrent EC No prior cytotoxic regimens	Erlotinib 150 mg PO qday	32	CR: 0 (0) PR: 4 (13) SD: 15 (47)	N/A	N/A
Trastuzumab[80]	Advanced/Recurrent EC HER2+	Trastuzumab 4 mg/kg IV day 1 and 2 mg/kg days 8,15, & 22 q28 d	33	CR: 0 (0) PR: 0 (0) SD: 12 (36)	1.8	7.8

Abbreviations: CR, complete response; EC, endometrial cancer; IV, intravenous; ORR, overall response rate; PR, partial response; SD, stable disease.
[a] Available only in abstract form.

Cell Surface Receptors

Activation of intracellular pathways leading to cell proliferation occurs through a variety of surface receptors, including VEGFR, PDGFR, EGFR, Her-2, FGFR, and IGF-IR, and thus has become a point of interest for regulating cellular growth in endometrial cancers. Overexpression of EGFR has been demonstrated in 38% of type I tumors and 70% of type II tumors.[76] The same study showed high rates of HER2 immunopositivity in both type I and II tumors, 60% and 58% respectively. In addition, both EGFR and HER2 overexpression were associated with an overall worse prognosis.[76,77] EGFR inhibitors gefitinib and erlotinib have been used to treat patients with recurrent or persistent endometrial cancer but unfortunately demonstrated limited RRs or failed to correlate response with EGFR mutations or gene amplification.[55,78] Trastuzumab was used in the treatment of HER2+ serous and endometrioid endometrial cancers. Results from these studies have been mixed with documented response in case reports but no objective response seen in a phase II trial.[79,80] Combinations with these agents and cytotoxic chemotherapy are the focus of ongoing investigations.

TP53

TP53 mutations are common in serous endometrial cancers (91%) and high-grade endometrioid tumors (25%).[5] Although frequently mutated, the type of TP53 mutation—wild-type (WT), gain-of-function (GOF), or loss-of-function (LOF)—was not defined in TCGA report. This is critically important because some p53 mutants are inconsequential and retain WT activity, whereas GOF p53 predicts aggressive tumor growth with poor response to treatment.[81] In fact, when comparing treatment outcomes between types of TP53 mutations in GOG 86P, a near doubling of PFS was seen for patients with LOF TP53 mutations in the bevacizumab group (19.6 months for LOF, 12.2 months for WT, and 10.6 months for GOF).[82] The improved survival among patients with LOF TP53 mutations was felt to be related to antiangiogenic blockade of subsequently activated p38 and abrogation of the G2/M checkpoint where damaged cells can transition into mitoses without repair and are sensitive to M-phase active cytotoxic chemotherapy (taxanes).[83] The identification of such actionable p53 mutations may facilitate selection of patients who stand to gain the greatest benefit from antiangiogenic agents.

SUMMARY

The incidence of endometrial cancer within the United States has reached epidemic proportions. Although patients diagnosed with type 1, early stage disease often have a favorable prognosis, those with advanced stage, recurrent, or high-grade histologies have much worse outcomes. Recent genomic characterization of endometrial tumors has identified several aberrant pathways and potential targetable mutations. Available targeted agents evaluated within clinical trials are summarized in **Table 3**. Unfortunately, to date there have been very few therapeutic agents that have led to durable remission in patients with recurrent or advanced disease. Studies exploring the role of novel agents such as poly (ADP-ribose) polymerase inhibitors, NSAIDs, metformin, and HDAC inhibitors, are ongoing. Many of the above strategies are promising, but more work is needed to identify pretreatment markers that predict treatment response and improve targeted therapy.

REFERENCES

1. Siegel RL, Miller KD, Jemal A. Cancer statistics, 2018. CA Cancer J Clin 2018;68: 7–30.

2. Creasman WT, Odicino F, Maisonneuve P, et al. Carcinoma of the corpus uteri. FIGO 26th annual report on the results of treatment in gynecological cancer. Int J Gynaecol Obstet 2006;95(Suppl 1):S105–43.

3. Sheikh MA, Althouse AD, Freese KE, et al. USA endometrial cancer projections to 2030: should we be concerned? Future Oncol 2014;10(16):2561–8.

4. Bokhman JV. Two pathogenetic types of endometrial carcinoma. Gynecol Oncol 1983;15(1):10–7.

5. The Cancer Genome Atlas Research Network. Integrated genomic characterization of endometrial carcinoma. Nature 2013;497(7447):67–73.

6. Calle EE, Rodriguez C, Walker-Thurmond K, et al. Overweight, obesity, and mortality from cancer in a prospectively studied cohort of U.S. adults. N Engl J Med 2003;348(17):1625–38.

7. Akhmedkhanov A, Zeleniuch-Jacquotte A, Toniolo P. Role of exogenous and endogenous hormones in endometrial cancer: review of the evidence and research perspectives. Ann N Y Acad Sci 2001;943:296–315.

8. Skandalis SS, Afratis N, Smirlaki G, et al. Cross-talk between estradiol receptor and EGFR/IGF-IR signaling pathways in estrogen-responsive breast cancers: Focus on the role and impact of proteoglycans. Matrix Biol 2014;35:182–93.

9. Luhn P, Dallal CM, Weiss JM, et al. Circulating adipokine levels and endometrial cancer risk in the Prostate, Lung, Colorectal and Ovarian Cancer Screening Trial. Cancer Epidemiol Biomarkers Prev 2013;22(7). https://doi.org/10.1158/1055-9965.EPI-13-0258.

10. Guerrero J, Tobar N, Cáceres M, et al. Soluble factors derived from tumor mammary cell lines induce a stromal mammary adipose reversion in human and mice adipose cells. Possible role of TGF-beta1 and TNF-alpha. Breast Cancer Res Treat 2010;119(2):497–508.

11. Sartipy P, Loskutoff DJ. Monocyte chemoattractant protein 1 in obesity and insulin resistance. Proc Natl Acad Sci U S A 2003;100(12):7265–70.

12. Gao J, Tian J, Lv Y, et al. Leptin induces functional activation of cyclooxygenase-2 through JAK2/STAT3, MAPK/ERK, and PI3K/AKT pathways in human endometrial cancer cells. Cancer Sci 2009;100(3):389–95.

13. Soliman PT, Wu D, Tortolero-Luna G, et al. Association between adiponectin, insulin resistance, and endometrial cancer. Cancer 2006;106(11):2376–81.

14. Slomovitz BM, Coleman RL. The PI3K/AKT/mTOR pathway as a therapeutic target in endometrial cancer. Clin Cancer Res 2012;18(21):5856–64.

15. Jabbour HN, Milne SA, Williams ARW, et al. Expression of COX-2 and PGE synthase and synthesis of PGE(2)in endometrial adenocarcinoma: a possible autocrine/paracrine regulation of neoplastic cell function via EP2/EP4 receptors. Br J Cancer 2001;85(7):1023–31.

16. Tsujii M, Kawano S, Tsuji S, et al. Cyclooxygenase regulates angiogenesis induced by colon cancer cells. Cell 1998;93(5):705–16.

17. Wang D, Dubois RN. Eicosanoids and cancer. Nat Rev Cancer 2010;10(3): 181–93.

18. Lentz SS, Brady MF, Major FJ, et al. High-dose megestrol acetate in advanced or recurrent endometrial carcinoma: a Gynecologic Oncology Group Study. J Clin Oncol 1996;14(2):357–61.

19. Whitney CW, Brunetto V, Zaino RJ, et al. Phase II study of medroxyprogesterone acetate plus tamoxifen in advanced endometrial carcinoma: a Gynecologic Oncology Group study. Gynecol Oncol 2004;92(1):4–9.

20. Fiorica JV, Brunetto V, Hanjani P, et al. Phase II trial of alternating courses of megestrol acetate and tamoxifen in advanced endometrial carcinoma: a Gynecologic Oncology Group study. Gynecol Oncol 2004;92(1):10–4.
21. Yang S, Xiao X, Jia Y, et al. Epigenetic modification restores functional PR expression in endometrial cancer cells. Curr Pharm Des 2014;20(11):1874–80.
22. Sasaki M, Kaneuchi M, Fujimoto S, et al. Hypermethylation can selectively silence multiple promoters of steroid receptors in cancers. Mol Cell Endocrinol 2003; 202(1–2):201–7.
23. Slomovitz BM, Jiang Y, Yates MS, et al. Phase II study of everolimus and letrozole in patients with recurrent endometrial carcinoma. J Clin Oncol 2015;33(8):930–6.
24. Soliman PT, Westin SN, Iglesias DA, et al. Phase II study of everolimus and letrozole in women with advanced/recurrent endometrial cancer. J Clin Oncol 2016; 34(15_suppl):5506.
25. Fleming GF, Filiaci VL, Marzullo B, et al. Temsirolimus with or without megestrol acetate and tamoxifen for endometrial cancer: a gynecologic oncology group study. Gynecol Oncol 2014;132(3):585–92.
26. Lambropoulou M, Alexiadis G, Limberis V, et al. Clinicopathologic and prognostic significance of cyclooxygenase-2 expression in endometrial carcinoma. Histol Histopathol 2005;20(3):753–9.
27. Rothwell PM, Price JF, Fowkes FG, et al. Short-term effects of daily aspirin on cancer incidence, mortality, and non-vascular death: analysis of the time course of risks and benefits in 51 randomised controlled trials. Lancet 2012;379(9826): 1602–12.
28. Neill AS, Nagle CM, Protani MM, et al. Aspirin, nonsteroidal anti-inflammatory drugs, paracetamol and risk of endometrial cancer: a case-control study, systematic review and meta-analysis. Int J Cancer 2013;132(5):1146–55.
29. Matsuo K, Cahoon SS, Yoshihara K, et al. Association of low-dose aspirin and survival of women with endometrial cancer. Obstet Gynecol 2016;128(1):127–37.
30. Brasky TM, Felix AS, Cohn DE, et al. Nonsteroidal anti-inflammatory drugs and endometrial carcinoma mortality and recurrence. J Natl Cancer Inst 2017; 109(3):1–10.
31. Evans JM, Donnelly LA, Emslie-Smith AM, et al. Metformin and reduced risk of cancer in diabetic patients. BMJ 2005;330(7503):1304–5.
32. Libby G, Donnelly LA, Donnan PT, et al. New users of metformin are at low risk of incident cancer: a cohort study among people with type 2 diabetes. Diabetes Care 2009;32(9):1620–5.
33. Cantrell LA, Zhou C, Mendivil A, et al. Metformin is a potent inhibitor of endometrial cancer cell proliferation–implications for a novel treatment strategy. Gynecol Oncol 2010;116(1):92–8.
34. Hanna RK, Zhou C, Malloy KM, et al. Metformin potentiates the effects of paclitaxel in endometrial cancer cells through inhibition of cell proliferation and modulation of the mTOR pathway. Gynecol Oncol 2012;125(2):458–69.
35. Watson P, Lynch HT. Extracolonic cancer in hereditary nonpolyposis colorectal cancer. Cancer 1993;71(3):677–85.
36. Moreira L, Balaguer F, Lindor N, et al. Identification of Lynch syndrome among patients with colorectal cancer. JAMA 2012;308(15):1555–65.
37. Provenzale D, Gupta S, Ahnen DJ, et al. Genetic/Familial High-Risk Assessment: Colorectal Version 1.2016, NCCN Clinical Practice Guidelines in Oncology. J Natl Compr Canc Netw 2016;14(8):1010–30.

38. Kakar S, Burgart LJ, Thibodeau SN, et al. Frequency of loss of hMLH1 expression in colorectal carcinoma increases with advancing age. Cancer 2003;97(6): 1421–7.
39. Esteller M, Levine R, Baylin SB, et al. MLH1 promoter hypermethylation is associated with the microsatellite instability phenotype in sporadic endometrial carcinomas. Oncogene 1998;17(18):2413–7.
40. Boyiadzis MM, Kirkwood JM, Marshall JL, et al. Significance and implications of FDA approval of pembrolizumab for biomarker-defined disease. J Immunother Cancer 2018;6(1):1–7.
41. Tamura M, Gu J, Matsumoto K, et al. Inhibition of cell migration, spreading, and focal adhesions by tumor suppressor PTEN. Science 1998;280(5369):1614–7.
42. Tashiro H, Blazes MS, Wu R, et al. Mutations in PTEN are frequent in endometrial carcinoma but rare in other common gynecological malignancies. Cancer Res 1997;57(18):3935–40.
43. McConechy MK, Ding J, Cheang MC, et al. Use of mutation profiles to refine the classification of endometrial carcinomas. J Pathol 2012;228(1):20–30.
44. Shu CA, Pike MC, Jotwani AR, et al. Uterine cancer after risk-reducing salpingo-oophorectomy without hysterectomy in women with BRCA mutations. JAMA Oncol 2016;2(11):1434–40.
45. Billingsley CC, Cohn DE, Mutch DG, et al. Polymerase varepsilon (POLE) mutations in endometrial cancer: clinical outcomes and implications for Lynch syndrome testing. Cancer 2015;121(3):386–94.
46. Cosgrove CM, Tritchler DL, Cohn DE, et al. An NRG Oncology/GOG study of molecular classification for risk prediction in endometrioid endometrial cancer. Gynecol Oncol 2018;148(1):174–80.
47. Bosse T, Nout RA, McAlpine JN, et al. Molecular classification of grade 3 endometrioid endometrial cancers identifies distinct prognostic subgroups. Am J Surg Pathol 2018;42(5):561–8.
48. Howitt BE, Shukla SA, Sholl LM, et al. Association of polymerase e-mutated and microsatellite-instable endometrial cancers with neoantigen load, number of tumor-infiltrating lymphocytes, and expression of PD-1 and PD-L1. JAMA Oncol 2015;1(9):1319–23.
49. Gatalica Z, Snyder C, Maney T, et al. Programmed cell death 1 (PD-1) and its ligand (PD-L1) in common cancers and their correlation with molecular cancer type. Cancer Epidemiol Biomarkers Prev 2014;23(12):2965–70.
50. Mehnert JM, Panda A, Zhong H, et al. Immune activation and response to pembrolizumab in POLE-mutant endometrial cancer. J Clin Invest 2016;126(6): 2334–40.
51. Hirai M, Nakagawara A, Oosaki T, et al. Expression of vascular endothelial growth factors (VEGF-A/VEGF-1 and VEGF-C/VEGF-2) in postmenopausal uterine endometrial carcinoma. Gynecol Oncol 2001;80(2):181–8.
52. Aghajanian C, Sill MW, Darcy KM, et al. Phase II trial of bevacizumab in recurrent or persistent endometrial cancer: a Gynecologic Oncology Group study. J Clin Oncol 2011;29(16):2259–65.
53. Bender D, Sill MW, Lankes HA, et al. A phase II evaluation of cediranib in the treatment of recurrent or persistent endometrial cancer: an NRG Oncology/Gynecologic Oncology Group study. Gynecol Oncol 2015;138(3):507–12.
54. McMeekin DS, Sill MW, Benbrook D, et al. A phase II trial of thalidomide in patients with refractory endometrial cancer and correlation with angiogenesis biomarkers: a Gynecologic Oncology Group study. Gynecol Oncol 2007;105(2): 508–16.

55. Leslie KK, Sill MW, Fischer E, et al. A phase II evaluation of gefitinib in the treatment of persistent or recurrent endometrial cancer: a Gynecologic Oncology Group study. Gynecol Oncol 2013;129(3):486–94.

56. Leslie KK, Sill MW, Lankes HA, et al. Lapatinib and potential prognostic value of EGFR mutations in a Gynecologic Oncology Group phase II trial of persistent or recurrent endometrial cancer. Gynecol Oncol 2012;127(2):345–50.

57. Coleman RL, Sill MW, Lankes HA, et al. A phase II evaluation of aflibercept in the treatment of recurrent or persistent endometrial cancer: a Gynecologic Oncology Group study. Gynecol Oncol 2012;127(3):538–43.

58. Aghajanian C, Filiaci VL, Dizon DS, et al. A randomized phase II study of paclitaxel/carboplatin/bevacizumab, paclitaxel/carboplatin/temsirolimus and ixabepilone/carboplatin/bevacizumab as initial therapy for measurable stage III or IVA, stage IVB or recurrent endometrial cancer, GOG-86P. J Clin Oncol 2015; 33(15_suppl):5500.

59. Lorusso D, Ferrandina G, Colombo N, et al. Randomized phase II trial of carboplatin-paclitaxel (CP) compared to carboplatin-paclitaxel-bevacizumab (CP-B) in advanced (stage III-IV) or recurrent endometrial cancer: The MITO END-2 trial. J Clin Oncol 2015;33(15_suppl):5502.

60. Alvarez EA, Brady WE, Walker JL, et al. Phase II trial of combination bevacizumab and temsirolimus in the treatment of recurrent or persistent endometrial carcinoma: a Gynecologic Oncology Group study. Gynecol Oncol 2013;129(1):22–7.

61. Mutter GL, Lin MC, Fitzgerald JT, et al. Altered PTEN expression as a diagnostic marker for the earliest endometrial precancers. J Natl Cancer Inst 2000;92(11): 924–30.

62. Ali IU. Gatekeeper for endometrium: the PTEN tumor suppressor gene. J Natl Cancer Inst 2000;92(11):861–3.

63. Dutt A, Salvesen HB, Greulich H, et al. Somatic mutations are present in all members of the AKT family in endometrial carcinoma. Br J Cancer 2009;101(7): 1218–9 [author reply: 1220–1].

64. Shoji K, Oda K, Nakagawa S, et al. The oncogenic mutation in the pleckstrin homology domain of AKT1 in endometrial carcinomas. Br J Cancer 2009;101(1): 145–8.

65. Oda K, Stokoe D, Taketani Y, et al. High frequency of coexistent mutations of PIK3CA and PTEN genes in endometrial carcinoma. Cancer Res 2005;65(23): 10669–73.

66. Hayes MP, Wang H, Espinal-Witter R, et al. PIK3CA and PTEN mutations in uterine endometrioid carcinoma and complex atypical hyperplasia. Clin Cancer Res 2006;12(20 Pt 1):5932–5.

67. Colombo N, McMeekin DS, Schwartz PE, et al. Ridaforolimus as a single agent in advanced endometrial cancer: results of a single-arm, phase 2 trial. Br J Cancer 2013;108(5):1021–6.

68. Oza AM, Pignata S, Poveda A, et al. Randomized phase II trial of ridaforolimus in advanced endometrial carcinoma. J Clin Oncol 2015;33(31):3576–82.

69. Ray-Coquard I, Favier L, Weber B, et al. Everolimus as second- or third-line treatment of advanced endometrial cancer: ENDORAD, a phase II trial of GINECO. Br J Cancer 2013;108(9):1771–7.

70. Caduff RF, Johnston CM, Frank TS. Mutations of the Ki-ras oncogene in carcinoma of the endometrium. Am J Pathol 1995;146(1):182–8.

71. Koul A, Willén R, Bendahl PO, et al. Distinct sets of gene alterations in endometrial carcinoma implicate alternate modes of tumorigenesis. Cancer 2002;94(9): 2369–79.

72. Duggan BD, Felix JC, Muderspach LI, et al. Early mutational activation of the c-Ki-ras oncogene in endometrial carcinoma. Cancer Res 1994;54(6):1604–7.

73. Coleman RL, Sill MW, Thaker PH, et al. A phase II evaluation of selumetinib (AZD6244, ARRY-142886), a selective MEK-1/2 inhibitor in the treatment of recurrent or persistent endometrial cancer: an NRG Oncology/Gynecologic Oncology Group study. Gynecol Oncol 2015;138(1):30–5.

74. Carracedo A, Ma L, Teruya-Feldstein J, et al. Inhibition of mTORC1 leads to MAPK pathway activation through a PI3K-dependent feedback loop in human cancer. J Clin Invest 2008;118(9):3065–74.

75. Westin SN, Sill MW, Coleman RL, et al. Limited access safety lead-in of the MEK inhibitor trametinib in combination with GSK2141795, an AKT inhibitor, in patients with recurrent or persistent endometrial cancer: A Gynecologic Oncology Group study. Gynecol Oncol 2016;141(S1):4–5.

76. Khalifa MA, Mannel RS, Haraway SD, et al. Expression of EGFR, HER-2/neu, P53, and PCNA in endometrioid, serous papillary, and clear cell endometrial adenocarcinomas. Gynecol Oncol 1994;53(1):84–92.

77. Hetzel DJ, Wilson TO, Keeney GL, et al. HER-2/neu expression: a major prognostic factor in endometrial cancer. Gynecol Oncol 1992;47(2):179–85.

78. Oza AM, Eisenhauer EA, Elit L, et al. Phase II study of erlotinib (OSI 774) in women with recurrent or metastatic endometrial cancer: NCIC CTG IND-148. J Clin Oncol 2008;26(26):4319–25.

79. Jewell E, Secord AA, Brotherton T, et al. Use of trastuzumab in the treatment of metastatic endometrial cancer. Int J Gynecol Cancer 2006;16(3):1370–3.

80. Fleming GF, Sill MW, Darcy KM, et al. Phase II trial of trastuzumab in women with advanced or recurrent, HER2-positive endometrial carcinoma: a Gynecologic Oncology Group study. Gynecol Oncol 2010;116(1):15–20.

81. Blandino G, Levine AJ, Oren M. Mutant p53 gain of function: differential effects of different p53 mutants on resistance of cultured cells to chemotherapy. Oncogene 1999;18(2):477–85.

82. Mallen AR, Filiaci VL, Levine DA, et al. Evidence for synthetic lethality between bevacizumab and chemotherapy in advanced, p53 null endometrial cancers. 2018 Society of Gynecologic Oncology Annual Meeting on Women's Cancer; March 24-27, 2018; New Orleans, LA. p. 47–8.

83. Meng X, Dizon DS, Yang S, et al. Strategies for molecularly enhanced chemotherapy to achieve synthetic lethality in endometrial tumors with mutant p53. Obstet Gynecol Int 2013;2013:828165.

(At Least) Once in Her Lifetime: Global Cervical Cancer Prevention

Philip E. Castle, PhD, MPH[a],*, Amanda Pierz, MS[b]

KEYWORDS

- Cervical cancer • Human papillomavirus (HPV) • Screening • Vaccination • Cytology
- Pap • Cervical intraepithelial neoplasia (CIN) • Global health

KEY POINTS

- Cervical cancer disproportionately burdens lower-resourced settings, in which nearly 90% of cervical cancer and cervical cancer–related deaths occur.
- Targeting human papillomavirus (HPV) by prophylactic HPV vaccination in young adolescent girls and HPV-based screening in mid-adult women offers the most cost-effective strategy to reduce cervical cancer burden worldwide and mitigate the health disparities in cervical cancer burden between low- and high-resourced settings.
- Political and social will, along with the necessary financial investments, will be necessary to realize the opportunity for significant global reductions in the cervical cancer burden.
- Perfect cervical cancer prevention (total eradication) is practically and financially unrealistic.

INTRODUCTION: THE BURDEN OF CERVICAL CANCER

There were approximately 528,000 cases of invasive cervical cancer (ICC) and 266,000 ICC-related deaths globally in 2012, making it the fourth most common cancer in women and the fourth leading cause of female cancer-related mortality.[1] The introduction of effective Papanicolaou (Pap)-based (cytology) screening in some, mostly high-income countries (HICs) in the mid to late twentieth century has led to a steady decreases in ICC incidence and mortality in those countries.[2,3] An estimated greater than 80% of all ICC occurs in low-income and middle-income countries

---

Competing Interests: Dr P.E. Castle has received cervical cancer tests and diagnostics for research at a reduced or no cost from Roche, Becton Dickinson, Cepheid, and Arbor Vita Corporation.

[a] Department of Epidemiology and Population Health, Albert Einstein College of Medicine, 1300 Morris Park Avenue, Belfer Building, Room 1308C, Bronx, NY 10461, USA; [b] Department of Epidemiology and Population Health, Albert Einstein College of Medicine, 1300 Morris Park Avenue, Belfer 1308A, Bronx, NY 10461, USA
* Corresponding author.
E-mail address: philip.castle@einstein.yu.edu

Obstet Gynecol Clin N Am 46 (2019) 107–123
https://doi.org/10.1016/j.ogc.2018.09.007
0889-8545/19/© 2018 Elsevier Inc. All rights reserved.

(LMICs),[4] where high-coverage, Pap-based screening has never been successfully implemented.[2,3] ICC is not only more common in LMICs, women with ICC are more likely to die from it due to absent cancer management services in LMICs (**Fig. 1**).

Africa, especially Sub-Saharan Africa (SSA), suffers the highest rates of ICC incidence and related mortality worldwide. Nearly 20% of ICC and ICC-related deaths globally occur in Africa.[1] More than 90% of ICC in Africa occurs in SSA, which has an age-standardized rate (ASR) of ICC incidence of 34.8 per 100,000 and mortality of 22.5 per 100,000,[1] approximately fivefold greater rates than the United States, western European countries, and Australia.[1] The high prevalence of human immunodeficiency virus (HIV) infection, a strong risk factor for ICC,[5] also contributes to the high rates of ICC in SSA. The global burden of ICC may be much greater than appreciated or accounted for based on cancer registries, which tend to have lesser quality data in the lower resource setting where ICC burden is greatest.[1]

ICC primarily afflicts women in their 30s, 40s, and 50s, when they are working and raising families, so the societal impact of ICC on a per-case basis is on average much greater than for other adult cancers, which tend to occur a decade or more later in life. Thus, there is a strong rationale for intervening globally to reduce the burden of ICC if it can be done efficiently and cost effectively.

NEW OPPORTUNITIES FOR CERVICAL CANCER PREVENTION: TARGETING HUMAN PAPILLOMAVIRUS

Since the discovery of human papillomavirus (HPV) in the tissue from ICC by Harold Zur Hausen (2008 Nobel Laureate in Medicine) and colleagues[6] 30 years ago, there have been rapid advances in our understanding of ICC and its cause. We now know that persistent cervical infections by certain types of HPV, designated as high-risk, carcinogenic, or cancer-associated, cause virtually all ICC everywhere in the world.[7] Even rare histologic types of ICC, such as neuroendocrine cancers, previously thought to be "HPV-negative" ICC, have been shown to be largely caused by

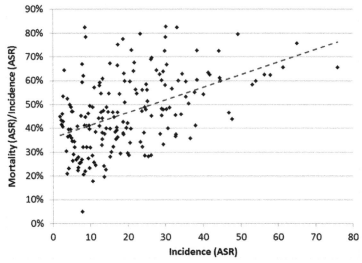

Fig. 1. Relationship of the ratio of the annual rate of mortality/incidence by the incidence rate for ICC by country. The red dotted line shows the linear correlation $(y = 0.0053x + 0.3621; R^2 = 0.2221)$.

HPV.[8] HPV also causes a significant number of vulvar, vaginal, anal, penile, and oropharyngeal cancers.[9] Approximately 5.2% of the human cancer burden is caused by HPV.[9] HPV16 causes approximately 60% of ICC, HPV18 causes approximately 10% to 15% of ICC.[10] Together, HPV16 and HPV18 account for approximately 70% of ICC, and the same 12 to 15 high-risk HPV (HPV) types cause 95% to 99% of ICC on all continents everywhere in the world.[10] Thus, an important corollary of these findings is that HPV does not discriminate by race or ethnicity and the same HPV-targeted prevention tools will be broadly protective. Thus, the only two important causes of ICC are persistent cervical infections by HPV genotypes AND a lack of access to preventive services.

The identification of HPV as the necessary cause of ICC has led to revolutionary advances in cervical cancer prevention that target it, including the development of prophylactic vaccines for primary prevention and sensitive, molecular HPV testing for cervical cancer screening for secondary prevention. HPV vaccination and testing are highly efficacious ($\geq$90%) for preventing infection and detection of cervical precancer and early cancer, respectively. If used in an age-optimized manner that takes into account the natural history of HPV and ICC, both interventions can be highly effective and cost-effective.

Fundamental to deciding at what age a specific intervention should be best used depends on the natural history of cervical carcinogenesis. In most populations, the peak prevalence of HPV happens approximately 5 years after the population median age of sexual initiation, approximately 15–17 years of age in many countries/cultures. Perhaps not surprisingly, most HPV infections that will ultimately cause ICC in the absence of intervention are acquired within a few years after population median age of sexual initiation; 50% and 75% of ICC-causing HPV infections are acquired by the age of 22 years and 32 years, respectively.[11] Thus, the benefits of HPV vaccination will decrease while those of screening, which detect prevalent HPV infection and associated disease, will increase with older ages. Notably, population screening primarily detects and treats prevalent and missed prevalent disease resulting from adolescent and early adulthood HPV infections.

PRIMARY PREVENTION: PROPHYLACTIC HUMAN PAPILLOMAVIRUS VACCINATION IN ADOLESCENTS/PRE-ADOLESCENTS
Efficacy

The first generation of HPV vaccines, Gardasil (Merck & Co, Kenilworth, NJ)[12] and Cervarix (GlaxoSmithKline, Wavre, Belgium),[13] targeted HPV16 and HPV18. Gardasil also targets HPV6 and HPV11, noncarcinogenic HPV types responsible for 90% of genital warts (*Condyloma acuminata*). Because Cervarix vaccination results in very high cross-protection against HPV31, 33, and 45,[14] it may achieve more than 70% cervical cancer prevention expected for vaccination against HPV16 and HPV18 in HPV-naïve populations. The next generation HPV vaccine, Gardasil 9 (Merck & Co),[15] targets HPV31, 33, 35, 52, and 58 in addition to HPV6, 11, 16 and HPV18 and is predicted to prevent approximately 90% of ICC. Thus, *if the protection offered by HPV vaccines is lifelong, the first-generation HPV vaccines may achieve as good as, and Gardasil 9 better than, the ICC prevention that the very best cervical cancer screening programs achieve over a lifetime of screening.*

Given that HPV vaccination is only prophylactic and not therapeutic, the ideal timing of HPV vaccination for effectiveness and therefore cost-effectiveness is before sexual initiation and exposure to HPV ie, HPV-naïve women. On a population level, this can be achieved by vaccinating a few years before the population median age of sexual initiation. As the median age of sexual initiation is 15 to 17 years in many populations, the World Health Organization (WHO) recommends vaccination programs to target 9- to 13-year-old girls,[16] and the Centers for Disease Control and Prevention (CDC) recommends routine HPV vaccination for girls (and boys) 11 to 12 years of age.[17] With older cohorts of women, prophylactic vaccine is equally efficacious but less effective because fewer women benefit from HPV vaccination, resulting in lower effectiveness and cost-effectiveness. Based on immunogenicity data, the WHO[18] and CDC[19] have recently endorsed the use of two-dose schedules for girls (and boys) younger than 15 years for all HPV vaccines.

The most successful strategy for delivering HPV vaccine to adolescents appears to be school-based vaccination programs.[20] As the percentage of dropouts increases with age, targeting women at younger ages might increase the efficiency of the program. The added advantage is that the age-specific anti-HPV antibody titers are higher with earlier age of vaccination that is the plateau of antibody titers that follows the peak titers immediately after the final vaccine dose will be higher with earlier age of HPV vaccination.

Effectiveness

Numerous reports from countries, including Australia,[21] Scotland,[22] Denmark,[23] and the United States,[24] have documented reductions in HPV infections and HPV-related diseases and abnormalities. As an illustrative example, Australia implemented vaccination with Gardasil in 2007, shortly after its approval by the Food and Drug Administration (FDA) and following a public awareness campaign. The HPV vaccination program achieved greater than 70% coverage in 2007 and has remained fairly constant over the first 10-year period.[25] Within several years after their national HPV vaccination was implemented, there was a significant decrease in genital warts, 90% of which is caused by HPV6 and HPV11, among women and heterosexual men (due to herd protection) but not among homosexual men.[26] Subsequently, there have been documented decreases in prevalence of HPV16 and HPV18 in vaccinated women[27] and now unvaccinated women (due to herd protection),[27] and high-grade cervical abnormalities, first in younger women[21] and now in slightly older women[28] as the vaccinated cohorts age. A recent study from Finland reported the first evidence that HPV vaccination prevents ICC.[29]

Safety

The safety of HPV vaccines remains controversial, despite strong reassurances of safety from the WHO,[30] European Medicines Agency,[31] and the CDC[32] among other international agencies and regulatory bodies based on reviews of the evidence and active surveillance data. Extensive reviews of safety studies have concluded that there is no evidence of increased risks of serious adverse events and minor increases in risk of minor adverse events, such as localized pain at the site of injection, headaches, and syncope,[33–35] which are consistent with other pediatric vaccines.

Dosing

Antibody titers appear to be robust to different immunization schedules, with increasing evidence that somewhat longer intervals between penultimate and last dose can improve the antibody titers.[36,37] Flexible schedules and fewer doses will simplify logistics of delivery and provide greater flexibility to tailor HPV vaccination to local realities. Given the inverse relationship of antibody titers with age and the duration of immune response now demonstrated, childhood priming followed a single booster shot in early adolescence seems like a plausible strategy for delivery and warrants investigation.

There are some observational data from clinical trials that a single dose of Cervarix[38] and Gardasil[39] are highly protective against infection of targeted HPV types. However, studies nested in populations receiving routine HPV vaccination have failed to show protection from one dose of Cervarix[22] or Gardasil.[40] As noted by the lead author of one trial,[39] "Data on long-term protection beyond 7 years against HPV infection and cervical precancerous lesions are needed before policy guidelines regarding a single dose can be formulated and implemented."

Global Uptake of Human Papillomavirus Vaccination

Although many HICs have implemented HPV vaccination either through national or opportunistic vaccination programs, few LMICs have implemented HPV vaccination, despite need and the numerous demonstration/feasibility projects that have been conducted since HPV vaccines became generally available (2007) and the addition of HPV vaccination to the roster of vaccines supported by GAVI in 2012. A pooled analysis of HPV vaccination coverage[41] found that of the more than 100 million women vaccinated against HPV by 2014, only 1% of them lived in LMICs. Since then, a number of LMICs have started or soon plan to start immunization with HPV vaccines.[42] However, because of delays in the introduction of HPV vaccination will likely result in millions of women acquiring and dying of cervical cancer, primarily women living in LMICs where screening is largely unavailable.

To make HPV vaccination more widely available, a global procurement strategy is needed to meet the needs of LMICs that are not GAVI-eligible. These upper middle, lower middle, and lower income countries may still lack the means to purchase the HPV vaccination at an affordable price. Although the Pan American Health Organization–negotiated price of $8.90 per dose is well below market price, it is still beyond the means of many non–GAVI-eligible LMICs in Latin America. Individual countries lack the leverage and the high-volume need that will make suppliers bring the prices down. Inevitably, negotiations between the consumer country and the supplier reach a stalemate: the consumer wants to know the price per unit before making a commitment to purchase a number of units and the supplier wants to know the commitment to purchase a number of units before setting a price.

SECONDARY PREVENTION: CERVICAL SCREENING USING HUMAN PAPILLOMAVIRUS TESTING IN ADULT WOMEN

Although prophylactic HPV vaccination may be the ultimate cervical cancer prevention strategy, current vaccines prevent infections but do not treat preexisting infections and conditions.[43,44] Therefore, even if universal female HPV vaccination could be rapidly deployed, there would still be several generations of at-risk, HPV-infected women who would not benefit from, and would be unlikely to be targeted for, HPV vaccination. Without robust screening, millions of women will die of ICC before the impact of HPV vaccines on ICC is observed.[45]

Efficacy

HPV testing is more sensitive[46–49] and reliable[50,51] for detection of CIN3, AIS, or invasive ICC ($\geq$CIN3) of the cervix than Pap testing. The increased sensitivity of HPV testing over Pap testing for $\geq$ CIN3 translates into 2 important benefits: (1) earlier detection of CIN3/AIS lesions that if treated would result in a reduced incidence of ICC within 4 to 5 years[52] and ICC-related death within 8 years[53] and (2) greater reassurance against cancer (lower cancer risk) following a negative result for many years,[52–54] which permits screening at an extended interval of 5 to 10 years, depending on the acceptable maximum cancer risk. Thus, using HPV testing for the primary ICC screen, women would need only one to a few screens in their lifetimes to significantly reduce the burden of ICC.[55] HPV testing offers other important advantages including objective (vs subjective) results, and easier implementation because these molecular tests do not require specialized medical training, that is, molecular tests are processed by machine and therefore do not require a large network staffed by cytopathologists. These advantages make the introduction of HPV testing for cervical cancer screening into LMICs more feasible than cytology.

The most important advantage of HPV testing is the possibility of using self-collected specimens. A recent meta-analysis concluded that self-collected specimens were equally accurate for the detection of cervical precancer and cancer when using polymerase chain reaction–based HPV testing and slightly less sensitive and specific when using a signal amplification-based HPV testing compared with using a provider-collected specimen.[56] However, most of those data on self-collection have been collected in a clinic-based, research setting. It is probably realistic to expect a small-to-modest decrement in performance of self-collected specimens versus provider-collected specimens, if for no other reason than women may not sample correctly or at all or forget to return their specimen. However, in low screening coverage settings, which are generally the case in LMICs, using self-collection to increase coverage will offset any small decrements in sensitivity using self-collected specimens may have.[57]

Self-collection offers a number of advantages over provider collection, including at-home collection in privacy without a pelvic examination. In most LMICs, there are probably insufficient numbers of clinics to support a nationwide clinic-based cervical cancer screening program so self-collection outside of the clinic is a necessity to expand coverage. There is ample evidence showing that unscreened/underscreened women living in LMICs[58] or in an impoverished region of developed countries[59] chose self-collection and HPV testing over a clinic-based Pap when offered through a community-outreach program. More unscreened/underscreened women living in developed countries chose self-collection over clinic-based Pap when offered passively to be screened (eg, mailed self-collection kits vs invitation letters).[60] There may also personal reluctance or cultural taboo for some women to undergo a pelvic examination in front of a male provider.[61,62]

A significant issue is the management of the HPV-positive women. There is a paucity of trained pathologists in many LMICs and especially in SSA, where there are typically 10-fold to 100-fold fewer pathologists per population than in England and the United States,[63] making scaled-up management and treatment algorithms–based biopsy diagnosis impossible. Thus, alternative methods of managing screen-positive women must be considered while gap in pathology services remains.

WHO has recommended either (1) treating all HPV-positive individuals or (2) using visual inspection after acetic acid (VIA) to triage the HPV-positive individuals for immediate treatment versus follow-up for evidence of persistent HPV infection.[64] Treating all HPV-positive individuals, Screen and Treat (S&T), will result in the greatest risk reduction (greatest programmatic sensitivity) (**Fig. 2**) and will reduce risk for almost 20 years at least. S&T will result in the most overtreatment (lowest programmatic specificity) but using an ablative therapy that is fairly benign and has very few complications. Ablative therapy also may reduce the cancer susceptibility of the cervix and thereby reduce the future risk of cancer.[65]

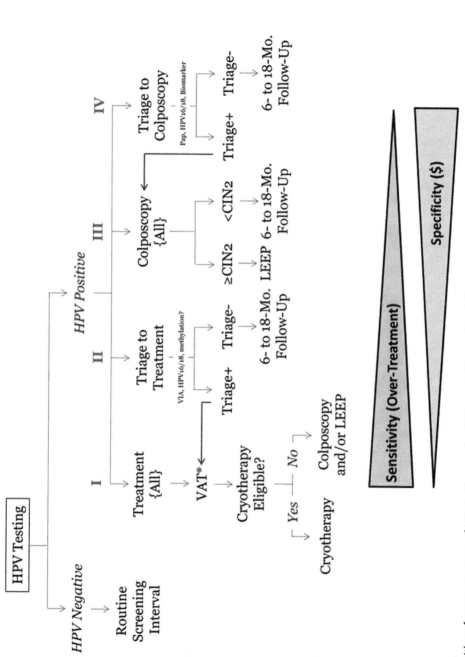

Fig. 2. Algorithms for management of HPV testing results. CIN2, cervical intraepithelial neoplasia grade 2; ≥CIN2, CIN2 or more severe diagnoses; <CIN2, less severe than CIN2 diagnoses; LEEP, loop electrosurgical procedure; VAT, visual assessment for treatment. * Like VIA, dilute acetic acid is applied to the cervix. However, the goal of VAT is decide the type of treatment rather than the goal of VIA, which is to decide whether they are screen or triage positive.

VIA triage may add specificity, that is, reduce overtreatment, but unless all un-treated, HPV-positive women return for their follow-up visit and care, the effectiveness of screening will be reduced. Another approach is the use partial HPV genotyping for triage. HPV16 and HPV18 or HPV16, HPV18, and HPV45 represent 70% to 80% of the cancer risk and many next-generation HPV tests provide concurrent partial HPV genotyping readout with the primary HPV test results (vs sequential testing).[66] A recent study in China using a lower-cost HPV DNA test with sequential triage using a research-only use test for a pool of HPV16, 18, and 45 have shown this to be very sensitive while reducing the number of positive individuals who needed immediate care.[67] Using higher viral load cutpoint[67] might also be considered. Other triage strategies, such as cytology and biomarkers (eg, host and/or viral methylation), are available but may not (yet) be applicable in most LMIC settings due to cost, logistics, or laboratory capacity.

The HPV S&T strategy without triage is logistically the simplest and most robust in the context of LMICs, which typically have weak health care delivery systems that cannot handle complex clinical algorithms, as well as its high programmatic sensitivity. Loss to follow-up of the HPV+/Triage− could undermine some of the health benefits of introducing HPV testing. Self-collected and/or provider-collected specimens could be used to implement such a program. Self-collection kits could be distributed via community health workers, who communicate results back to the women and could serve as patient navigators for the HPV-positive women to ensure good follow-up and completion of the intervention. A provider collection might offer the opportunity to complete the HPV S&T in a single clinical visit, reducing the losses to follow-up, and deliver other health care services. Although overtreatment by an HPV S&T approach might be viewed as a barrier, it should be seen in the context of the lifetime risk of treatment in a more traditional screen-diagnose-treat program, which probably results in approximately 10% to 20% of women being treated versus a lifetime risk of ICC without screening of approximately 2%.

Target Age

WHO recommends screening for women aged 30 to 49 years, with the upper range of ages overlapping the typical peak of ICC incidence. The question then becomes what ages should be targeted for screening because screen detection of cancers without the ability to provide appropriate care raises moral and ethical dilemmas in many cultures, even if the overall population benefits from the screening intervention because some cancers are prevented. One strategy that might be deployed to minimize the number of screen-detected cancers is through age restriction. Restricting screening to younger ages (eg, 30–34, 30–39, 35–39, or 35–44 years) places a greater emphasis on early detection and treatment of cervical precancers and reduces the number of screen-detected cancers that are mostly unmanageable in LMICs at this time.

Catch-up Phase of the Screening Program

Another reason to restrict further the target age of screening, at least at first, is simply the overwhelming number of adult women who would be the target of screening if a national program targeted women aged 30 to 49 years as recommended by WHO.[64] In most countries, approximately 15% to 20% of all women are ages 30 to 49 years. In the next 10 years, women who are 20 to 29 years now, will reach the age of screening, most of whom will also not have access to screening. Therefore, the number of women aged 30 to 49 years now or in the next 10 years is approximately

22% to 30% of the total number of women living in that country now and would be beyond the resources and capacity of most LMICs to implement. As a result, the program could become paralyzed by the overwhelming task to screen more than one-fourth of the female population even in a 10-year timeframe.

Very simply, countries could start with once-in-a-lifetime screen at the optimal year of age, between 30 and 35 years, and just continue with 1-year age cohorts; for example, women at or reaching the age of 30 years get their once-in-a-lifetime screen henceforth. Using this strategy, approximately 1% of the population, those reaching that target age of screening, are screened, which is a more manageable number on an annual basis. Public education campaigns and birthday notifications for countries with an established birth registry would remind women of their screening. If and when additional resources became available and the program had become facile and could handle larger numbers of women, screening could then be expanded to include a wider age range.

Simplified algorithms of S&T may be the only realistic approach, at least until screening program transitions from this "catch-up" phase into the maintenance phase, when adding more specificity to reduce overtreatment might be more practical and affordable. Practically speaking, to have the greatest immediate impact on the global burden of ICC, targeting high numbers of unscreened women in densely populated areas should be a priority. High-throughput HPV testing at a centralized laboratory could be coupled with specimens collected using either "spoke-and-wheel" model in which specimens are collected from surrounding clinics and transported to the testing center or use a campaign strategy. In these high-volume scenarios, same-day testing and treatment are unlikely and therefore require data systems and strategies to achieve good follow-up of the screen-positive women, a well-known challenge in the LMIC settings,[68] which is critical for effectiveness. For equal access for remote, rural populations, either the spoke-and-wheel model will need to be extended or low-cost point-of-care (POC) HPV testing used, when the latter becomes available.

Community health workers, nurses, and/or midwives are likely the key personnel to execute an effective screening program. They can (1) provide the education, (2) enroll women into getting screening, (3) deliver the self-collection kit and assist or collect the specimen as well as transport a set of specimens to the testing laboratory or provide POC testing, and (4) serve as the patient navigator for the screen-positive individuals to get management/treatment in a timely fashion. In most LMICs, they are the primary health care providers, especially for women's health care needs like maternal and child care. Community health workers, nurses, and/or midwives are trusted and known health care providers, and also female, making participation and compliance by the women in need of screening much more likely.

Sustained Phase of the Screening Program

Once the catch-up phase of the screening program is completed, the program enters a sustained phase. The annual numbers of women who need their once-in-a-lifetime screen declines significantly, approximately 5% of the catch-up numbers. After catch-up, if 1-year age cohorts reaching the age of screening can be screened and managed within a year, every year, the program reaches a steady state. Much of the workforce required for the catch-up phase will need to be "repurposed" to provide other health care needs and also can be tasked to increase coverage of the cervical cancer screening program to nonparticipants and hard-to-reach populations, if it is cost-effective to do so.

Current Availability of Human Papillomavirus Testing

The commercially available HPV tests have been previously reviewed,[69] but the market and available products are rapidly evolving. Currently, there are 5 FDA-approved HPV tests: Hybrid Capture 2 (hc2; Qiagen, Germantown, MD, USA) (approved in 2003), Cervista (Hologic, Bedford, MA, USA) (approved in 2009), cobas4800 (cobas; Roche Molecular Systems, Pleasanton, CA, USA) (approved in 2011), Aptima (Gen-Probe/Hologic, San Diego, CA, USA) (approved in 2011), and Onclarity (Becton Dickinson, Franklin Lakes, NY, USA) (approved in 2018). The FDA recently approved 2 HPV tests, cobas[70] and Onclarity,[71] for primary cervical screening. A number of other tests have received other regulatory approvals and/or have met international standards for clinical validation.[72]

Although these tests may be considered too expensive or too complex for many low-resource settings, it is worth noting that current validated HPV tests are now being purchased by organized screening programs in Europe for less than $10 per test: the Netherlands and Sweden are using the cobas HPV test (Roche Molecular Systems, Pleasanton, CA) and Italy is using Hybrid Capture 2. High-volume, coordinated purchasing by a funding organization such as the World Bank, Global Fund, or establishing a new, GAVI-like organization for procurement of in vitro diagnostics could further reduce the price of these tests. Given that once-in-a-lifetime HPV testing will make a large impact on ICC incidence and mortality and is cost-effective or highly cost-effective, financing strategies to take advantage of the current capacities should be initiated.

The complexity of these tests is no greater than the complexity of the tests that are used for HIV diagnosis and management by the US President's Emergency Plan for AIDS Relief program.[73] In fact, the Xpert test is a rapid ($\sim$1 hour), laboratory-in-a-cartridge HPV DNA test that requires only 3 testing steps: load the sample in the testing cartridge, insert the cartridge, and start the test. careHPV (Qiagen, Gaithersburg, MD) is the first widely available, commercialized lower-cost DNA test for a pool of 14 HPV genotypes. Although careHPV is based on the same technology as HC2, it costs only $5 per test (including sampler and buffer) and designed to be simpler to use than HC2. careHPV is being implemented in El Salvador.[74] Preliminary studies of careHPV have shown sensitivity and specificity that can approach that of HC2 but its performance appears to be more variable, unlike HC2, and is significantly lower when self-collected specimens are used instead of provider-collected specimens like HC2.[75,76]

BARRIERS FOR GLOBAL CERVICAL CANCER PREVENTION

The biggest barrier to implementation of cervical cancer prevention remains the lack of real commitment of resources globally, 7 years after the United Nations Political Declaration on Non-Communicable Diseases,[77] from which cervical cancer prevention considered a priority. Key investments should be in developing global procurement strategies for HPV tests for LMICs and HPV vaccines for non–GAVI-eligible LMICs. Such organized strategies with volume purchasing at lower prices per test and vaccine doses, along with subsidizing the costs for the least-resources countries, might go a long way to significant global reductions in ICC. Additional investments in health systems would be necessary but there would be significant value added for the prevention and control of other, higher-burden diseases such as cardiovascular disease and diabetes. Indeed, breaking down "disease silos" and developing a coordinated effort to address major noncommunicable diseases will have the greatest return on investment. Finally, microfinancing could be used to jumpstart the development of high-coverage supply chain and companies to provide training, maintenance, and repair of equipment locally.

However, simply investing resources will not be enough. Advocacy and education will be critical to make this a sufficiently high priority for policy makers and raise awareness and widespread acceptance among women of all nationalities, races/ethnicities, and belief systems. Cancer registries and data systems will need to be greatly improved, including standardization of data collection, to measure the impact of these interventions to secure the political will to sustain these programs and to track female individuals in follow-up, for example, second doses of vaccine or management of a positive-screening result.

Establishing national HPV vaccination programs requires farsightedness because the approximately 15-year to 20-year delay between implementation and return on investment in terms of cancer prevention. That is, those who implement an HPV vaccination program in their country are unlikely to still be in the leadership and may not even be alive when these "seeds bear fruit,"

The development of a $1 POCT test will be transformative but that alone is not enough. More affordable and robust HPV testing must be accompanied by better management and treatment tools. That is, screening must be inclusive of the downstream care or it is just testing and will not prevent cancer. In addition, although promising developments are in progress, it will take some years to validate, commercialize, and reach the market place. In the meantime, one woman will get ICC every minute and one woman will die from ICC every 2 minutes worldwide.

We therefore must make use of the highly effective HPV tests and treatments that are already available to start reducing the burden of ICC now. Streamlining the WHO prequalification process to include FDA-approved tests would be one step. Another step in the right direction is the development of a WHO Model List of Essential In Vitro Diagnostics,[78] to complement the Model List of Essential Medicines,[79] which includes HPV testing in its first iteration. Together, these developments might catalyze global procurement strategies that will increase access to high-quality HPV tests at lower costs.

FINAL COMMENTS

As shown by Kim and colleagues,[80] as the program approaches total elimination (100% cervical cancer prevention), the incremental gains in cervical cancer prevention become extraordinarily expensive on per ICC averted basis that is 1 per >$1,000,000. Thus, perfect cervical cancer prevention is unrealistic, unless Gardasil-9 unexpectedly shows cross-protection against nontargeted types or a new multivalent, "pan-HPV vaccine" is developed by combining the nine HPV types of virus like particles (VLPs) included in Gardasil-9 with AS04 adjuvant in Cervarix to induce purposefully cross-protection against nontargeted HPV types.

In LMICs, the decision to do any or more cervical cancer prevention, even if it is a great value, must be weighed against other competing public health and medical needs. Thus, how much ICC reduction is desirable is both a global and local policy decision. At the global level, actions must be taken on societal, political, and market levels to overcome global inequities on access to the best prevention tools. Locally, the prevention of cervical cancer must be weighed against other competing needs, some of which are quite basic, for example, healthy food, clean water, and sanitation, which can save many more lives than cervical cancer prevention. In the LMIC settings, discussions of HPV vaccination and screening in younger cohorts and screening and HPV vaccination (FASTER HPV[81]) and/or multi-rounds of screening in older cohorts are "putting the cart before the horse." The primary goal should be to get 1 high-quality intervention into all women, vaccination in preadolescent and early adolescent girls, and screening in mid-adult women, and move toward greater global equity for cervical cancer prevention.

Finally, should there be true global mobilization around cervical cancer prevention, realistic expectations are a must. As modeled by Simms and colleagues (submitted), with high-coverage HPV vaccination and twice-in-a-lifetime screening, the total global burden of ICC will not go down for decades, even if the annual incidence rates will. There are two good reasons for the long lag time between intervention and reduction in the total burden of ICC: (1) population growth and (2) the slow development of ICC from the causal infection, preventing infection today will not meaningfully impact ICC rates for several decades. Moreover, these models assume an aggressive global introduction that is probably not feasible both logistically and politically, especially in LMICs. Therefore, even if there is a global mobilization for cervical cancer prevention on an unprecedented scale, benefits will not be seen for the foreseeable future and certain not by those who implemented the policies to act. In addition, words like "eradication" and "elimination" preferably are not used but if they are, must be used cautiously and tempered with a careful explanation that they do not mean 100% prevention. Unrealistic expectations lead to overutilization (eg, screening of adolescent females, screening of women aged 65 and older with negative screening histories, and vaccination of older women), cost inefficiencies (eg, HPV and cytology cotesting vs primary HPV screening), and medicolegal consequences.

Thus, the real challenge ahead for cervical cancer prevention may be "staying the course" politically, socially, and economically over several decades to glean the benefits of intervening on this largely preventable, major cause of morbidity and mortality in women globally.

ACKNOWLEDGMENTS

Due to word limits, many relevant publications could not be cited in this article. We apologize to those authors for the exclusion of their works from the bibliography.

REFERENCES

1. Ferlay J, Soerjomataram I, Ervik M, et al. GLOBOCAN 2012 v1.0, cancer incidence and mortality worldwide: IARC CancerBase No. 11. Lyon (France): International Agency for Research on Cancer; 2013.
2. Cervix cancer screening. IARC Press, IARC Handbooks of Cancer Prevention, Volume 10. 2005.
3. Kitchener HC, Castle PE, Cox JT. Chapter 7: achievements and limitations of cervical cytology screening. Vaccine 2006;24(Suppl 3):S3/63-70.
4. Ferlay J, Shin HR, Bray F, et al. GLOBOCAN 2008 v2.0, cancer incidence and mortality worldwide: IARC CancerBase No. 10. Lyon (France): International Agency for Research on Cancer; 2010.
5. Grulich AE, van Leeuwen MT, Falster MO, et al. Incidence of cancers in people with HIV/AIDS compared with immunosuppressed transplant recipients: a meta-analysis. Lancet 2007;370:59–67.
6. Durst M, Gissmann L, Ikenberg H, et al. A papillomavirus DNA from a cervical carcinoma and its prevalence in cancer biopsy samples from different geographic regions. Proc Natl Acad Sci U S A 1983;80:3812–5.
7. Schiffman M, Castle PE, Jeronimo J, et al. Human papillomavirus and cervical cancer. Lancet 2007;370:890–907.

8. Castle PE, Pierz A, Stoler MH. A systematic review and meta-analysis on the attribution of human papillomavirus (HPV) in neuroendocrine cancers of the cervix. Gynecol Oncol 2018;148:422–9.

9. Forman D, de MC, Lacey CJ, et al. Global burden of human papillomavirus and related diseases. Vaccine 2012;30(Suppl 5):F12–23.

10. de SS, Quint WG, Alemany L, et al. Human papillomavirus genotype attribution in invasive cervical cancer: a retrospective cross-sectional worldwide study. Lancet Oncol 2010;11:1048–56.

11. Burger EA, Kim JJ, Sy S, et al. Age of acquiring causal human papillomavirus (HPV) infections: leveraging simulation models to explore the natural history of HPV-induced cervical cancer. Clin Infect Dis 2017;65:893–9.

12. Munoz N, Kjaer SK, Sigurdsson K, et al. Impact of human papillomavirus (HPV)-6/11/16/18 vaccine on all HPV-associated genital diseases in young women. J Natl Cancer Inst 2010;102:325–39.

13. Lehtinen M, Paavonen J, Wheeler CM, et al. Overall efficacy of HPV-16/18 AS04-adjuvanted vaccine against grade 3 or greater cervical intraepithelial neoplasia: 4-year end-of-study analysis of the randomised, double-blind PATRICIA trial. Lancet Oncol 2012;13:89–99.

14. Malagon T, Drolet M, Boily MC, et al. Cross-protective efficacy of two human papillomavirus vaccines: a systematic review and meta-analysis. Lancet Infect Dis 2012;12:781–9.

15. Joura EA, Giuliano AR, Iversen OE, et al. A 9-valent HPV vaccine against infection and intraepithelial neoplasia in women. N Engl J Med 2015;372:711–23.

16. Human papillomavirus vaccines: WHO position paper, October 2014. Geneva (Switzerland): WHO; 2014. Weekly Epidemiological Record. Available at: http://www.who.int/wer.

17. Centers for Disease Control and Prevention (CDC). FDA licensure of quadrivalent human papillomavirus vaccine (HPV4, Gardasil) for use in males and guidance from the Advisory Committee on Immunization Practices (ACIP). MMWR Morb Mortal Wkly Rep 2010;59:630–2.

18. World Health Organization. Immunization, vaccines and biologicals: human papillomavirus (HPV). 2018. Available at: http://www.who.int/immunization/diseases/hpv/en/. Accessed March 27, 2018.

19. Centers for Disease Control and Prevention. CDC recommends only two HPV shots for younger adolescents. 2016. Available at: https://www.cdc.gov/media/releases/2016/p1020-hpv-shots.html. Accessed March 27, 2018.

20. Das JK, Salam RA, Arshad A, et al. Systematic review and meta-analysis of interventions to improve access and coverage of adolescent immunizations. J Adolesc Health 2016;59:S40–8.

21. Gertig DM, Brotherton JM, Budd AC, et al. Impact of a population-based HPV vaccination program on cervical abnormalities: a data linkage study. BMC Med 2013;11:227.

22. Kavanagh K, Pollock KG, Cuschieri K, et al. Changes in the prevalence of human papillomavirus following a national bivalent human papillomavirus vaccination programme in Scotland: a 7-year cross-sectional study. Lancet Infect Dis 2017;17:1293–302.

23. Baldur-Felskov B, Dehlendorff C, Munk C, et al. Early impact of human papillomavirus vaccination on cervical neoplasia—nationwide follow-up of young Danish women. J Natl Cancer Inst 2014;106:djt460.

24. Oliver SE, Unger ER, Lewis R, et al. Prevalence of human papillomavirus among females after vaccine introduction-national health and nutrition examination survey, United States, 2003-2014. J Infect Dis 2017;216:594–603.
25. National HPV Vaccination Program Register. Coverage Data. 2018. Available at: http://www.hpvregister.org.au/research/coverage-data. Accessed March 27, 2018.
26. Donovan B, Franklin N, Guy R, et al. Quadrivalent human papillomavirus vaccination and trends in genital warts in Australia: analysis of national sentinel surveillance data. Lancet Infect Dis 2011;11:39–44.
27. Machalek DA, Garland SM, Brotherton JML, et al. Very low prevalence of vaccine human papillomavirus (HPV) types among 18 to 35 year old Australian women, nine years following implementation of vaccination. J Infect Dis 2018;217(10):1590–600.
28. Brotherton JM, Gertig DM, May C, et al. HPV vaccine impact in Australian women: ready for an HPV-based screening program. Med J Aust 2016;204:184–184e1.
29. Luostarinen T, Apter D, Dillner J, et al. Vaccination protects against invasive HPV-associated cancers. Int J Cancer 2018;142:2186–7.
30. Global Advisory Committee on Vaccine Safety (GACVS). Safety update of HPV vaccines. Geneva (Switzerland): World Health Organization; 2017. Available at: http://www.who.int/vaccine_safety/committee/topics/hpv/June_2017/en/. Accessed April 9, 2018.
31. European Medicines Agency. Human papillomavirus vaccines. London: European Medicines Agency; 2016. Available at: https://www.ema.europa.eu/medicines/human/referrals/human-papillomavirus-vaccines-cervarix-gardasil-gardasil-9-silgard. Accessed April 9, 2018.
32. Centers for Disease Control and Prevention. Human papillomavirus (HPV) vaccine safety. Atlanta (GA): Centers for Disease Control and Prevention; 2018. Available at: https://www.cdc.gov/hpv/parents/vaccinesafety.html. Accessed April 9, 2018.
33. Phillips A, Patel C, Pillsbury A, et al. Safety of human papillomavirus vaccines: an updated review. Drug Saf 2018;41:329–46.
34. Costa APF, Cobucci RNO, da Silva JM, et al. Safety of human papillomavirus 9-valent vaccine: a meta-analysis of randomized trials. J Immunol Res 2017;2017:3736201.
35. Ogawa Y, Takei H, Ogawa R, et al. Safety of human papillomavirus vaccines in healthy young women: a meta-analysis of 24 controlled studies. J Pharm Health Care Sci 2017;3:18.
36. Widdice LE, Unger ER, Panicker G, et al. Antibody responses among adolescent females receiving two or three quadrivalent human papillomavirus vaccine doses at standard and prolonged intervals. Vaccine 2018;36:881–9.
37. Neuzil KM, Canh DG, Thiem VD, et al. Immunogenicity and reactogenicity of alternative schedules of HPV vaccine in Vietnam: a cluster randomized noninferiority trial. JAMA 2011;305:1424–31.
38. Kreimer AR, Struyf F, Del Rosario-Raymundo MR, et al. Efficacy of fewer than three doses of an HPV-16/18 AS04-adjuvanted vaccine: combined analysis of data from the Costa Rica Vaccine and PATRICIA trials. Lancet Oncol 2015;16(7):775–86.
39. Sankaranarayanan R, Joshi S, Muwonge R, et al. Can a single dose of human papillomavirus (HPV) vaccine prevent cervical cancer? Early findings from an Indian study. Vaccine 2018;36(32 Pt A):4783–91.
40. Crowe E, Pandeya N, Brotherton JM, et al. Effectiveness of quadrivalent human papillomavirus vaccine for the prevention of cervical abnormalities: case-control study nested within a population based screening programme in Australia. BMJ 2014;348:g1458.

41. Bruni L, Diaz M, Barrionuevo-Rosas L, et al. Global estimates of human papillomavirus vaccination coverage by region and income level: a pooled analysis. Lancet Glob Health 2016;4:e453–63.
42. LaMontagne DS, Bloem PJN, Brotherton JML, et al. Progress in HPV vaccination in low- and lower-middle-income countries. Int J Gynaecol Obstet 2017; 138(Suppl 1):7–14.
43. Garland SM, Hernandez-Avila M, Wheeler CM, et al. Quadrivalent vaccine against human papillomavirus to prevent anogenital diseases. N Engl J Med 2007;356:1928–43.
44. Hildesheim A, Herrero R, Wacholder S, et al. Effect of human papillomavirus 16/18 L1 viruslike particle vaccine among young women with preexisting infection: a randomized trial. JAMA 2007;298:743–53.
45. Gage JC, Castle PE. Preventing cervical cancer globally by acting locally: if not now, when? J Natl Cancer Inst 2010;102:1524–7.
46. Cuzick J, Clavel C, Petry KU, et al. Overview of the European and North American studies on HPV testing in primary cervical cancer screening. Int J Cancer 2006; 119:1095–101.
47. Rijkaart DC, Berkhof J, Rozendaal L, et al. Human papillomavirus testing for the detection of high-grade cervical intraepithelial neoplasia and cancer: final results of the POBASCAM randomised controlled trial. Lancet Oncol 2012;13:78–88.
48. Ronco G, Giorgi-Rossi P, Carozzi F, et al. Efficacy of human papillomavirus testing for the detection of invasive cervical cancers and cervical intraepithelial neoplasia: a randomised controlled trial. Lancet Oncol 2010;11(3):249–57.
49. Castle PE, Stoler MH, Wright TC Jr, et al. Performance of carcinogenic human papillomavirus (HPV) testing and HPV16 or HPV18 genotyping for cervical cancer screening of women aged 25 years and older: a subanalysis of the ATHENA study. Lancet Oncol 2011;12:880–90.
50. Castle PE, Wheeler CM, Solomon D, et al. Interlaboratory reliability of hybrid capture 2. Am J Clin Pathol 2004;122:238–45.
51. Carozzi FM, Del Mistro A, Confortini M, et al. Reproducibility of HPV DNA testing by hybrid capture 2 in a screening setting. Am J Clin Pathol 2005;124:716–21.
52. Ronco G, Dillner J, Elfstrom KM, et al. Efficacy of HPV-based screening for prevention of invasive cervical cancer: follow-up of four European randomised controlled trials. Lancet 2013;383(9916):524–32.
53. Sankaranarayanan R, Nene BM, Shastri SS, et al. HPV screening for cervical cancer in rural India. N Engl J Med 2009;360:1385–94.
54. Dillner J, Rebolj M, Birembaut P, et al. Long term predictive values of cytology and human papillomavirus testing in cervical cancer screening: joint European cohort study. BMJ 2008;337:a1754.
55. Schiffman M, Castle PE. The promise of global cervical-cancer prevention. N Engl J Med 2005;353:2101–4.
56. Arbyn M, Verdoodt F, Snijders PJ, et al. Accuracy of human papillomavirus testing on self-collected versus clinician-collected samples: a meta-analysis. Lancet Oncol 2014;15:172–83.
57. Campos NG, Castle PE, Wright TC Jr, et al. Cervical cancer screening in low-resource settings: a cost-effectiveness framework for valuing tradeoffs between test performance and program coverage. Int J Cancer 2015;137(9):2208–19.
58. Arrossi S, Thouyaret L, Herrero R, et al. Effect of self-collection of HPV DNA offered by community health workers at home visits on uptake of screening for cervical cancer (the EMA study): a population-based cluster-randomised trial. Lancet Glob Health 2015;3:e85–94.

59. Castle PE, Rausa A, Walls T, et al. Comparative community outreach to increase cervical cancer screening in the Mississippi Delta. Prev Med 2011;52:452–5.

60. Verdoodt F, Jentschke M, Hillemanns P, et al. Reaching women who do not participate in the regular cervical cancer screening programme by offering self-sampling kits: a systematic review and meta-analysis of randomised trials. Eur J Cancer 2015;51:2375–85.

61. Munthali AC, Ngwira BM, Taulo F. Exploring barriers to the delivery of cervical cancer screening and early treatment services in Malawi: some views from service providers. Patient Prefer Adherence 2015;9:501–8.

62. Rosser JI, Hamisi S, Njoroge B, et al. Barriers to cervical cancer screening in rural Kenya: perspectives from a provider survey. J Community Health 2015;40:756–61.

63. Adesina A, Chumba D, Nelson AM, et al. Improvement of pathology in sub-Saharan Africa. Lancet Oncol 2013;14:e152–7.

64. World Health Organization. New guidelines on screening and treatment for cervical cancer. Geneva (Switzerland): World Health Organization; 2013.

65. Herfs M, Yamamoto Y, Laury A, et al. A discrete population of squamocolumnar junction cells implicated in the pathogenesis of cervical cancer. Proc Natl Acad Sci U S A 2012;109:10516–21.

66. Kunckler M, Schumacher F, Kenfack B, et al. Cervical cancer screening in a low-resource setting: a pilot study on an HPV-based screen-and-treat approach. Cancer Med 2017;6:1752–61.

67. Qiao YL, Jeronimo J, Zhao FH, et al. Lower cost strategies for triage of human papillomavirus DNA-positive women. Int J Cancer 2014;134:2891–901.

68. Sherris J, Wittet S, Kleine A, et al. Evidence-based, alternative cervical cancer screening approaches in low-resource settings. Int Perspect Sex Reprod Health 2009;35:147–54.

69. Schiffman M, Wentzensen N, Wacholder S, et al. Human papillomavirus testing in the prevention of cervical cancer. J Natl Cancer Inst 2011;103:368–83.

70. FDA approves first human papillomavirus test for primary cervical cancer screening. Rockville (MD): FDA News Release; 2014.

71. U.S. Food and Drug Administration. BD Onclarity HPV assay - P160037. Rockville (MD): U S Food and Drug Administration; 2018. Available at: https://www.fda.gov/MedicalDevices/ProductsandMedicalProcedures/DeviceApprovalsandClearances/Recently-ApprovedDevices/ucm598991.htm. Accessed May 4, 2018.

72. Arbyn M, Snijders PJ, Meijer CJ, et al. Which high-risk HPV assays fulfil criteria for use in primary cervical cancer screening? Clin Microbiol Infect 2015;21:817–26.

73. Goosby E, Dybul M, Fauci AS, et al. The United States president's emergency plan for AIDS relief: a story of partnerships and smart investments to turn the tide of the global AIDS pandemic. J Acquir Immune Defic Syndr 2012;60(Suppl 3):S51–6.

74. Cremer M, Maza M, Alfaro K, et al. Scale-up of an human papillomavirus testing implementation program in El salvador. J Low Genit Tract Dis 2017;21:26–32.

75. Jeronimo J, Bansil P, Lim J, et al. A multicountry evaluation of careHPV testing, visual inspection with acetic acid, and papanicolaou testing for the detection of cervical cancer. Int J Gynecol Cancer 2014;24:576–85.

76. Qiao YL, Sellors JW, Eder PS, et al. A new HPV-DNA test for cervical-cancer screening in developing regions: a cross-sectional study of clinical accuracy in rural China. Lancet Oncol 2008;9:929–36.

77. United Nations. UN political declaration on NCDs. New York: United Nations; 2011. Available at: http://www.who.int/nmh/events/un_ncd_summit2011/political_ declaration_en.pdf. Accessed May 8, 2018.
78. Schroeder LF, Guarner J, Elbireer A, et al. Time for a model list of essential diagnostics. N Engl J Med 2016;374:2511–4.
79. World Health Organization. World Health Organization model list of essential in vitro diagnostics. 1st edition. Geneva (Switzerland): World Health Organization; 2018. Available at: http://www.who.int/medical_devices/diagnostics/WHO_EDL_ 2018.pdf. Accessed November 1, 2018.
80. Kim JJ, Burger EA, Sy S, et al. Optimal cervical cancer screening in women vaccinated against human papillomavirus. J Natl Cancer Inst 2016;109: djw216.
81. Bosch FX, Robles C, Diaz M, et al. HPV-FASTER: broadening the scope for prevention of HPV-related cancer. Nat Rev Clin Oncol 2016;13:119–32.

Vulvar Cancer

Daniel Weinberg, MD*, Ricardo A. Gomez-Martinez, MD

KEYWORDS

- Vulvar cancer • Squamous cell carcinoma • Melanoma • Paget disease • Surgery
- Chemotherapy • Radiation

KEY POINTS

- Vulvar cancer is an uncommon gynecologic malignancy that arises from both human papillomavirus (HPV)-mediated and HPV-independent pathways. Most patients with squamous cell carcinoma (SCC) of the vulva present with early stage disease.
- Surgery remains the backbone of therapy for SCC, with primary chemoradiation playing a prominent role in advanced disease.
- Patients with vulvar melanoma more commonly present with advanced disease than other patients with cutaneous melanoma. Patients with vulvar melanoma should be treated in consultation with a melanoma specialist.
- The vulva is the most common site of extramammary Paget disease. This condition is rarely lethal, but recurrence is common.

There will be an estimated 6190 new cases of vulvar cancer in 2018, accounting for 0.4% of all cancers. This is primarily a disease of the elderly with a median age at diagnosis of 68 years. Incidence of vulvar cancer has been increasing by an average of 0.6% per year for the past 10 years, whereas relative survival seems to be decreasing.[1,2] Squamous cell carcinoma (SCC) accounts for greater than 90% of vulvar cancers. Dysplastic lesions generally precede SCC. Melanoma is the second most common type of vulvar cancer. The remaining cases consist of adenocarcinoma, basal cell carcinoma, sarcoma, and undifferentiated carcinoma. Extramammary Paget disease (EMPD) is most commonly localized to the vulva and is a uniquely challenging entity.

VULVAR ANATOMY

The vulva comprises the external female genitalia and includes the labia majora, labia minora, vestibule, clitoris, vaginal introitus, and urethral meatus. The internal and external pudendal arteries are responsible for most of the vulvar supply, whereas

Disclosure Statement: The authors have no disclosures.
Department of Obstetrics and Gynecology, University of New Mexico, MSC10 5580, 1 University of New Mexico, Albuquerque, NM 87131, USA
* Corresponding author.
E-mail address: dweinberg@salud.unm.edu

Obstet Gynecol Clin N Am 46 (2019) 125–135
https://doi.org/10.1016/j.ogc.2018.09.008
0889-8545/19/© 2018 Elsevier Inc. All rights reserved.

obgyn.theclinics.com

the ilioinguinal, genitofemoral, and pudendal nerves innervate the tissue. Given the importance of lymph node status in vulvar cancer staging and management, understanding the lymphatic drainage of the vulva is critical. The vast majority of vulvar lymphatic drainage is through the inguinal lymph nodes—first the superficial inguinal nodes, then traversing the cribriform fascia to the deep inguinal nodes, then follows the iliac vasculature to the external iliac nodes, and ultimately the paraaortic nodes. Drainage from the clitoris can sometimes proceed directly to the deep inguinal nodes, and less commonly, the external iliac nodes (pelvic nodes).[3]

SQUAMOUS CELL CARCINOMA

SCC accounts for nearly 90% of cases of vulvar cancer. Vulvar SCC can be broadly classified as HPV-mediated and non–HPV-mediated and is generally preceded by noninvasive vulvar intraepithelial neoplasia (VIN). Fifty nine percent of patients present with localized disease, 30% with spread to regional lymph nodes, 6% with distant metastases, and 5% unstaged. Overall survival at 5 years is 71%.[1]

Preinvasive Disease

The introduction of the Lower Anogenital Squamous Terminology in 2012 unified terminology for all HPV-associated squamous lesions of the lower anogenital tract and recommended the use of the terms Low-Grade Squamous Intraepithelial Lesion (LSIL) and High-Grade Squamous Intraepithelial Lesion (HSIL).[4] This approach was endorsed by the International Society for the Study of Vulvovaginal Disease (ISSVD), American Society for Colposcopy and Cervical Pathology, and the College of American Pathologists. In 2014, the World Health Organization Classification of Tumors of the Vulva subdivided squamous intraepithelial lesions as LSIL, HSIL, and differentiated-type VIN (dVIN). This terminology was adopted nearly in full by the ISSVD in 2015, with minor modifications (**Box 1**).[5]

HSIL sometimes referred to as VIN usual type (uVIN) is caused by HPV, whereas VIN that is associated with chronic inflammatory lesions of the vulva, most importantly lichen sclerosus, is referred to as dVIN. HPV-mediated disease is found in younger women, accounts for most of the cases of VIN, and its prevalence continues to increase.[6–8] HPV 16 is associated with greater than 77% of cases of HSIL, whereas HPV 33 and 18 are associated with 11% and 2.6% of cases, respectively.[9] Additional risk factors include smoking, multiple sexual partners, young age of first intercourse, and immunosuppression.[9,10] Less than 5% of uVIN progresses to invasive SCC; however, HPV-associated carcinoma accounts for 40% of all vulvar SCC and is believed to be the cause of the recent increase worldwide.[11] HSIL lesions are often asymptomatic and vulvoscopy with biopsy is recommended for any

---

Box 1
2015 ISSVD terminology of vulvar squamous intraepithelial lesions

Low-grade squamous intraepithelial lesion (flat condyloma or HPV effect)

High-grade squamous intraepithelial lesion (VIN usual type)

Vulvar intraepithelial neoplasia, differentiated-type

From Bornstein J, Bogliatto F, Haefner HK, et al. The 2015 International Society for the Study of Vulvovaginal Disease (ISSVD) terminology of vulvar squamous intraepithelial lesions. Obstet Gynecol 2016;127(2):267; with permission.

symptomatic women or women with a suspicious lesion. Quadrivalent and nonavalent HPV vaccines have been proved efficacious in preventing HSIL, and universal vaccination of young girls and boys is recommended by ACOG.[12–14] Wide local excision with gross lateral margins of at least 0.5 cm and a depth of 4 mm should be considered first choice in treatment.[15] Although the safest minimum margin is unclear, positive margins are associated with significantly greater risk of recurrence.[16] Laser ablation is preferred for treating extensive disease or multifocal lesions.[17] Medical management with topical agents is generally preferred for the treatment of younger patients, recurrent lesions, and patients who are poor surgical candidates. Imiquimod 5% applied 3 times weekly for 16 weeks is the most commonly used topical agent, with partial response rates of 80% and complete response rates of 50%.[18–21] Cidofovir 1% applied 3 times weekly for 16 to 24 weeks is another commonly used topical agent that has demonstrated response rates similar to that of imiquimod. 5-Fluourouracil (5-FU) is another topical agent that has demonstrated response rates of up to 75%; however, its use has been limited by higher rates of local side effects than imiquimod and cidofovir.[22]

Although dVIN accounts for less than 10% of preinvasive vulvar lesions, it has a higher rate of malignant transformation than uVIN and is thought to be the immediate precursor to up to 80% of cases of vulvar SCC.[23] Women with dVIN are older and more likely to harbor P53 mutations.[24] The low prevalence of dVIN is thought to be due to rapid progression of this lesion to invasive carcinoma and underdiagnosis.[25] This lesion arises within the context of lichen sclerosus, a chronic, inflammatory, mucocutaneous lesion that is most commonly found on the genital skin. Lichen sclerosus most commonly presents with itching, but patients may experience pain, voiding dysfunction, sexual dysfunction, and bleeding. Diagnosis is primarily clinical: lichen sclerosus classically begins on the clitoral hood and progresses to the labia minora, vestibule, perineal, and perianal areas to form the characteristic figure-of-eight distribution. The skin is fragile, resulting in fissures and frequent scarring that ultimately destroy the labial architecture. Topical clobetasol propionate 0.05% results in symptomatic improvement in nearly all patients and complete remission in 70% of patients after a 12-week treatment course, whereas low-potency steroids can be used for maintenance.[26] Patients undergoing surveillance should be biopsied if there are areas with persistent keratosis, erosion, erythema, warty or papular lesions, no response to therapy, or if second-line treatment is to be used.[27]

Invasive Cancer

Diagnosis
Most vulvar cancers present symptomatically as either a palpable lump or a visible lesion with or without associated pruritus, dysuria, discharge, or bleeding. Visualization can be difficult due to distortion of labial architecture from atrophy or inflammatory dermatoses. Any suspicious lesion should be biopsied to the level of the underlying stroma.[28]

Pathology
SCC is classified into 3 primary histologic subtypes: warty, basaloid, and keratinizing. Warty and basaloid account for the minority of cases, are found in younger women, and are HPV mediated. Keratinizing SCC accounts for 65% to 80% of SCC subtypes, is found in older patients, and arises from the HPV-independent pathway.[29] Stage at diagnosis, and more specifically, nodal metastasis, is the most important prognostic factor. Additional important clinicopathologic factors for nodal disease and recurrence include presence of vascular space invasion, depth of invasion, and histologic and cytologic grade.[30,31]

Staging

Nonmelanoma vulvar carcinomas are staged surgically using a hybrid classification system that combines the TNM system defined by the American Joint Committee on Cancer (AJCC) 7th Staging Edition and the Federation International de Gynecology et Obstetrique (FIGO) 2009 revision.[32,33]

Several methods for assessing depth of invasion have been proposed; however, currently depth of invasion is measured from the epithelial junction of the most superficial dermal papilla to the deepest point of tumor invasion.[34,35] Multiple aspects of the FIGO staging system have been questioned and include the prognostic value of FIGO stage 1 and 2 disease because they do not differ in disease-specific survival and the uses of pelvic lymph node metastasis to define stage IVB disease.[36,37]

Management

All patients should have a complete history and physical examination, complete blood count, assessment of liver and renal function, and evaluation of the vagina and cervix with cytologic smears. Performance of computed tomography (CT), PET/CT, and MRI may aid in determining extent of tumor as well as pelvic and distant metastases, especially in the setting of locally advanced tumors.[34]

Management of SCC of the vulva is determined by disease stage. In general, small tumors that are clinically IA can be treated with local surgery. Larger lesions, especially those measuring greater than 2 cm, have an increased risk of lymph node metastasis.[38] Radical surgery, lymphadenectomy, and adjunctive radiation and chemotherapy are mainstay therapies for regionally advanced disease. Treatment for disseminated disease is generally palliative.

Early Stage Tumors

Stage IA disease is treated surgically. This approach achieves high cure rates due to the extremely low risk of nodal metastasis when tumor depth of invasion is less than 1 mm.[39] The goal of excision is to achieve 1 to 2 cm negative margins. Risk of recurrence is associated with depth of invasion, presence of carcinoma at the surgical margin, and histologic grade; however, recent evidence suggests that patients with close but negative margins (1–10 mm) may not benefit from repeat excision due to increased operative morbidity and low yield of carcinoma in repeat excision.[40,41]

When tumor depth is greater than 1 mm or the tumor diameter exceeds 2 cm in diameter, radical resection (deep margin extending to the deep perineal fascia of the urogenital diaphragm) combined with lymph node assessment should be performed. This is due to the 20% to 30% risk of occult nodal metastases.[42,43] Primary surgical management is generally preferred over primary pelvic radiotherapy, because there seems to be a survival benefit and lower rate of nodal recurrence with surgery; however, randomized data to support this are limited.[44,45] Small (<2 cm) and unilateral (>1 cm from the midline) tumors are at low risk of metastasizing to contralateral groin nodes and can therefore be treated with ipsilateral inguinofemoral lymphadenectomy. Larger lesions and tumors located near the clitoris and labia minora are more likely to have bilateral lymph node spread and should be treated with bilateral inguinofemoral lymphadenectomy.[46] Uncertainty remains as to the optimal number of lymph nodes resected and risk of recurrence.[47] The 3-incision technique remains the standard of care for radical vulvectomy with bilateral inguinofemoral lymphadenectomy due to good locoregional control and acceptable surgical morbidity.[48,49]

Adjuvant radiation therapy (with or without chemotherapy) improves locoregional control and survival following discovery of positive inguinofemoral lymph nodes on surgical pathology.[50–52]

Sentinel Lymph Node Biopsy

The principles of lymph node exploration noted earlier remain a viable option for surgical management of vulvar tumors; however, utilization of sentinel lymph node (SLN) biopsy is becoming the standard of care for initial surgical management of vulvar tumors up to 4 cm in diameter with clinically negative inguinofemoral lymph nodes. SLN dissection has demonstrated high sensitivity and specificity for the identification of occult groin lymph node metastases in clinically early stage vulvar SCCs.[53] Unilateral tumors greater than 2 cm from the midline can be managed with ipsilateral sentinel lymph node dissection, whereas bilateral SLN dissection should be carried out for midline tumors.[54] If an SLN is not detected, complete inguinofemoral lymphadenectomy should be performed.

Groin node recurrence is low (2.3%–3%) in patients with SLNs negative for metastatic disease compared with patients with positive SLNs (8%).[55,56] This correlates to a high disease-specific survival rate of nearly 97%. In addition, patients undergoing SLN dissection experience less short- and long-term morbidity than patients undergoing inguinal lymphadenectomy.[55] The GROINSS-V trial was able to further demonstrate that size of SLN metastases correlates with disease-specific survival: 94.4% for metastases 2 mm or smaller versus 69.5% for metastases greater than 2 mm.[57]

The optimal management of a positive SLN is unclear and completion lymphadenectomy or external beam radiation therapy (EBRT) should be considered. It is also recommended that the contralateral groin should be evaluated surgically or treated with EBRT in the event of a positive ipsilateral SLN.[34] The ongoing GROINSS-V-II trial is assessing whether radiation therapy is safe in patients with SLN metastases less than or equal to 2 mm instead of performing completion lymphadenectomy.

Locally Advanced Disease

Radical resection was historically the standard of care for the treatment of locally advanced disease; however, treatment has moved toward more conservative approaches that optimize oncologic outcomes while reducing treatment morbidity. GOG 101 demonstrated that only 3% of patients with T3 and T4 tumors had residual unresectable tumors following chemoradiation.[58] Follow-up to GOG 101 demonstrated high rates of nodal control in patients with N2/N3 disease who underwent preoperative chemoradiation.[59] GOG 205 further demonstrated complete clinical response amongst patients with T3/T4 tumors following chemoradiation, with 78% of patients achieving complete clinical response.[60] Primary chemoradiation has become the initial treatment of choice for locally advanced disease followed by resection of residual tumor.

Patients presenting with large T2 and T3 tumors should undergo additional radiographic workup to assess for nodal disease. If there is no radiographic evidence of nodal disease, inguinofemoral lymph node dissection should be performed. If no nodal metastases are found on pathology, EBRT can be confined to the primary tumor. If there is no radiographic evidence of nodal metastases, but lymph node dissection is not carried out, then it is recommended to irradiate the primary tumor as well as the groin and pelvic nodal beds. If enlarged inguinofemoral or pelvic nodes are detected on imaging, fine-needle aspiration of enlarged nodes can be considered to confirm presence of metastatic disease. Radiation of the primary tumor as well as groin and pelvic nodes is again recommended in this setting. Results of GOG 205 and similar studies have raised the question of whether definitive chemoradiation therapy can be recommended in patients with locally advanced disease with nodal metastases.[61] This is being explored within the ongoing GOG 279 trial.

Extrapelvic Metastatic Disease

The management of patients with distant metastatic disease focuses on palliative care and improvement of quality of life. Chemoradiation can be used for symptom relief at the primary tumor site and pelvis. Systemic chemotherapy can be used; however, much of the literature guiding use is from cervical cancer. Supportive care remains an important alternative.[36]

Surveillance

Given high recurrence rates of 12% to 39.5% across all patients with vulvar SCC, routine surveillance is recommended following primary treatment.[62,63] Most recurrences occur within the first 2 years after treatment: 32.7% of patients with node-positive cancer and 5.1% amongst women with negative nodes.[63] Patients with nodal metastatic disease recur at the groin on average at 10.5 months.[56] After 2 years posttreatment, the annual risk of recurrence for node-positive and node-negative cancers approximate one another and cumulative recurrence risk continues to increase after 5 years posttreatment.[43,56,63]

The Society of Gynecologic Oncologists and the NCCN recommend surveillance with history and detailed physical examination every 3 months for the first 2 years following treatment. This interval can then be spaced out depending on initial disease features and patient characteristics for a total of 5 years of surveillance. Because vulvar SCC is often HPV mediated, it is important to assess the cervix, vagina, and anus for evidence of preinvasive or invasive disease. Laboratory and imaging studies should be performed based on clinical indications.[34,63] Biopsies should be performed to all suspicious lesions.

Recurrence

Recurrent disease confined to the vulva can be treated with surgical resection only with cure rates of 20% to 79%. Pelvic exenteration is an option for patients with large local recurrences for whom other treatments are not an option. This is a highly morbid procedure with median survival of 11 months and overall survival of 57% at 2 years. Adjuvant radiotherapy is an option for some patients; however, indications and survival benefit over surgery alone are unclear.[62]

Nodal recurrence has long been regarded as nearly universally fatal; however, a recent cohort of 30 patients with groin recurrence reported 5-year survival of 50% with combination of surgery and chemoradiation.[62,64] Although the generalizability of these findings is unclear, this study highlights the importance of early detection of disease recurrence and the use of multimodal therapy. Systemic chemotherapy is reserved for radiosensitization and palliative therapy.

MELANOMA

Melanoma accounts for up to 10% of invasive vulvar cancers.[65,66] The median age of diagnosis for vulvar and vaginal melanoma is 68 years. It is more common among whites compared with nonwhites. Approximately half of patients present with localized disease and 8.4% present with advanced disease. Median survival for black patients is 16 months compared with 39 months for nonblacks. Vulvar melanoma is far rarer than cutaneous melanoma, is diagnosed at an older age with more advanced stage, and has significantly worse survival.[67] Melanoma classically presents as an asymmetrical black macule, papule, or nodule, with irregular borders extending greater than 7 mm in diameter, most commonly on the labia majora, labia minora, and clitoral hood. Amelanotic melanoma accounts for up to 25% of vulvar melanomas and presents as an erythematous lesion.[22,68]

Treatment for localized melanoma is primarily surgical. First-line systemic therapy for stage III disease (nodal metastases) includes anti-PD-1 checkpoint immunotherapy with nivolumab, pembrolizumab, or nivolumab/pembrolizumab combination therapy. Patients with metastatic tumors harboring BRAF mutations should be treated with BRAF/MEK inhibitor combination therapy with debrafenib/trametinib or vemurafenib/cobimetinib or single-agent BRAF inhibitor therapy with vermurafenib or dabrafenib. Second-line therapies include high-dose interleukin 2 (IL-2), biochemotherapy (combination of high-dose interferon, IL-2, and cytotoxic chemotherapy), and imatinib for tumors with *c-KIT* mutations. Clinical trials should be offered to any patient with advanced disease. Given the rarity of vulvar melanoma and the complexity of its treatment, the authors recommend coordination of care with a melanoma specialist.[69]

EXTRAMAMMARY PAGET DISEASE

EMPD is an intraepidermal adenocarcinoma that is most commonly found on the vulva and accounts for 1% to 2% of vulvar malignancies. Primary EMPD arises from the intraepidermal component of apocrine sweat glands and is associated with an underlying adenocarcinoma of dermal apocrine glands in approximately 9% of cases.[68] Dermal invasion can occur in 4% to 19% of primary EMPD.[70] Secondary EMPD is associated with an underlying anal or rectal adenocarcinoma, urothelial carcinoma, or distant adenocarcinoma.[71] Primary EMPD is most common among white women in their 60s and is classically characterized as a sharply demarcated, painful, and erythematous rash over the labia majora.[68] The visual borders do not correspond to the histopathologic extent of disease, which likely accounts for the high rate of recurrence after primary resection.[68] Use of Mohs micrographic surgery is associated with a significantly lower recurrence rate than wide local excision.[72] Surgical resection remains the mainstay primary therapy for invasive disease and may consist of simple vulvectomy or radical vulvectomy with or without inguinofemoral lymphadenectomy depending on the extent of disease.[70] Radiation therapy has been described with a limited role. Topical therapies with 5-FU and imiquimod as well as chemotherapy with trastuzumab and/or pacitaxel, vincristine, cisplatin, carboplatin, 5-FU, etoposide, and docetaxel have been described as well.[68,70,73] SEER data places 5-year survival for invasive EMPD at 94.9% for localized disease, 84.9% for regional disease, and 52.5% for distant disease.[73]

REFERENCES

1. Vulvar cancer - cancer stat facts. Available at: https://seer.cancer.gov/statfacts/html/vulva.html. Accessed August 29, 2018.
2. Akhtar-Danesh N, Elit L, Lytwyn A. Trends in incidence and survival of women with invasive vulvar cancer in the United States and Canada: a population-based study. Gynecol Oncol 2014;134(2):314–8.
3. Moore KL, Dalley AF, Agur AMR. Clinically oriented anatomy. Baltimore (MD): Lippincott Williams & Wilkins; 2013. p. 1171.
4. Darragh TM, Colgan TJ, Cox JT, et al. The lower anogenital squamous terminology standardization project for HPV-associated lesions: background and consensus recommendations from the College of American Pathologists and the American Society for Colposcopy and Cervical Pathology. Arch Pathol Lab Med 2012;136(10):1266–97.
5. Bornstein J, Bogliatto F, Haefner HK, et al. The 2015 International Society for the Study of Vulvovaginal Disease (ISSVD) terminology of vulvar squamous intraepithelial lesions. Obstet Gynecol 2016;127(2):264–8.

6. Jones RW, Rowan DM, Stewart AW. Vulvar intraepithelial neoplasia: aspects of the natural history and outcome in 405 women. Obstet Gynecol 2005;106(6): 1319–26.

7. Judson PL, Habermann EB, Baxter NN, et al. Trends in the incidence of invasive and in situ vulvar carcinoma. Obstet Gynecol 2006;107(5):1018–22.

8. Baandrup L, Varbo A, Munk C, et al. In situ and invasive squamous cell carcinoma of the vulva in Denmark 1978-2007-a nationwide population-based study. Gynecol Oncol 2011;122(1):45–9.

9. Léonard B, Kridelka F, Delbecque K, et al. A clinical and pathological overview of vulvar condyloma acuminatum, intraepithelial neoplasia, and squamous cell carcinoma. Biomed Res Int 2014;2014:480573.

10. Reyes MC, Cooper K. An update on vulvar intraepithelial neoplasia: terminology and a practical approach to diagnosis. J Clin Pathol 2014;67(4):290–4.

11. Forman D, de Martel C, Lacey CJ, et al. Global burden of human papillomavirus and related diseases. Vaccine 2012;30(Suppl 5):F12–23.

12. Muñoz N, Kjaer SK, Sigurdsson K, et al. Impact of human papillomavirus (HPV)-6/11/16/18 vaccine on all HPV-associated genital diseases in young women. J Natl Cancer Inst 2010;102(5):325–39.

13. Immunization Expert Work Group, Committee on Adolescent Health Care. Committee opinion no. 704: human papillomavirus vaccination. Obstet Gynecol 2017; 129(6):e173–8.

14. Oliver SE, Unger ER, Lewis R, et al. Prevalence of human papillomavirus among females after vaccine introduction-national health and nutrition examination survey, United States, 2003-2014. J Infect Dis 2017;216(5):594–603.

15. Preti M, Scurry J, Marchitelli CE, et al. Vulvar intraepithelial neoplasia. Best Pract Res Clin Obstet Gynaecol 2014;28(7):1051–62.

16. Wallbillich JJ, Rhodes HE, Milbourne AM, et al. Vulvar intraepithelial neoplasia (VIN 2/3): comparing clinical outcomes and evaluating risk factors for recurrence. Gynecol Oncol 2012;127(2):312–5.

17. Baggish MS. Improved laser techniques for the elimination of genital and extragenital warts. Am J Obstet Gynecol 1985;153(5):545–50.

18. Lawrie TA, Nordin A, Chakrabarti M, et al. Medical and surgical interventions for the treatment of usual-type vulval intraepithelial neoplasia. Cochrane Database Syst Rev 2016;(1):CD011837.

19. Mathiesen O, Buus SK, Cramers M. Topical imiquimod can reverse vulvar intraepithelial neoplasia: a randomised, double-blinded study. Gynecol Oncol 2007; 107(2):219–22.

20. van Seters M, van Beurden M, ten Kate FJW, et al. Treatment of vulvar intraepithelial neoplasia with topical imiquimod. N Engl J Med 2008;358(14):1465–73.

21. Westermann C, Fischer A, Clad A. Treatment of vulvar intraepithelial neoplasia with topical 5% imiquimod cream. Int J Gynaecol Obstet 2013;120(3):266–70.

22. Carter JS, Downs LS. Vulvar and vaginal cancer. Obstet Gynecol Clin North Am 2012;39(2):213–31.

23. van de Nieuwenhof HP, van Kempen LCLT, de Hullu JA, et al. The etiologic role of HPV in vulvar squamous cell carcinoma fine tuned. Cancer Epidemiol Biomarkers Prev 2009;18(7):2061–7.

24. Hoang LN, Park KJ, Soslow RA, et al. Squamous precursor lesions of the vulva: current classification and diagnostic challenges. Pathology 2016;48(4):291–302.

25. Micheletti L, Preti M, Radici G, et al. Vulvar lichen sclerosus and neoplastic transformation: a retrospective study of 976 cases. J Low Genit Tract Dis 2016;20(2): 180–3.

26. Fistarol SK, Itin PH. Diagnosis and treatment of lichen sclerosus: an update. Am J Clin Dermatol 2013;14(1):27–47.

27. Neill SM, Lewis FM, Tatnall FM, et al, British Association of Dermatologists. British Association of Dermatologists' guidelines for the management of lichen sclerosus 2010. Br J Dermatol 2010;163(4):672–82.

28. Zweizig S, Korets S, Cain JM. Key concepts in management of vulvar cancer. Best Pract Res Clin Obstet Gynaecol 2014;28(7):959–66.

29. Alkatout I, Schubert M, Garbrecht N, et al. Vulvar cancer: epidemiology, clinical presentation, and management options. Int J Womens Health 2015;7:305–13.

30. Gómez Rueda N, Vighi S, Garcia A, et al. Histologic predictive factors. Therapeutic impact in vulvar cancer. J Reprod Med 1994;39(2):71–6.

31. Sznurkowski JJ, Milczek T, Emerich J. Prognostic factors and a value of 2009 FIGO staging system in vulvar cancer. Arch Gynecol Obstet 2013;287(6):1211–8.

32. Pecorelli S. Revised FIGO staging for carcinoma of the vulva, cervix, and endometrium. Int J Gynaecol Obstet 2009;105(2):103–4.

33. FIGO Committee on Gynecologic Oncology. FIGO staging for carcinoma of the vulva, cervix, and corpus uteri. Int J Gynaecol Obstet 2014;125(2):97–8.

34. Koh W-J, Dorigo O, Mutch D. NCCN guidelines index table of contents discussion. Squamous Cell Carcinoma 2017;53.

35. Wilkinson EJ, Kneale B, Lynch PJ. Report of the ISSVD terminology committee. J Reprod Med 1986;31(10):973–4.

36. Tabbaa ZM, Gonzalez J, Sznurkowski JJ, et al. Impact of the new FIGO 2009 staging classification for vulvar cancer on prognosis and stage distribution. Gynecol Oncol 2012;127(1):147–52.

37. Thaker NG, Klopp AH, Jhingran A, et al. Survival outcomes for patients with stage IVB vulvar cancer with grossly positive pelvic lymph nodes: time to reconsider the FIGO staging system? Gynecol Oncol 2015;136(2):269–73.

38. Homesley HD, Bundy BN, Sedlis A, et al. Prognostic factors for groin node metastasis in squamous cell carcinoma of the vulva (a Gynecologic Oncology Group study). Gynecol Oncol 1993;49(3):279–83.

39. Magrina JF, Gonzalez-Bosquet J, Weaver AL, et al. Squamous cell carcinoma of the vulva stage IA: long-term results. Gynecol Oncol 2000;76(1):24–7.

40. Yoder BJ, Rufforny I, Massoll NA, et al. Stage IA vulvar squamous cell carcinoma: an analysis of tumor invasive characteristics and risk. Am J Surg Pathol 2008; 32(5):765–72.

41. Ioffe YJ, Erickson BK, Foster KE, et al. Low yield of residual vulvar carcinoma and dysplasia upon re-excision for close or positive margins. Gynecol Oncol 2013; 129(3):528–32.

42. Gonzalez Bosquet J, Kinney WK, Russell AH, et al. Risk of occult inguinofemoral lymph node metastasis from squamous carcinoma of the vulva. Int J Radiat Oncol Biol Phys 2003;57(2):419–24.

43. Gonzalez Bosquet J, Magrina JF, Gaffey TA, et al. Long-term survival and disease recurrence in patients with primary squamous cell carcinoma of the vulva. Gynecol Oncol 2005;97(3):828–33.

44. Stehman FB, Bundy BN, Ball H, et al. Sites of failure and times to failure in carcinoma of the vulva treated conservatively: a Gynecologic Oncology Group study. Am J Obstet Gynecol 1996;174(4):1128–32 [discussion: 1132–3].

45. van der Velden J, Fons G, Lawrie TA. Primary groin irradiation versus primary groin surgery for early vulvar cancer. Cochrane Database Syst Rev 2011;(5):CD002224.

46. Gonzalez Bosquet J, Magrina JF, Magtibay PM, et al. Patterns of inguinal groin metastases in squamous cell carcinoma of the vulva. Gynecol Oncol 2007; 105(3):742–6.

47. Diehl A, Volland R, Kirn V, et al. The number of removed lymph nodes by inguinofemoral lymphadenectomy: impact on recurrence rates in patients with vulva carcinoma. Arch Gynecol Obstet 2016;294(1):131–6.

48. Farias-Eisner R, Cirisano FD, Grouse D, et al. Conservative and individualized surgery for early squamous carcinoma of the vulva: the treatment of choice for stage I and II (T1-2N0-1M0) disease. Gynecol Oncol 1994;53(1):55–8.

49. Siller BS, Alvarez RD, Conner WD, et al. T2/3 vulva cancer: a case-control study of triple incision versus en bloc radical vulvectomy and inguinal lymphadenectomy. Gynecol Oncol 1995;57(3):335–9.

50. Mahner S, Jueckstock J, Hilpert F, et al. Adjuvant therapy in lymph node-positive vulvar cancer: the AGO-CaRE-1 study. J Natl Cancer Inst 2015;107(3).

51. Gill BS, Bernard ME, Lin JF, et al. Impact of adjuvant chemotherapy with radiation for node-positive vulvar cancer: a National Cancer Data Base (NCDB) analysis. Gynecol Oncol 2015;137(3):365–72.

52. Ignatov T, Eggemann H, Burger E, et al. Adjuvant radiotherapy for vulvar cancer with close or positive surgical margins. J Cancer Res Clin Oncol 2016;142(2): 489–95.

53. Levenback CF, Ali S, Coleman RL, et al. Lymphatic mapping and sentinel lymph node biopsy in women with squamous cell carcinoma of the vulva: a gynecologic oncology group study. J Clin Oncol 2012;30(31):3786–91.

54. Coleman RL, Ali S, Levenback CF, et al. Is bilateral lymphadenectomy for midline squamous carcinoma of the vulva always necessary? An analysis from Gynecologic Oncology Group (GOG) 173. Gynecol Oncol 2013;128(2):155–9.

55. Levenback CF, van der Zee AGJ, Rob L, et al. Sentinel lymph node biopsy in patients with gynecologic cancers expert panel statement from the International Sentinel Node Society Meeting, February 21, 2008. Gynecol Oncol 2009; 114(2):151–6.

56. Te Grootenhuis NC, van der Zee AGJ, van Doorn HC, et al. Sentinel nodes in vulvar cancer: Long-term follow-up of the GROningen INternational Study on Sentinel nodes in Vulvar cancer (GROINSS-V) I. Gynecol Oncol 2016;140(1): 8–14.

57. Oonk MH, van Hemel BM, Hollema H, et al. Size of sentinel-node metastasis and chances of non-sentinel-node involvement and survival in early stage vulvar cancer: results from GROINSS-V, a multicentre observational study. Lancet Oncol 2010;11(7):646–52.

58. Moore DH, Thomas GM, Montana GS, et al. Preoperative chemoradiation for advanced vulvar cancer: a phase II study of the Gynecologic Oncology Group. Int J Radiat Oncol Biol Phys 1998;42(1):79–85.

59. Montana GS, Thomas GM, Moore DH, et al. Preoperative chemo-radiation for carcinoma of the vulva with N2/N3 nodes: a gynecologic oncology group study. Int J Radiat Oncol Biol Phys 2000;48(4):1007–13.

60. Moore DH, Ali S, Koh W-J, et al. A phase II trial of radiation therapy and weekly cisplatin chemotherapy for the treatment of locally-advanced squamous cell carcinoma of the vulva: a gynecologic oncology group study. Gynecol Oncol 2012; 124(3):529–33.

61. Rao YJ, Chundury A, Schwarz JK, et al. Intensity modulated radiation therapy for squamous cell carcinoma of the vulva: Treatment technique and outcomes. Adv Radiat Oncol 2017;2(2):148–58.

62. Nooij LS, Brand FAM, Gaarenstroom KN, et al. Risk factors and treatment for recurrent vulvar squamous cell carcinoma. Crit Rev Oncol Hematol 2016;106: 1–13.

63. Salani R, Khanna N, Frimer M, et al. An update on post-treatment surveillance and diagnosis of recurrence in women with gynecologic malignancies: Society of Gynecologic Oncology (SGO) recommendations. Gynecol Oncol 2017; 146(1):3–10.

64. Frey JN, Hampl M, Mueller MD, et al. Should groin recurrence still be considered as a palliative situation in vulvar cancer patients?: A brief report. Int J Gynecol Cancer 2016;26(3):575–9.

65. Moxley KM, Fader AN, Rose PG, et al. Malignant melanoma of the vulva: an extension of cutaneous melanoma? Gynecol Oncol 2011;122(3):612–7.

66. Murzaku EC, Penn LA, Hale CS, et al. Vulvar nevi, melanosis, and melanoma: an epidemiologic, clinical, and histopathologic review. J Am Acad Dermatol 2014; 71(6):1241–9.

67. Mert I, Semaan A, Winer I, et al. Vulvar/vaginal melanoma: an updated surveillance epidemiology and end results database review, comparison with cutaneous melanoma and significance of racial disparities. Int J Gynecol Cancer 2013;23(6):1118–25.

68. Clinician's update on the benign, premalignant, and malignant skin tumours of the vulva: the dermatologist's view. - PubMed - NCBI. Available at: https://www.ncbi. nlm.nih.gov/pubmed/28812059. August 30, 2018.

69. Coit DG, Thompson JA, Algazi A, et al. NCCN guidelines insights: melanoma, version 3.2018. J Natl Compr Canc Netw 2016;14(8):945–58.

70. Borghi C, Bogani G, Ditto A, et al. Invasive paget disease of the vulva. Int J Gynecol Cancer 2018;28(1):176–82.

71. Wilkinson EJ, Brown HM. Vulvar Paget disease of urothelial origin: a report of three cases and a proposed classification of vulvar Paget disease. Hum Pathol 2002;33(5):549–54.

72. Bae JM, Choi YY, Kim H, et al. Mohs micrographic surgery for extramammary Paget disease: a pooled analysis of individual patient data. J Am Acad Dermatol 2013;68(4):632–7.

73. Karam A, Dorigo O. Treatment outcomes in a large cohort of patients with invasive Extramammary Paget's disease. Gynecol Oncol 2012;125(2):346–51.

Chemotherapy, Biologic, and Immunotherapy Breakthroughs in Cancer Care

Christine Rojas, MD[a], Yovanni Casablanca, MD[b],*

KEYWORDS

- Chemotherapy • Antiangiogenic therapy • Tyrosine kinase inhibitors (TKI)
- Immunotherapy • PARP inhibitors • Targeted therapy • Toxicity

KEY POINTS

- Greater understanding of the molecular pathways activated in cancer has led to the development of novel targeted therapies.
- Antiangiogenesis agents, tyrosine kinase inhibitors, and poly adenosine 5'-diphosphate ribose polymerase inhibitors are active in gynecologic cancer and can be used to treat selective patients.
- Immunotherapy has been a recent breakthrough in the treatment of many cancer types and is currently under investigation in gynecologic cancer in clinical trials.
- Personalized treatment of gynecologic cancer should incorporate targeted therapy, with selection and dosing based on the patient's history, disease type, molecular assessment, and ability to tolerate toxicities.

Cancer has been defined as "unregulated cell growth and the invasion and spread of cells from the site of origin."[1] Ten cancer hallmarks have been described: growth signal autonomy, evasion of growth inhibitory signals, avoidance of immune destruction, unlimited replicative potential, tumor production of inflammation, invasion, metastasis, angiogenesis, genome instability, evasion of cell death, and reprogramming of energy metabolism.[1] Traditionally, chemotherapy agents have exerted their

Disclosure Statement: The authors have no commercial or financial disclosures related to topics in this work. The opinions or assertions contained herein are the private ones of the author/speaker and are not to be construed as official or reflecting the views of the Department of Defense, the Uniformed Services University of the Health Sciences, or any other agency of the US Government.

[a] Gynecologic Cancer Center of Excellence, Murtha Cancer Center, Walter Reed National Military Medical Center, Building 19, 3rd Floor, Room 3462, 4954 North Palmer Road, Bethesda, MD 20889-5630, USA; [b] Department of Obstetrics and Gynecology, Uniformed Services University of the Health Sciences, 9618 Alta Vista Terrace, Bethesda, MD 20814, USA
* Corresponding author.
E-mail address: yovanni.casablanca.mil@mail.mil

Obstet Gynecol Clin N Am 46 (2019) 137–154
https://doi.org/10.1016/j.ogc.2018.09.009
0889-8545/19/Published by Elsevier Inc.

effects by disrupting the cell cycle, thus reducing replicative potential. However, as seen clinically, there are various mechanisms that cancer cells use to develop chemo-resistance. Advancements in the understanding of cancer's molecular complexity have led to the development of many new treatment strategies and therapies. In the field of Gynecology Oncology, use of antiangiogenic agents, tyrosine kinase inhibitors (TKIs), poly adenosine 5'-diphosphate (ADP) ribose polymerase (PARP) inhibitors, monoclonal antibody drugs, and immunotherapy agents has emerged as novel alter-native therapies in the last decade. These new therapies are expanding the weaponry available to combat gynecologic disease either on their own or in combination with established chemotherapy regimens.

ANTIANGIOGENIC THERAPY

Cancer cells stimulate angiogenesis for tumor survival and expansion.[1] The regulation of angiogenesis involves a balance between angiogenic inducers and inhibitors. Anti-angiogenic therapies, such as bevacizumab, are designed to reduce the ability of the cancer to create blood supply for itself, leading to either reduction or stabilization of disease. Bevacizumab is a monoclonal antibody that blocks angiogenesis by inhibiting the binding of the vascular endothelial growth factor (VEGF) ligand to its receptor[2] (**Fig. 1**). In the past decade, the International Collaborative Ovarian Neoplasm Group trial (ICON-7), the Gynecologic Oncology Group trials (GOG-218 and GOG-213), and OCEANS and AURELIA trials revealed that inhibiting VEGF signaling with

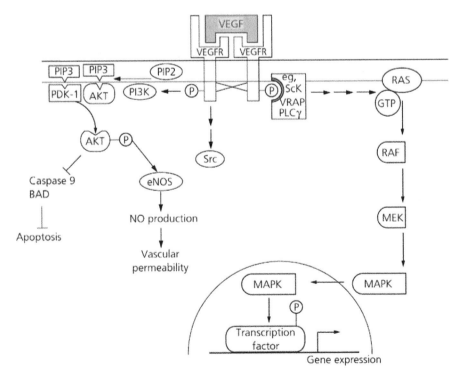

Fig. 1. The VEGF signal transduction pathway. FGFR, fibroblast growth factor receptors. (*From* Pecorino, L. Molecular biology of cancer: mechanisms, targets and therapeutics. 3rd Ed. New York: Oxford University Press; 2012. By permission of Oxford University Press www.oup.com.)

bevacizumab is associated with improvements of progression-free survival (PFS) in patients with ovarian cancer in the primary treatment and recurrence setting (**Table 1**).

In the ICON-7 trial, 1528 women with any stage of ovarian cancer requiring adjuvant therapy were randomized to one of 2 regimens following upfront surgery: (1) standard chemotherapy with 6 cycles of carboplatin and paclitaxel or (2) standard chemotherapy plus concurrent bevacizumab followed by up to 12 cycles of additional bevacizumab.[3] At 42 months, PFS was 22.4 months with standard therapy compared with 24.1 months when bevacizumab was added.[3] However, patients at higher risk for progression (International Federation of Gynecology and Obstetrics [FIGO] stage IV disease or stage III disease with >1 cm gross residual) displayed a greater benefit from bevacizumab with a PFS at 42 months of 18.1 months with bevacizumab versus 14.5 months without. This subgroup also had a significantly improved overall survival (OS) of 39.3 months with bevacizumab versus 34.5 months with standard treatment.[4] Bevacizumab treatment was associated with greater adverse effects however (see **Table 1**).

GOG-218 evaluated the use of bevacizumab in 1873 women with stage III or IV ovarian cancer following primary surgical cytoreduction.[5] Patients were randomized to one of 3 treatment arms: (1) standard therapy with intravenous carboplatin and paclitaxel, (2) standard therapy plus concurrent bevacizumab, and (3) standard therapy, concurrent bevacizumab, and continued bevacizumab for up to an additional 16 cycles. This phase 3 trial revealed that the median PFS improved by 3.8 months (10.3 months in arm 1 vs 14.1 months in arm 3) with the addition of bevacizumab during and following chemotherapy.[5] However, there was no significant difference in OS between the 3 arms (39 months).[5] A subsequent subgroup analysis demonstrated that treatment with bevacizumab improved both PFS and OS in women with ascites.[6] Use of intravenous and intraperitoneal bevacizumab has also been shown to provide symptomatic relief for patients with malignant ascites, leading to no further need for paracentesis in some cases.[7,8] Based on the results of GOG-218, the Food and Drug Administration (FDA) has recently approved the use of bevacizumab in combination with carboplatin and paclitaxel for primary treatment of patients with epithelial ovarian, fallopian tube, or primary peritoneal cancer.[9]

The OCEANS phase 3 trial sought to compare the efficacy and safety of bevacizumab with gemcitabine and carboplatin (GC) to GC alone in 484 patients with platinum-sensitive recurrent ovarian, primary peritoneal, or fallopian tube cancer.[10] Similar to GOG 218, the OCEANS trial found a 4-month improvement in median PFS in patients who received bevacizumab with GC and continued on maintenance bevacizumab, with a reported PFS of 12.4 months compared with 8.4 months for the control group.[10] OS was comparable between the 2 arms.[11]

In the GOG 213 trial, 674 women with platinum-sensitive recurrent ovarian cancer were randomly assigned to undergo (or not) secondary cytoreduction and separately to 2 different chemotherapy arms: (1) carboplatin and paclitaxel, (2) carboplatin and paclitaxel with concurrent bevacizumab and continued bevacizumab until progression.[12] In this trial, bevacizumab improved PFS by 4 months again (10 vs 14 months); however, unlike the trials in the upfront setting, there was also a significant OS benefit of 5 months seen (37 vs 42 months).[12] As a result of these data, in 2016, bevacizumab was approved by the FDA for use with chemotherapy for platinum-sensitive recurrent ovarian cancer.

Bevacizumab has also been shown to be effective in platinum-resistant ovarian cancer. In the AURELIA study, 361 patients were randomized to receive bevacizumab or placebo in addition to single-agent chemotherapy (paclitaxel, liposomal doxorubicin, or topotecan). PFS was improved in the bevacizumab-containing therapy with a survival of 6.7 months compared with 3.4 months in the chemotherapy-alone group.[13] OS

Table 1
Landmark trials of bevacizumab in gynecologic cancer

Trial or Author	Setting	Phase	n	Treatment Groups	Results	Toxicities with Bevacizumab
Cannistra et al[63]	Recurrent disease (ovarian cancer)	2	44	Single group: single agent bevacizumab every 21 d	Partial response in 15.9%	Grade 3–4 hypertension (HTN; 9.1%), proteinuria (15.9%), bleeding (2.3%), wound-healing complications (2.3%), GI perforation (11.4%), arterial thromboembolic events (6.8%)
GOG 218	First line (ovarian cancer)	3	1873	Carboplatin/paclitaxel PLUS a. Placebo cycle 2–22 b. Bevacizumab 15 mg/kg q 3 wk for cycles 2–6, then placebo for cycles 7–22 c. Bevacizumab cycles 2–22	PFS a. 10.3 mo b. 11.2 mo c. 14.1 mo	HTN (16.5% in Bev initiation group; 22.9% in throughout group), GI wall disruption (2.8%)
ICON 7	First line (ovarian cancer)	3	1528	Carboplatin/paclitaxel a. Placebo b. Bevacizumab, 7.5 mg/kg q 3 wk	PFS a. 20.3 mo b. 21.8 mo	Grade 2 HTN (18%), grade ≥3 thrombotic event (7%), GI perforation (3%)
OCEANS	Recurrent disease (ovarian cancer)	3	484	a. Carboplatin/gemcitabine plus placebo b. Carboplatin/gemcitabine plus bevacizumab	PFS a. 8.4 mo b. 12.4 mo	Grade ≥3 HTN (17.4%), proteinuria (8.5%), VTE (4.0%), neutropenia (20.6%)
AURELIA	Recurrent disease (ovarian cancer)	3	361	Single-agent chemotherapy (liposomal doxorubicin, topotecan, or paclitaxel) a. Placebo b. Bevacizumab (10 mg/kg q wk or 15 mg/kg q 3 wk)	PFS a. 3.4 mo b. 6.7 mo	Grade ≥2 HTN (20.1%), grade ≥2 proteinuria (10.6%), grade ≥2 GI perforation (2.2%), grade ≥2 fistula/abscess 2.2%, bleeding 1.1%, thromboembolic event (2.8%)

Trial	Disease	Phase	N	Regimen	Outcome	Adverse events
GOG 213	Recurrent disease (ovarian cancer)	3	674	Carboplatin/paclitaxel a. Placebo b. Bevacizumab 15 mg/kg followed by maintenance with or without bevacizumab	OS a. 37.3 mo b. 42.2 mo	HTN (12%), fatigue (8%), proteinuria (8%)
MITO-END2	Recurrent/advanced disease (endometrial cancer)	2	108	Carboplatin and paclitaxel (6–8 cycles) a. Placebo b. Bevacizumab followed by bevacizumab maintenance	PFS a. 8.7 mo b. 13 mo	VTE (5.7%), arterial thrombosis (5.7%), neutropenic fever (5.7%), grade 3 diarrhea (1.9%)
GOG 240	Recurrent/advanced disease (cervical cancer)	3	452	Cisplatin and paclitaxel (or topotecan) a. Placebo b. Bevacizumab	PFS OS a. 6.0 mo a. 13.3 mo b. 8.2 mo b. 16.8 mo	Fistula (15%, all previously irradiated)

Abbreviation: VTE, venous thromboemblism.

was not significantly different; however, the PFS improvement was enough to achieve FDA approval for bevacizumab for platinum-resistant recurrent ovarian cancer in November 2014.

The use of bevacizumab has also expanded to other gynecologic cancer sites, specifically cervical cancer, as a result of a phase 3 trial of advanced cervical cancer (GOG-240). In this study, 452 women with metastatic, persistent, or recurrent cervical cancer were randomized to chemotherapy (paclitaxel with cisplatin or topotecan) with or without bevacizumab. A higher response rate (48% vs 36%) and significant improvement in PFS (8.2 vs 6.0 months) and OS (16.8 vs 13.3 months) were seen in the chemotherapy plus bevacizumab group compared with the chemotherapy-only group.[14] The addition of bevacizumab did significantly increase the incidence of adverse events (see **Table 1**), but as a result of the OS benefit, the FDA expanded the indication for bevacizumab to first-line treatment of metastatic cervical cancer in August 2014.

In endometrial cancer, VEGF expression is associated with higher histologic grade, lymphovascular space invasion, lymph node metastasis, and deep myometrial invasion.[15] In GOG-229, a phase 2 trial of bevacizumab in women with recurrent or persistent endometrial cancer, 14% of the 52 women who received bevacizumab experienced clinical response and 40% survived progression free for at least 6 months.[16] Furthermore, in the phase 2 MITO-END 2 trial, patients with advanced or recurrent disease were given carboplatin and paclitaxel chemotherapy and randomized to receive bevacizumab concurrently with continuation as a single agent until progression or toxicity. As seen in other trials, bevacizumab added an additional 4 months to PFS in this study (8.7 months vs 13.0 months).[17]

The fusion protein VEGF Trap, also named Aflibercept, consists of native vascular endothelial growth factor receptor (VEGFR) sequences and, by binding with VEGF, prevents VEGFR activation on the tumor endothelial cells. Phase 2 studies have shown it to be effective for patients with ovarian cancer for symptom management of recurrent ascites.[18] However, assessment for objective disease response has not met endpoints.[19] It is currently being studied in the phase 1 setting in combination with immunotherapy agents in a variety of solid tumors.[20]

Trebananib, an angiopoietin (Ang) 1 and 2 neutralizing peptibody, prevents the interaction of the angiopoietins with their target tie 2 receptors.[21] The phase 3 TRINOVA-1 study randomized 919 patients with recurrent ovarian cancer to weekly paclitaxel with trebananib or placebo. PFS was improved by 2 months with trebananib (7.2 vs 5.4 months). OS was not improved overall; however, in patients with ascites, there was a 2-month OS improvement (14.5 vs 12.3 months). In the TRINOVA-2 study, trebananib was paired with liposomal doxorubicin in the same patient population, and it did not improve PFS.[22]

Toxicity

VEGF inhibition by both monoclonal antibodies and TKIs (as seen in the next section) includes cardiovascular effects (hypertension, venous thromboembolism, left ventricular dysfunction) and noncardiovascular effects (proteinuria, bleeding, delayed wound healing, gastrointestinal [GI] perforation, fatigue, and dysphoria; see **Table 1**).

TYROSINE KINASE INHIBITORS

Kinases play a crucial role in major cell functions, such as cell-cycle progression, signal transduction, and transcription. As a result, small-molecule TKIs have become an important target for therapeutic development.[1] Specifically, TKIs interfere with intracellular signaling pathways by preventing kinases from catalyzing the transfer of the γ phosphate group from adenosine triphosphate to target proteins.[23] Multiple oral TKIs have become available for a variety of tumors, including gynecologic cancers (**Table 2**).

AGO-OVAR16 used pazopanib, a TKI targeting the VEGF, platelet-derived growth factor (PDGF), and c-kit receptors. In this phase 3 study, 940 patients with epithelial ovarian cancer were randomized to either pazopanib or placebo following a complete or partial remission after primary treatment. Pazopanib prolonged PFS in this setting by 17.9 months compared with 12.3 months in the placebo group.[24] OS was equivalent, and treatment with pazopanib was also correlated with significant adverse effects (see **Table 2**).

Pazopanib has also shown activity in phase 2 trials of patients with soft tissue sarcomas, including leiomyosarcoma.[25] In the European Organization for Research and Treatment of Cancer phase 3 PALETTE trial, pazopanib was used in patients with progressive sarcoma and increased PFS significantly (4.6 vs 1.6 months) but did not have an OS effect.[25] Despite toxicity, because of the poor prognosis from this disease, pazopanib was approved by the FDA for treatment of patients with advanced soft tissue sarcoma who have received at least one line of prior chemotherapy in April 2012.[26]

Another phase 3 trial, AGO-OVAR12, evaluated the use of nintedanib, a TKI that inhibits VEGF, PDGF, and fibroblast growth factor (FGF) receptors, in the primary treatment of advanced ovarian cancer. One thousand three hundred sixty-six patients were randomly assigned to receive 6 cycles of carboplatin and paclitaxel in addition to either oral nintedanib or placebo.[27] The addition of nintedanib resulted in a modest improvement in PFS, with a median of 17.3 months compared with 16.6 months in the placebo group.[27]

Similarly, in recurrent or persistent endometrial cancer, the phase 2 GOG-229J trial showed the safety and efficacy of cediranib, a TKI targeting VEGF, PDGF, and FGF receptors.[28] A trend toward improved PFS was observed in patients who received cediranib and who expressed microvessel density. The median OS in patients who received cediranib was 12.5 months with no grade 4 or 5 toxicities noted.[28] Cediranib was also evaluated in the ICON6 trial, where 450 patients with recurrent ovarian cancer were treated with platinum-based chemotherapy with and without concurrent cediranib as well as an arm with maintenance cediranib. The median PFS was improved with maintenance cediranib at 11.0 months versus 8.7 months, albeit with toxic effects.[29] Cediranib is also being evaluated currently in combination with olaparib (a PARP inhibitor) in phase 2 and 3 trials for patients with recurrent platinum-sensitive and platinum-resistant/refractory ovarian cancer.

Toxicity

Antiangiogenic TKIs have the classic side effects and toxicities seen with VEGF inhibition but also have additional side effects, often referred to as "off-target" effects due to their affinity to multiple receptor sites (see **Table 2**).

POLY ADENOSINE 5'-DIPHOSPHATE RIBOSE POLYMERASE INHIBITORS

PARP is a key enzyme involved in repair of DNA single-strand breaks. By inhibiting repair of single-stand breaks, PARP inhibitors lead to the formation of double-strand breaks when replication ensues. In patients with a synchronous homologous repair deficiency (HRD), such as those with a BRCA 1 or 2 pathogenic mutation, these double-strand DNA breaks are also not able to be repaired, leading to cell apoptosis. This strategy is termed "synthetic lethality" and has been shown to render PARP

Table 2
Landmark trials of tyrosine kinase inhibitors in gynecologic cancer

Trial	Setting	Phase	n	Treatment Groups	Results	Toxicities with TKIs
AGO-OVAR 12	First line (ovarian cancer)	3	1366	Carboplatin/paclitaxel a. Placebo b. Nintedanib (200 mg) twice daily on days 2–21 of every 3-wk cycle	PFS a. 16.6 mo b. 17.3 mo	Diarrhea (22%), neutropenia (42%), anemia (12%), thrombocytopenia (12%)
AGO-OVAR 16	Maintenance (ovarian cancer)	3	940	Maintenance a. Placebo b. Pazopanib (800 mg) daily × 24 mo	PFS a. 12.3 mo b. 17.9 mo	Serious adverse events (26%), HTN (30%), diarrhea (8.2%), nausea, headache, hepatotoxicity (94%), neutropenia (9.9%), 3 fatal adverse events
MITO 11	Recurrent disease (ovarian cancer)	2	74	Weekly paclitaxel 80 mg/m² with a. Placebo b. Pazopanib 800 mg daily	PFS a. 3.49 mo b. 6.35 mo	Grade 3–4 neutropenia (30%), HTN (8%), anemia (5%), ileal perforation (2.7%), transaminitis (8%), fatigue (11%), leukopenia (11%)
PALETTE	Progressive disease (sarcoma)	3	369	a. Placebo b. Pazopanib 800 mg daily	PFS a. 1.6 mo b. 4.6 mo	Fatigue (65%), diarrhea (58%), nausea (54%), weight loss (48%), HTN (41%)
ICON-6	Recurrent disease (ovarian cancer)	3	456	Carboplatin/paclitaxel 6 cycles a. Placebo b. Concurrent cediranib 20 mg once daily and then placebo maintenance c. Concurrent cediranib 20 mg once daily and then maintenance with cediranib 20 mg once daily	PFS a. 8.7 mo b. 9.9 mo c. 11.0 mo	Diarrhea, neutropenia, hypertension, voice changes, hypothyroidism

inhibitor therapy to be quite effective for treatment of patients with HRD.[1] In the setting of ovarian cancer, PARP inhibitors have been evaluated in the setting of maintenance treatment after primary therapy as well as in all recurrent settings and have been shown to be active, even in patients without HRD (**Fig. 2**).

In 2014, olaparib became the first PARP inhibitor approved by the FDA for monotherapy for patients with deleterious germline BRCA mutated ovarian cancer following 3 or more prior lines of chemotherapy. The approval was based on data from a single-arm phase 2 study in 137 patients meeting these criteria demonstrating an overall response rate of 34% with a median duration of response of 7.9 months.[30]

Furthermore, olaparib has been studied as maintenance therapy for patients with platinum-sensitive recurrent disease regardless of the presence or absence of a BRCA mutation in Study 19 and in women with BRCA mutation in the SOLO2 trial. In the phase 2 Study 19 trial, 265 women with platinum-sensitive recurrent epithelial ovarian cancer were assigned to either olaparib maintenance treatment or placebo following partial or complete response to chemotherapy. An improvement in PFS of 8.4 months was notable in the olaparib group versus 4.8 months in the placebo group.[31] Similar results were observed in the phase 3 SOLO2/ENGOT-Ov21 trial, wherein 295 women with platinum-sensitive recurrent ovarian cancer and germline BRCA mutations received either olaparib or placebo.[32] Patients who received olaparib showed improved PFS compared with placebo, 19.1 versus 5.5 months, respectively.[32] There was no OS benefit seen in Study 19, and SOLO2 OS data are still immature (**Table 3**).

Most recently, another PARP inhibitor, rucaparib, has shown efficacy in both BRCA and non-BRCA mutated cancers. ARIEL 2 was a multicenter 2-part, phase 2 trial that evaluated rucaparib in patients with platinum-sensitive ovarian cancer. Patients were stratified into 3 subgroups based on next-generation sequencing results: BRCA mutant (germline or somatic mutation), BRCA wild-type, and high loss of heterozygosity (LOH), or BRCA wild-type and low LOH. Genomic LOH was considered representative of homologous recombination defect (HRD). The median PFS was statistically longer with rucaparib for patients with BRCA mutant (12.8 months) or high LOH

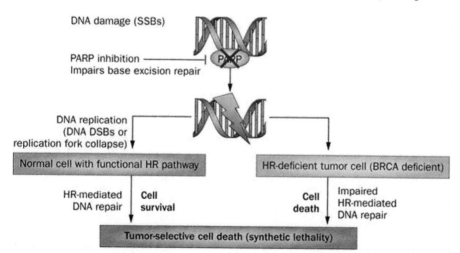

Fig. 2. The mechanism of synthetic lethal interactions: PARP inhibitors. DSB, double-strand break; HR, homologous recombination; SSB, single-strand break. (*From* Banerjee S, Kaye SB, Ashworth A. Making the best of PARP inhibitors in ovarian cancer. Nat Rev Clin Oncol 2010;7:508–19; with permission.)

Table 3
Landmark poly adenosine 5'-diphosphate ribose polymerase inhibitor trials in gynecologic cancer

Trial or Author	Setting	Phase	n	Treatment Groups	Results	Toxicities with PARP Inhibitors
Study 19	Maintenance (ovarian cancer)	2	265	Maintenance with either a. Placebo b. Olaparib 400 mg twice daily	PFS a. 4.8 mo b. 8.4 mo	Nausea (68%), fatigue (49%), vomiting (32%), anemia (17%)

ARIEL-3	Maintenance (ovarian cancer)	3	564	Maintenance with either
				a. Placebo
				b. Rucaparib 600 mg twice daily
				  i. BRCA mutated (germline or somatic)
				  ii. BRCA wild-type/LOH high
				  iii. BRCA wild-type/LOH low
					PFS
					a. 5.4 mo
					b. i. 16.6 mo
					  ii. 13.6 mo
					  iii. 10.8 mo
						Anemia (19%), transaminitis (10%)

NOVA trial	Recurrent disease (ovarian cancer)	3	490	Cohort 1: germline BRCA mutation carriers Cohort 2: no germline BRCA mutation carriers Randomize to either a. Placebo b. Niraparib	For germline mutations: PFS a. 5.5 mo b. 21.0 mo For no germline mutations, PFS a. 3.9 mo b. 9.3 mo	Thrombocytopenia (33.8%), anemia (25.3%), neutropenia (19.6%)
SOLO-2/ENGOT-Ov21	Recurrent disease (ovarian cancer)	3	295	Maintenance with either a. Placebo b. Olaparib 300 mg twice daily	PFS a. 5.5 mo b. 30.2 mo	Grade 3 or 4 anemia (19%), fatigue (4%), neutropenia (5%), intestinal obstruction (2%)
ARIEL-2	Recurrent disease (ovarian cancer)	3	206	Rucaparib (600 mg) twice daily in a. BRCA mutated (germline or somatic) b. BRCA wild-type/LOH high c. BRCA wild-type/LOH low	PFS a. 12.8 mo b. 5.7 mo c. 5.2 mo	Intestinal obstruction (5%), malignant neoplasm progression (5%), anemia (4%), transaminitis (12%)
Liu et al,[37] 2017	Recurrent disease (ovarian cancer)	2	90	a. Olaparib 400 mg twice daily b. Olaparib 200 mg twice daily + cediranib 300 mg daily	PFS a. 9.2 mo b. 17.7 mo	Grade 3 and 4 adverse events more common with combination therapy: fatigue (27%), diarrhea (22%), HTN (41%)

(5.7 months) compared with patients with BRCA wild-type and low LOH (5.2 months).[33] The investigators suggest that LOH testing might help extend rucaparib treatment to those patients with BRCA wild-type status.

ARIEL3 evaluated the use of rucaparib maintenance treatment in 561 patients with recurrent epithelial ovarian, fallopian tube, or primary peritoneal cancer following complete or partial remission after at least 2 prior lines of platinum-based chemotherapy.[34] This trial demonstrated a statistically significant improvement in median PFS for patients randomized to rucaparib in all patients (10.8 vs 5.4 months). In the patients with HRD, characterized by LOH high, the difference in PFS was even more pronounced (13.6 vs 5.4 months) and greatest in the BRCA mutant subgroup (16.6 vs 5.4 months).

Niraparib was also found to be an effective maintenance treatment option for patients with platinum-sensitive, recurrent ovarian cancer. In the phase 3 ENGOT-OV16/NOVA trial, patients were classified into 2 cohorts (gBRCA or non-gBRCA) based on the presence of a germline BRCA mutation. After chemotherapy completion, patients were randomized to receive niraparib or placebo until disease progression. PFS improved significantly in patients who received niraparib in both cohorts, 21.0 versus 5.5 months, respectively, in the gBRCA cohort, and 12.9 versus 3.8 months, respectively, in the non-gBRCA cohort.[35]

As a result of these series of studies, olaparib, rucaparib, and niraparib are now approved by the FDA for maintenance treatment of patients with platinum-sensitive recurrent epithelial ovarian, fallopian tube, or primary peritoneal cancer following a complete or partial response to platinum-based chemotherapy.[36] Approval is not only for patients with a BRCA mutation or HRD; however, cost-effectiveness is highest when used for these patients.[37] At current prices, no PARP meets standard ICER (incremental cost-effectiveness ratio) standards; however, niraparib appears to be the most cost-effective PARP when analyzed by progression-free life-years saved except for patients with germline BRCA mutations, where olaparib is slightly more cost-effective.[37] Compared with bevacizumab, PARPs are more cost-effective, and selection may be based on not only mutation status and cost but also toxicity profile in the context of clinical and patient factors.

Toxicities

PARP inhibitors have low rates of side effects but include nausea, fatigue, and GI upset, because they are oral agents. At higher doses, there are also myelosuppression, anemia, and neutropenia, but overall, they are generally well tolerated (see **Table 3**).

IMMUNOTHERAPY AGENTS

In addition to the prior discussed therapeutic strategies, immunotherapy has recently gained interest in gynecologic cancer treatment. One of the hallmarks of cancer is the significant ability to evade immune surveillance. Schreiber and colleagues[38] described 3 phases of "cancer immunoediting":

1. The elimination phase by which innate and adaptive response is triggered to specific tumor-associated antigens,
2. The equilibrium phase by which a balance between immune-mediated destruction and persistence of rare malignant clones is created, and
3. Immunologic escape by which the malignant clones are able to evade the adaptive immune system.[38]

Tumors may also evade immune surveillance with other mechanisms, such as loss or alteration of specific antigens or antigenic machinery, promotion of an immune-tolerant microenvironment by manipulation of cytokines, and upregulation of immune checkpoint molecules such as programmed cell death-1 (PD-1) and programmed cell death ligand-1 (PDL-1).[39–43]

The programmed cell death receptor (PD-1) protein found on the cell surface of lymphocytes and the interaction with its ligand, PDL-1, result in a cascade of downregulation of immune response.[44] Cancer cells upregulate PD-1/PDL-1 signaling, thus enabling tumors to turn off T cells and evade immune recognition.[44] Immunotherapy is aimed to increase the immune system's ability to recognize tumor cells. Immune checkpoint inhibitors work by preventing tumor cells from attaching or "turning off" T-cell recognition (**Fig. 3**).

Pembrolizumab is a monoclonal antibody to PD-1 and has been shown to be effective in many advanced solid tumors, specifically those that have mismatch repair deficiency (dMMR) or microsatellite instability (MSI). The FDA has approved pembrolizumab for women with dMMR or MSI endometrial cancer who have not responded to platinum-based chemotherapy. The PD-1/PDL-1 complex is expressed on tumor-infiltrating immune cells of 60% to 80% of primary endometrial cancers and in 100% of metastatic endometrial cancer.[15] In a phase 2 trial in patients with colorectal cancer, an immune-related PFS rate of 78% was seen in patients with MMR-deficient cancer and 11% in patients with MMR-proficient cancer, thus showing that MMR status predicts the clinical benefit of pembrolizumab.[45]

In 2017, the multicenter, phase 1b, KEYNOTE-028 trial published their findings regarding the safety and efficacy of pembrolizumab in women with PDL-1-positive cervical cancer. In the trial, 24 women with metastatic or recurrent disease received pembrolizumab every 2 weeks for 24 months. The overall response rate was 17%, and median

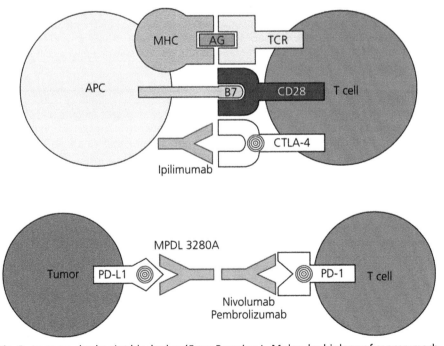

Fig. 3. Immune checkpoint blockades. (*From* Pecorino L. Molecular biology of cancer: mechanisms, targets, and therapeutics. 4th Ed. New York: Oxford University Press; 2016. By permission of Oxford University Press www.oup.com.)

duration of response was 5.4 months.[46] As a result of this trial, in June 2018, the FDA granted accelerated approval for pembrolizumab for patients with PDL-1 positive recurrent or metastatic cervical cancer with disease progression on or after chemotherapy.[47]

Nivolumab, an anti-PD-1 antibody, was shown to have activity in platinum-resistant ovarian cancer in a small phase 2 study. Twenty patients treated were seen to have a response rate of 15% with a disease control rate of 45%.[48] Avelumab, a monoclonal antibody to PD-L1, is being studied in a phase 2 fashion along with carboplatin and paclitaxel in advanced or recurrent endometrial cancer in the soon to be recruiting MITO-END 3 trial.[49]

Another immune checkpoint that may be exploited for immunotherapy is the cytotoxic T-lymphocyte associated protein 4 (CTLA-4), which negatively regulates T-cell effector responses. Ipilimumab is a monoclonal antibody that blocks the interaction between CTLA-4 and its ligands, thereby promoting antitumor responses through T-cell activation and tumor infiltration. It has been shown to be an active drug in melanoma and prostate cancer and is being studied in gynecologic cancer currently in combination with nivolumab.[50]

Finally, adoptive cell therapy, such as chimeric antigen receptor (CAR) T-cell treatment, is also under development in gynecologic cancer.[51] In this therapy, T cells are extracted from a patient's serum, and a CAR is added to the cell surface. This receptor is designed to recognize a specific tumor antigen and becomes activated when the CAR is bound to the cancer cell. Downstream signaling within the T cell then leads to immune cell activation and cytotoxic activity.

Toxicities

Systemic adverse events of fatigue (16%–24%) and infusion-related reactions (25%) are common for patients receiving immunotherapy (anti-PD-1 or anti-PD-L1 agents).[52] Additional side effects include skin and mucosal manifestations, GI effects (diarrhea/colitis), hepatotoxicity, pneumonitis, and thyroid dysfunction. Estimates of 30% to 40% of dermatologic complication have been reported with pembrolizumab.[53] Typically, diarrhea/colitis manifests 6 weeks into immunotherapy treatment with rates approximately 30%.[52] Although pneumonitis is rare, identification is important because it can be a potentially fatal complication. Thyroid function should be evaluated because incidence rates can range from 3.8% to 13.2%, based on the type of immunotherapy given.[54]

OTHER TARGETED THERAPIES

A phase 2 study of stage III/IV patients with uterine serous cancer demonstrated that trastuzumab, a monoclonal antibody to the HER2 receptor, when added to chemotherapy increased PFS for patients with advanced HER2/neu-positive uterine serous carcinoma to 12.6 months compared with 8.0 months if only chemotherapy was given.[55]

Mammalian target of rapamycin (mTOR) inhibitors have been used for recurrent epithelial ovarian cancer. mTOR is a serine/threonine kinase involved in protein synthesis.[56] Prior published studies have shown that the mTOR pathway is upregulated in cancers, and its inhibition may provide an effective strategy.[56–58] A vastly studied mTOR inhibitor is temsirolimus, which is involved in decreased expression of mRNAs essential for cell-cycle progression.[59] As a result, cells are arrested in the G1 phase of the cell cycle.[59] The GOG conducted a phase 2 trial evaluating temsirolimus in 60 patients with persistent/recurrent epithelial ovarian cancer.[56] Out of the 54 eligible patients, modest activity of temsirolimus was notable with 24% of patients progressing $\geq$6 months and 9.3% achieving partial response.[56] The common adverse events that were reported included fatigue and GI and metabolic abnormalities. However, the PFS was insufficient to justify further study in a phase 3 trial.[56] In 2016, the German Gynecological Oncology Group reported results of administering weekly temsirolimus 25 mg to both refractory/resistant ovarian cancer and advanced/recurrent endometrial carcinoma patients.[60,61] After 8 weeks of treatment, 4.5% achieved partial response and 31.8% reached stable disease.[61] Although there are preliminary phase 2 trials showing response to temsirolimus, there have been no reported mTOR inhibitor phase 3 trials in ovarian cancer.

Toxicities

Reported toxicities of mTOR inhibitors have involved hematologic effects, GI manifestations, respiratory symptoms, and kidney abnormalities. Specifically, anemia has been reported in 19% to 57% and thrombocytopenia in 8% to 30% of patients. The most common GI manifestations include constipation (28%–36%), diarrhea (25%–42%), nausea (25%–36%), and vomiting (19%–25%).[62]

SUMMARY

The development of drug resistance to standard chemotherapy leads to persistent and progressive disease in many patients with cancer. Expanding the understanding of the molecular signaling that cancer uses to promote reproduction and propagation is essential for developing novel therapy. The incorporation of next-generation sequencing to identify mutations unique to refractory cancers may potentially lead to matched targeted therapies. These targeted therapies, such as antiangiogenic agents, TKIs, PARP inhibitors, and immunotherapy agents, have been explored in gynecologic cancer and show various amounts of promise. Increasing knowledge in cancer biology will allow the development of new treatments tailored to a particular signaling pathway, while minimizing toxic side effects. The last decade has provided remarkable progress in therapeutic development in the field of Gynecologic Oncology and will lead to continued clinical improvements in the future.

REFERENCES

1. Pecorino L. Molecular biology of cancer: mechanisms, targets, and therapeutics. 3rd edition. Oxford (United Kingdom): Oxford University Press; 2012.
2. Shaw D, Clamp A, Jayson GC. Angiogenesis as a target for the treatment of ovarian cancer. Curr Opin Oncol 2013;25(5):558–65.
3. Perren TJ, Swart AM, Pfisterer J, et al. A phase 3 trial of bevacizumab in ovarian cancer. N Engl J Med 2011;365(26):2484–96.
4. Oza AM, Cook AD, Pfisterer J, et al. Standard chemotherapy with or without bevacizumab for women with newly diagnosed ovarian cancer (ICON7): overall survival results of a phase 3 randomised trial. Lancet Oncol 2015;16(8):928–36.
5. Burger RA, Brady MF, Bookman MA, et al. Incorporation of bevacizumab in the primary treatment of ovarian cancer. N Engl J Med 2011;365(26):2473–83.
6. Ferriss JS, Java JJ, Bookman MA, et al. Ascites predicts treatment benefit of bevacizumab in front-line therapy of advanced epithelial ovarian, fallopian tube and peritoneal cancers: an NRG Oncology/GOG study. Gynecol Oncol 2015;139(1): 17–22.
7. Numnum TM, Rocconi RP, Whitworth J, et al. The use of bevacizumab to palliate symptomatic ascites in patients with refractory ovarian carcinoma. Gynecol Oncol 2006;102(3):425–8.

8. Hamilton CA, Maxwell GL, Chernofsky MR, et al. Intraperitoneal bevacizumab for the palliation of malignant ascites in refractory ovarian cancer. Gynecol Oncol 2008;111(3):530–2.

9. FDA approves bevacizumab in combination with chemotherapy for ovarian cancer. US Food & Drug Administration; 2018. Available at: https://www.fda.gov/drugs/informationondrugs/approveddrugs/ucm610664.htm.

10. Aghajanian C, Blank SV, Goff BA, et al. OCEANS: a randomized, double-blind, placebo-controlled phase III trial of chemotherapy with or without bevacizumab in patients with platinum-sensitive recurrent epithelial ovarian, primary peritoneal, or fallopian tube cancer. J Clin Oncol 2012;30(17):2039–45.

11. Aghajanian C, Goff B, Nycum LR, et al. Final overall survival and safety analysis of OCEANS, a phase 3 trial of chemotherapy with or without bevacizumab in patients with platinum-sensitive recurrent ovarian cancer. Gynecol Oncol 2015; 139(1):10–6.

12. Coleman RL, Brady MF, Herzog TJ, et al. Bevacizumab and paclitaxel-carboplatin chemotherapy and secondary cytoreduction in recurrent, platinum-sensitive ovarian cancer (NRG Oncology/Gynecologic Oncology Group study GOG-0213): a multicentre, open-label, randomised, phase 3 trial. Lancet Oncol 2017;18(6):779–91.

13. Pujade-Lauraine E, Hilpert F, Weber B, et al. Bevacizumab combined with chemotherapy for platinum-resistant recurrent ovarian cancer: The AURELIA open-label randomized phase III trial. J Clin Oncol 2014;32(13):1302–8.

14. Tewari KS, Sill MW, Penson RT, et al. Bevacizumab for advanced cervical cancer: final overall survival and adverse event analysis of a randomised, controlled, open-label, phase 3 trial (Gynecologic Oncology Group 240). Lancet 2017; 390(10103):1654–63.

15. Makker V, Green AK, Wenham RM, et al. New therapies for advanced, recurrent, and metastatic endometrial cancers. Gynecol Oncol Res Pract 2017;4:19.

16. Aghajanian C, Sill MW, Darcy KM, et al. Phase II trial of bevacizumab in recurrent or persistent endometrial cancer: a Gynecologic Oncology Group study. J Clin Oncol 2011;29(16):2259–65.

17. Lorusso D, Ferrandina G, Colombo N, et al. Randomized phase II trial of carboplatin-paclitaxel (CP) compared to carboplatin-paclitaxel-bevacizumab (CP-B) in advanced (Stage III-IV) or recurrent endometrial cancer: MITO END-2 Trial. 2015 ASCO Annual Meeting. Chicago, May 29–June 2, 2015. [Abstract: 5502].

18. Colombo N, Mangili G, Mammoliti S, et al. A phase II study of aflibercept in patients with advanced epithelial ovarian cancer and symptomatic malignant ascites. Gynecol Oncol 2012;125(1):42–7.

19. Tew WP, Colombo N, Ray-Coquard I, et al. Intravenous aflibercept in patients with platinum-resistant, advanced ovarian cancer: results of a randomized, double-blind, phase 2, parallel-arm study. Cancer 2014;120(3):335–43.

20. Pembrolizumab and Ziv-aflibercept in treating patients with advanced solid tumors (NCT02298959). Available at: www.clinicaltrials.gov. Accessed November 1, 2018.

21. Monk BJ, Poveda A, Vergote I, et al. Final results of a phase 3 study of trebananib plus weekly paclitaxel in recurrent ovarian cancer (TRINOVA-1): long-term survival, impact of ascites, and progression-free survival-2. Gynecol Oncol 2016; 143(1):27–34.

22. Marth C, Vergote I, Scambia G, et al. ENGOT-ov-6/TRINOVA-2: randomised, double-blind, phase 3 study of pegylated liposomal doxorubicin plus trebananib

or placebo in women with recurrent partially platinum-sensitive or resistant ovarian cancer. Eur J Cancer 2017;70:111–21.

23. Arora A, Scholar EM. Role of tyrosine kinase inhibitors in cancer therapy. J Pharmacol Exp Ther 2005;315(3):971–9.

24. Floquet A, Vergote I, Colombo N, et al. Progression-free survival by local investigator versus independent central review: comparative analysis of the AGO-OVAR16 Trial. Gynecol Oncol 2015;136(1):37–42.

25. van der Graaf WT, Blay JY, Chawla SP, et al. Pazopanib for metastatic soft-tissue sarcoma (PALETTE): a randomised, double-blind, placebo-controlled phase 3 trial. Lancet 2012;379(9829):1879–86.

26. Heudel P, Cassier P, Derbel O, et al. Pazopanib for the treatment of soft-tissue sarcoma. Clin Pharm 2012;4:65–70.

27. du Bois A, Kristensen G, Ray-Coquard I, et al. Standard first-line chemotherapy with or without nintedanib for advanced ovarian cancer (AGO-OVAR 12): a randomised, double-blind, placebo-controlled phase 3 trial. Lancet Oncol 2016;17(1):78–89.

28. Bender D, Sill MW, Lankes HA, et al. A phase II evaluation of cediranib in the treatment of recurrent or persistent endometrial cancer: an NRG Oncology/Gynecologic Oncology Group study. Gynecol Oncol 2015;138(3):507–12.

29. Ledermann JA, Embleton AC, Raja F, et al. Cediranib in patients with relapsed platinum-sensitive ovarian cancer (ICON6): a randomised, double-blind, placebo-controlled phase 3 trial. Lancet 2016;387(10023):1066–74.

30. Kaufman B, Shapira-Frommer R, Schmutzler RK, et al. Olaparib monotherapy in patients with advanced cancer and a germline BRCA1/2 mutation. J Clin Oncol 2015;33(3):244–50.

31. Ledermann J, Harter P, Gourley C, et al. Olaparib maintenance therapy in platinum-sensitive relapsed ovarian cancer. N Engl J Med 2012;366(15):1382–92.

32. Pujade-Lauraine E, Ledermann JA, Selle F, et al. Olaparib tablets as maintenance therapy in patients with platinum-sensitive, relapsed ovarian cancer and a BRCA1/2 mutation (SOLO2/ENGOT-Ov21): a double-blind, randomised, placebo-controlled, phase 3 trial. Lancet Oncol 2017;18(9):1274–84.

33. Swisher EM, Lin KK, Oza AM, et al. Rucaparib in relapsed, platinum-sensitive high-grade ovarian carcinoma (ARIEL2 Part 1): an international, multicentre, open-label, phase 2 trial. Lancet Oncol 2017;18(1):75–87.

34. Coleman RL, Oza AM, Lorusso D, et al. Rucaparib maintenance treatment for recurrent ovarian carcinoma after response to platinum therapy (ARIEL3): a randomised, double-blind, placebo-controlled, phase 3 trial. Lancet 2017; 390(10106):1949–61.

35. Mirza MR, Monk BJ, Herrstedt J, et al. Niraparib maintenance therapy in platinum-sensitive, recurrent ovarian cancer. N Engl J Med 2016;375(22): 2154–64.

36. Sabatucci I, Maltese G, Lepori S, et al. Rucaparib: a new treatment option for ovarian cancer. Expert Opin Pharmacother 2018;19(7):765–71.

37. Liu AY, Cohen JG, Walsh CS, et al. A cost-effectiveness analysis of three PARP inhibitors for maintenance therapy in platinum-sensitive recurrent ovarian cancer. Gynecol Oncol 2017;147(1):196.

38. Schreiber RD, Old LJ, Smyth MJ. Cancer immunoediting: integrating immunity's roles in cancer suppression and promotion. Science 2011;331(6024):1565–70.

39. Shoushtari AN, WJ, Hellman M. Principles of cancer immunotherapy. 2018. Available at: https://www.uptodate.com/contents/principles-of-cancer-immunotherapy. Accessed February 18, 2018.

40. Johnsen AK, Templeton DJ, Sy M, et al. Deficiency of transporter for antigen presentation (TAP) in tumor cells allows evasion of immune surveillance and increases tumorigenesis. J Immunol 1999;163(8):4224–31.

41. Donia M, Andersen R, Kjeldsen JW, et al. Aberrant expression of MHC Class II in melanoma attracts inflammatory tumor-specific CD4+ T- cells, which dampen CD8+ T-cell antitumor reactivity. Cancer Res 2015;75(18):3747–59.

42. Guo F, Wang Y, Liu J, et al. CXCL12/CXCR4: a symbiotic bridge linking cancer cells and their stromal neighbors in oncogenic communication networks. Oncogene 2016;35(7):816–26.

43. Tumeh PC, Harview CL, Yearley JH, et al. PD-1 blockade induces responses by inhibiting adaptive immune resistance. Nature 2014;515(7528):568–71.

44. Udall M, Rizzo M, Kenny J, et al. PD-L1 diagnostic tests: a systematic literature review of scoring algorithms and test-validation metrics. Diagn Pathol 2018; 13(1):12.

45. Le DT, Uram JN, Wang H, et al. PD-1 blockade in tumors with mismatch-repair deficiency. N Engl J Med 2015;372(26):2509–20.

46. Frenel JS, Le Tourneau C, O'Neil B, et al. Safety and efficacy of pembrolizumab in advanced, programmed death ligand 1-positive cervical cancer: results from the phase Ib KEYNOTE-028 trial. J Clin Oncol 2017;35(36):4035–41.

47. FDA approves pembrolizumab for advanced cervical cancer with disease progression during or after chemotherapy. 2018. Available at: https://www.fda.gov/drugs/informationondrugs/approveddrugs/ucm610572.htm. Accessed November 1, 2018.

48. Hamanishi JM, Mandai M, Ikeda T. et al. Efficacy and safety of anti-PD-1 antibody (Nivolumab:BMS-936558,ONO-4538) in patients with platinum-resistant ovarian cancer. 2014 ASCO Annual Meeting. Chicago, May 30–June 2, 2014. [Abstract: 5511].

49. Carboplatin, paclitaxel with or without avelumab in advanced or recurrent endometrial cancer (MITO END-3) (NCT03503786). Available at: www.clinicaltrials.gov. Accessed June 1, 2018.

50. Combination of nivolumab and ipilimumab in breast, ovarian and gastric cancer patients (NCT03342417). 2017. Available at: www.clinicaltrials.gov. Accessed June 1, 2018.

51. Zhu X, Cai H, Zhao L, et al. CAR-T cell therapy in ovarian cancer: from the bench to the bedside. Oncotarget 2017;8(38):64607–21.

52. Hodi FS, O'Day SJ, McDermott DF, et al. Improved survival with ipilimumab in patients with metastatic melanoma. N Engl J Med 2010;363(8):711–23.

53. Naidoo J, Page DB, Li BT, et al. Toxicities of the anti-PD-1 and anti-PD-L1 immune checkpoint antibodies. Ann Oncol 2015;26(12):2375–91.

54. Barroso-Sousa R, Barry WT, Garrido-Castro AC, et al. Incidence of endocrine dysfunction following the use of different immune checkpoint inhibitor regimens: a systematic review and meta-analysis. JAMA Oncol 2018;4(2):173–82.

55. Fader AN, Roque DM, Siegel E, et al. Randomized phase II trial of carboplatin-paclitaxel versus carboplatin-paclitaxel-trastuzumab in uterine serous carcinomas that overexpress human epidermal growth factor receptor 2/neu. J Clin Oncol 2018;36(20):2044–51.

56. Behbakht K, Sill MW, Darcy KM, et al. Phase II trial of the mTOR inhibitor, temsirolimus and evaluation of circulating tumor cells and tumor biomarkers in persistent and recurrent epithelial ovarian and primary peritoneal malignancies: a Gynecologic Oncology Group study. Gynecol Oncol 2011;123(1):19–26.

57. Yuan R, Kay A, Berg WJ, et al. Targeting tumorigenesis: development and use of mTOR inhibitors in cancer therapy. J Hematol Oncol 2009;2:45.

58. Mabuchi S, Kawase C, Altomare DA, et al. mTOR is a promising therapeutic target both in cisplatin-sensitive and cisplatin-resistant clear cell carcinoma of the ovary. Clin Cancer Res 2009;15(17):5404–13.

59. Benoit MF, Williams-Brown MY, Edwards CL. Gynecologic oncology handbook: an evidence based clinical guide. 2nd edition. New York: Springer Publishing Company; 2018.

60. Gasparri ML, Bardhi E, Ruscito I, et al. PI3K/AKT/mTOR pathway in ovarian cancer treatment: are we on the right track? Geburtshilfe Frauenheilkd 2017;77(10): 1095–103.

61. Emons G, Kurzeder C, Schmalfeldt B, et al. Temsirolimus in women with platinum-refractory/resistant ovarian cancer or advanced/recurrent endometrial carcinoma. A phase II study of the AGO-study group (AGO-GYN8). Gynecol Oncol 2016;140(3):450–6.

62. Euvrard S, Morelon E, Rostaing L, et al. Sirolimus and secondary skin-cancer prevention in kidney transplantation. N Engl J Med 2012;367(4):329–39.

63. Cannistra SA, Matulonis UA, Penson RT, et al. Phase II study of bevacizumab in patients with platinum-resistant ovarian cancer or peritoneal serous cancer. J Clin Oncol 2008;26(10):1773.

Personalized Medicine in Gynecologic Cancer
Fact or Fiction?

Logan Corey, MD[a],*, Ana Valente, MD[a,1], Katrina Wade, MD[b]

KEYWORDS

- Personalized medicine • Precision medicine • Targeted therapies
- Gynecologic malignancies

KEY POINTS

- Personalized medicine is an evolving concept that centers around treating cancers based on tumor molecular profiling rather than location of origin.
- Tumor molecular profiling has allowed for several driver mutations to be identified in gynecologic malignancies and subsequent targeted therapies to be created.
- With direct to consumer marketing, patient demand for personalized medicine is increasing.

INTRODUCTION TO PERSONALIZED MEDICINE

Personalized medicine, also known as "precision medicine," is the science of individualizing cancer care by treating tumors based on their genetic makeup rather than their location of origin.[1] Both gene expressional profiling and genome-wide sequencing have played significant roles in making this possible.[2] Knowing a tumor's molecular sequence has allowed for creation of targeted therapies. Examples of current successful oncologic therapies include BRAF inhibitors (vemurafenib) used in melanoma treatment, RET inhibitors (sorafenib) used in advanced renal and hepatocellular carcinomas, and epidermal growth factor receptor or anaplastic lymphoma kinase inhibitors used in non–small-cell lung cancer.[3]

In gynecologic oncology, the application of personalized medicine is still a work in progress. Genetic offenders or "driver mutations" have been identified in ovarian cancer (BRCA mutations, NOTCH, P13 K, BRAS/MEK, FOX 1, p53),

Disclosure Statement: The authors have nothing to disclose.
[a] Department of Obstetrics and Gynecology, Ochsner Clinic Foundation, 2700 Napoleon Avenue, New Orleans, LA 70115, USA; [b] Department of Gynecologic Oncology, Ochsner Clinic Foundation, 2700 Napoleon Avenue, New Orleans, LA 70115, USA
[1] Present address: 1520 Saint Mary Street, Unit D, New Orleans, LA 70130.
* Corresponding author. 209 North Dupre Street, New Orleans, LA 70118.
E-mail address: logan.corey@ochsner.org

endometrial cancer (TP53, PTEN, P1K3CA, and KRAS) and cervical cancers (P1K3CA, TP53, RB1).[1] Therapies that target these molecules are being developed and are effective by various mechanisms, including interruption of tumor cell stroma, vasculature, and aberrant signaling mechanisms.[4] Several of these mutations and therapies and their use and challenges are discussed in this article, as we explore the intricacies of personalized medicine in gynecologic malignancy: is it fact or fiction?

DRIVER MUTATIONS

Oncogenic mutations belong to 1 of 2 groups of proteins: oncogenes or tumor suppressor genes. Mutations to oncogenes cause cancer growth, whereas mutations to tumor suppressor genes cause failure of inhibition of cell growth, and therefore indirectly lead to cancer. These oncogenic mutations are known as "driver mutations." Individual oncogenes also contain genetic alterations such as substitutions, insertions, deletions, rearrangements, and loss of heterozygosity. These "passenger mutations" are mutations that are commonly associated with driver mutations that do not themselves cause cancer. Interestingly, there is recent evidence proposed that passenger mutations in cumulative may not be benign bystanders within or around cancer genes and can be harmful to cancer cells.[5]

Identification of driver mutations is of interest because it stands to reason that if either type of driver mutations could be identified and countered, the cancer would be cured or slowed. Successes in such endeavors in other oncology subspecialties, for example, use of the Philadelphia mutation as a target and the use of imatinib in the treatment of chronic myelogenous leukemia, have encouraged expansion of this body of work into other fields including gynecology oncology.[6] Furthermore, the relatively recent capability of researchers to sequence entire cancer genomes in a cost-effective way has allowed for a rapid broadening of the search for driver mutations and the exploration of their utility as possible targets in cancer treatment. Strategies include prediction of function models, machine learning models, and models that are based on the difference in mutation frequencies between driver and passenger mutations.[7] Tumor suppressor genes are generally more difficult to identify as driver mutations than oncogenes. It is much simpler to insert an oncogene into a cell line and evaluate for cancer growth than it is to remove a tumor suppressor gene from a cell line and monitor for cancer growth (ie, knockout models). Occasionally, a single cancer will have multiple driver mutations. This is consistent with the suggestion that some common cancers are thought to require 5 to 7 rate-limiting events on the way to becoming cancerous.[8]

Other ways of identifying driver mutations involve looking for similar mutations in cancers that are present at increased frequency relative to the background genome. This was demonstrated in a large study by the Cancer Genome Atlas that examined more than 400 high-grade serous ovarian adenocarcinomas that used the previous method and found more than 96% of these tumors were characterized by p53 mutations. Additional mutations were identified by cross-referencing other databases. Multiple other mutations were found in most of the tumors along with the p53 mutations, including mutations in *BRAF* (N581S), *PIK3CA* (E545 K and H1047 R), *KRAS* (G12D), and *NRAS* (Q61 R).[8]

Isolating driver mutations in gynecologic cancer has proven difficult. This is most likely due to the complexity and ubiquitous nature of the pathways involved. Multiple pathways are of intense interest at the moment and seem to play a role in development of other cancer types including breast, gastrointestinal, and lung cancers.

TUMOR HETEROGENEITY

Tumor heterogeneity is one of the greatest challenges in the era of personalized medicine. Although studies such as The Cancer Genome Atlas Project (TCGA) and the NCI-Match have helped in our understanding of the molecular basis of gynecologic cancers, they have also highlighted both intertumor and intratumor heterogeneity.[9,10] Intratumor heterogeneity is the concept that multiple biopsies of a single tumor may contain genetic variation and multiple subclonal populations. Studies have highlighted that such extreme molecular diversity can exist in solid tumor biopsies, even when they are collected from the same patient.[11] Whole genome and whole exosome studies have also highlighted genomic heterogeneity during transition from primary tumor to recurrence to metastasis.[12] This presents a unique challenge, especially in attempts to identify curative treatment for advanced disease.[13]

CURRENT TARGETED THERAPIES
Antiangiogenic Therapies

Angiogenesis, or the creation of new vascular supply, plays a key role in successful tumorigenesis. It is a process driven by vascular endothelial growth factor (VEGF). Overexpression of VEGF leads to increased blood supply and subsequent increase in delivery of nutrients and oxygen to tumor beds.[14] Antiangiogenesis therapies target and inhibit VEGF. Bevacizumab is the most studied antiangiogenic agent used in gynecologic cancer treatment.[1] It is a recombinant monoclonal antibody and is the only antiangiogenic therapy approved by the Food and Drug Administration (FDA).[15] Several clinical trials have investigated bevacizumab and demonstrated its efficacy in the treatment of ovarian cancer,[16,17] although overall survival benefit is seen only when bevacizumab is used in combination with standard cytotoxic chemo and then followed by bevacizumab maintenance.[18] In addition, the GOG240 has shown improved progression-free and overall survival when bevacizumab is added to standard chemotherapy in advanced or recurrent cervical cancer.[19]

Poly-ADP-Ribose Polymerase Inhibitors

Poly-ADP-ribose polymerase (PARP) inhibitors are agents that interfere with DNA damage repair. Typically, PARP repairs single-strand DNA breaks.[20] If single-strand DNA breaks are unable to be repaired due to PARP inhibition and accumulate, the DNA replication fork is stalled. In this situation, the cell must rely on double-strand break repair (via the homologous recombination [HR] pathway) to be able to survive, a mechanism that is notoriously absent in BRCA-mutated cells.[1,20] This leads to BRCA-deficient cells being incredibly vulnerable to PARP inhibitors and likewise confers their sensitivity to platinum as HR is required to repair platinum-induced intrastrand and interstrand DNA cross links. Several clinical studies have confirmed PARP inhibitors are effective,[21,22] and have shown significant increase in progression-free survival with their use.[23] Currently, 3 PARP inhibitors are FDA approved: olaparib, rucaparib, and niraparib. The study of PARP inhibitors is still currently under way and the future holds promise that they will not only be reserved for patients with BRCA mutations but may also be used in patients whose tumors have functional defects in other DNA repair proteins.[14]

PHOSPHATIDYL INOSITOL 3-KINASE/AKT/MAMMALIAN TARGET OF RAPAMYCIN/ PHOSPHATASE AND TENSIN HOMOLOG

The phosphatidyl inositol 3-kinase (PI3K)/AKT/mammalian target of rapamycin (mTOR) pathway plays a critical role in the malignant transformation of human tumors and their subsequent growth, proliferation, and metastasis, including ovarian cancers.[24] Characteristic of cell cycle control pathways, there is a normal balance to the activators and inhibitors within these complex pathways and the PI3K/AKT/ mTOR pathway is no different. These interactions are currently being studied for their theoretic druggable and targetable proteins. At the most basic level, the checks and balances are summarized as the following.

Activated PI3K leads to downstream effects to activate AKT. Then AKT can directly activate mTORC1 or indirectly through phosphorylating Tuberin, which inhibits TSC1/TSC2 complex, which itself is an inhibitor of mTORC1. Activated mTORC1 leads to downstream effects encoding ribosomal proteins, elongation factors, and other proteins required for transition from G1 phase to S phase of cell cycle. Phosphatase and tensin homolog (PTEN) has a role to play in this pathway as a tumor suppressor. PTEN is a negative regulator of the PI3K-dependent AKT signaling and acts as an antagonist of phosphorylation of PIP2 to PIP3.[25]

The understanding of this pathway lends to understanding the separation of targets into 4 main categories: mTOR inhibitors, PI3K inhibitors, dual mTOR/PI3K inhibitors, and AKT inhibitors. Many phase 1 and phase 2 trials are being undertaken with the modest success. A phase III trial by GOG 170-I showed higher response rate to temsirolimus in patients with tumors that exhibited mTOR activity than patients with tumors without mTOR activity. Unfortunately, there seems to be possibility for resistance to inhibitors of the PI3K/AKT/mTOR pathway. The mechanism is unknown but speculated to involve loss of negative feedback loops normally induced when the pathway is active. Proposed mechanisms for combating this is combining these inhibitors with other agents that inhibit at different points of the pathway (**Fig. 1**).[24]

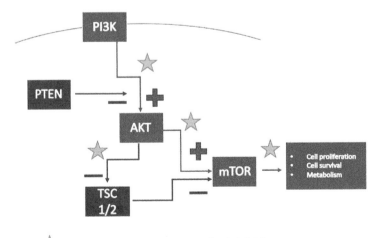

⭐ = Possible pathway targets for inhibition

Fig. 1. Simplified PI3K/AKT/mTOR pathway and possible points for inhibition.

Last, loss of function of PTEN has been detected in ovarian cancer as well as other cancers (eg, Cowden syndrome). This is of interest in PI3K/AKT/mTOR pathway because it is believed the ovarian cancer in PTEN knockout mouse models is caused through loss of inhibition of this pathway. Thus, inhibitors of PI3K/AKT/mTOR pathway may be beneficial as chemoprevention in selected patients with known PTEN mutations. It is especially hard to characterize the exact role of PTEN mutations in oncogenesis, as the protein acts in the cytoplasm as well as nucleus, and is also suspected to have antitumor effects by maintaining chromosomal stability, DNA double-strand break repair, and maintaining genome integrity.[26]

Consumer Marketing

The idea of personalized medicine began branching into the consumer market in the mid-2000s (DTC or Direct to Consumer). With the availability of high-throughput genomic sequencing, the price of testing an individual's genomic makeup reached a level affordable to the single consumer. Most of these tests are as simple as buccal or salivary swabs that are sent through the mail to the commercial laboratory. These private genetic laboratories offer testing for simple single-gene disorders (eg, cystic fibrosis) as well as pharmacogenomic tests to individualize drug treatment, including guidance for specific mutation-targeted treatment decisions for patients with cancers. They also include predictive genomic testing for complex disorders and traits such as hypertension and osteoporosis.[27] DTC marketing has become a popular among patients of all fields of medicine and the number of consumers of 23andMe and other similar DTC tests was more than 12 million in 2017. Most pertinent to our field, in March of 2018, the FDA authorized agencies to tell consumers whether they possess 1 of 3 germline mutations in the BRCA1 and BRCA2 genes.[28] **Table 1** lists just a few of the commercially available tumor sequencing assays.

Understanding and knowing BRCA1 and BRCA2 mutations, along with DNA mismatch repair genes of other hereditary cancer syndromes (eg, MLH1, MSH2,

Table 1
Examples of commercially available tumor gene sequencing tests

Tumor Test/Manufacturer	Targets Tested	Tissue	FDA Approval
FD1CDx	BRCA 1/2	Ovary	Yes
MSK-IMPACT	Varied, entire gene sequencing	Multiple	Yes[a]
SOLiD	Varied, entire gene sequencing	Multiple	Yes
Oncomine Dx Target Test	EGFR, BRAF, and ROS1	Lung	Yes
PathVysion	Her2/neu	Breast	Yes
PharmDx	Her2/neu	Breast	Yes
INFORM	Her2/neu	Breast	Yes
Dako	PD-L1	Lung	Yes
MI Profile	Many	Colon, lung	Yes
Solid Tumor Mutation Panel	Many	Multiple	Yes
SmartGenomics	Many	Multiple	Yes
Pervenio Lung NGS Assay	Many	Lung	Yes

Abbreviations: EGFR, epidermal growth factor receptor; FDA, Food and Drug Administration.
[a] Only at Sloan Kettering Memorial.

MSH6, and PMS2) presents significant opportunities in the treatment and prevention of some gynecologic cancers, including Lynch and Cowden, for example. This information can lead to alterations in screening and treatment plans. However, the availability of large population testing of these syndromes due to the DTC genetic testing leads to the idea that in general, the more genes tested, the more nonspecific the results, and the more variants of unknown significance will be found. Genetic counselors are a strained and poorly used source by the users of these genetic testing services. In one study, only 4% reported getting genetic counseling after receiving their genetic sequencing results, and 38% would have seen genetic counseling if one had been available. The risks of testing include increased anxiety or depression from positive results, uncertainty over inconclusive results, financial costs of testing, and difficulty navigating landscape of available testing modalities. Benefits of DTC genomic testing are narrow at this point, but by all accounts have a bright future. Current known benefits include more personalized prognosis, enhanced risk assessment, and improved triage to targeted therapies, such as using PARP inhibitors for BRCA carriers.

Treatment of gynecologic cancer with proprietary drugs, specific cancer therapies, and even specific hospital systems, is also affected by consumer directed advertisers. This is known as cancer related-direct to consumer advertisement (CR-DTCA).[29] CR-DTCA is particularly at risk for not clearly explaining costs, toxicity, and alternatives to patients as demonstrated in a retrospective review of warning letters sent by the FDA for not being fair and balanced, with the most (22%) being sent to CR-DTCA companies. Cancer therapy advertisement has the potential for wide-ranging affects including influencing treatment decisions and affecting the physician-patient relationship. In addition, gynecologic cancer presents challenges for clear information from advertisers to patients and oncologists, as within one general type of cancer (eg, ovarian cancer) there may be multiple potential targets, none of which seem to be singularly better than the other. This is in contrast to other cancers (eg, imatinib in patients with chronic myeloid leukemia with Philadelphia mutation) that have clear and successful treatment targets.

Overall, DTC affects oncologists as much or even more compared with other fields of medicine. Acceptance of the technology allowing for patient-obtained genetic information is necessary to help guide the conversation and inform patients and it would be "futile to try to reverse the course and reduce patients' access."[27] Personalized genetic sequencing tools currently have a role in BRCA and other DNA repair gene identification and can help with risk prediction as well as guide potential roles of chemoprevention. Expansion to more known genetic causes of gynecologic cancers, such as PTEN gene mutations and other homologous recombination-deficient genes, should be future goals of these sequencing tools.

The limiting factor in the usefulness of genetic sequencing tools seems to be with interpretation of the information for the consumers as well as the physicians. This is largely driven by lack of access to genetic counselors. Telemedicine, video chats, or requiring genetic counseling to be offered with the DTC genomic sequencing products may help increase access. Last, CR-DTCA seems to be more susceptible to bias information from marketers than other medical fields. The FDA is already monitoring advertisers but more scrutiny may be required in the future to ensure fair and balanced understanding of cancer therapies advertised to the general public.

PERSONALIZED TUMOR VACCINES

Personalized tumor vaccination is an aspect of treatment in gynecologic malignancies that has come in to play in recent years as we have gained knowledge that tumors may be largely immunogenic. Several studies have highlighted that host antitumor immune response plays a significant role in patient outcomes.[30,31] In ovarian cancer, the presence of tumor infiltrating lymphocytes (TILs) has been associated with increased progression-free survival and overall survival in patients with advanced disease.[30] Specifically, presence of CD-8 TILs has been found to correlate with survival in all stages and histologic types of ovary cancer.

Ovarian cancers are known to express tumor antigens that can serve as targets for peptide vaccination.[32] Peptide vaccinations are designed to target a variety of these antigens including NY-ESO-1, p53, WT-1, HER-2, and VEGF. They are often coadministered with GM-CSF to enhance immune response.[33,34] Whole tumor antigen vaccination is another option in personalized tumor vaccine development that provides for a wider range of tumor antigens.[35]

Dendritic cells (DCs) play a key role in development of cancer vaccination, as they serve as very potent antigen-presenting cells. We have seen in vitro that exposure of T cells to DCs pulsed with ovarian cancer antigens has resulted in the capability to kill autologous tumor cells.[36] Recently, a pilot clinical trial testing a personalized vaccine created by autologous DCs pulsed with oxidized autologous whole tumor lysate found personalized vaccination to induce T-cell response to autologous tumor antigen and increase survival.[37]

SUMMARY

In conclusion, personalized medicine in gynecologic oncology remains an evolving science. In recent years, the rapid advances in identification of the molecular drivers of gynecologic malignancies and the promise of targeted therapies have led to great enthusiasm. Although some of these therapies have been shown to have significant impact on outcomes (ie, PARP inhibitors in BRCA-mutated patients), others are still in need of additional research to identify when pathways may be most vulnerable to specific treatments (ie, PI3K in endometrial cancer). Tumor heterogeneity and tumor resistance contribute to the complexity of developing effective personalized therapies, as several studies have highlighted that tumor sampling may vary even among the same patient. We must continue to dedicate clinical research efforts to understanding how targeted therapies will be most applicable to patient care, especially as genetic testing becomes more available to patients through DTC markets.

REFERENCES

1. Barroilhet L, Matulonis U. The NCI-MATCH trial and precision medicine in gynecologic malignancy. Gynecol Oncol 2018;148(3):585–90.
2. Wiener C. Harrison's principles of internal medicine. New York: McGraw-Hill, Medical Pub. Division; 2008.
3. Coyne GO, Takebe N, Chen AP. Defining precision: the precision medicine initiative trials NCI-IMPACT and NCI-match. Curr Probl Cancer 2017;41(3):182–93.
4. Horwitz N, Matulonis U. New biologic agents for the treatment of gynecologic cancers. Hematol Oncol Clin North Am 2012;26:133–56.
5. McFarland CD, Korolev KS, Kryukov GV, et al. Impact of deleterious passenger mutations on cancer progression. Proc Natl Acad Sci U S A 2013;110(8):2910–5.
6. Druker BJ. Translation of the Philadelphia chromosome into therapy for CML. Blood 2008;112(13):4808–17.
7. Zhang J, Liu J, Sun J, et al. Identifying driver mutations from sequencing data of heterogeneous tumors in the era of personalized genome sequencing. Brief Bioinform 2014;15(2):244–55.

8. Michael S. The cancer genome. Nature 2009;458:719–24.

9. Getz G, Gabriel SB, Cibulskis K, et al. Integrated genomic characterization of endometrial carcinoma. Nature 2013;497(7447):67–73.

10. Integrated genomic analysis of ovarian carcinoma. Nature 2011;474(7573): 609–15.

11. Bashashati A, Ha G, Tone A. Distinct evolutionary trajectories of primary high-grade serous ovarian cancers revealed through spatial mutational profiling. J Pathol 2013;231(1):21–34.

12. Rodda E, Chapman J. Genomic insights in gynecologic cancer. Curr Probl Cancer 2017;41:8–36.

13. Testa U, Petrucci E, Pasquinin L, et al. Ovarian cancers: genetic abnormalities, tumor heterogeneity and progression, clonal evolution and cancer stem cells. Medicines (Basel) 2018;5(1) [pii:E16].

14. Berek J, Hacker N. Gynecologic oncology. 6th edition. Philadelphia: Lippincott Williams & Wilkins; 2014.

15. Liu J, Matulonis U. New strategies in ovarian cancer: translating the molecular complexity of ovarian cancer into treatment advances. Clin Cancer Res 2014; 20(20):5150–6.

16. Aghajanian C, Blank SV, Goff B, et al. OCEANS: a randomized, double blind, placebo-controlled phase III trial of chemotherapy with or without bevacizumab in patients with platinum sensitive recurrent epithelial ovarian, primary peritoneal or fallopian tube cancer. J Clin Oncol 2012;30(17):2039–45.

17. Pujade-Lauraine E, Hilpert F, Weber N, et al. Bevacizumab combined with chemotherapy for platinum resistant recurrent ovarian cancer: the AURELIA open-label randomized phase III trial. J Clin Oncol 2014;32(13):1302–8.

18. Coleman R, Brady M, Herzog T. Bevacizumab and paclitaxel-carboplatin chemo-therapy and secondary cytoreduction in recurrent, platinum-sensitive ovarian cancer (MRG Oncology/Gynecologic Oncology Group study GOG-0213): a mul-ticentre, open label randomized phase 3 trial. Lancet Oncol 2017;18(6):779–91.

19. Tewari K, Sill M, Long H, et al. Improved survival with bevacizumab in advanced cervical cancer. N Engl J Med 2014;370(8):734–43.

20. Liu J, Westin S. Rational selection of biomarker driver therapies for gynecologic cancers: the more we know, the more we know we don't know. Gyncol Oncol 2016;141:65–71.

21. Audeh M, Carmichael K, Penson R, et al. Oral poly(ADP-ribose) polymerase in-hibitor olaparib in patients with BRCA 1 or BRCA2 mutations and recurrent ovarian cancer: a proof of concept trial. Lancet 2010;376(9737):245–51.

22. Coleman R, sill M, Bell K, et al. A phase II evaluation of the potent highly selective PARP inhibitor veliparib in the treatment of persistent or recurrent epithelial ovarian, fallopian tube or primary peritoneal cancer in patients who carry germ-line BRCA 1 or 2 mutation. An NRG Oncology/Gynecologic Oncology Group study. Gynecol Oncol 2015;137(3):386–91.

23. Oza AM, Cibula D, Oaknin A, et al. Olaparib plus paclitaxel and carboplatin (P/C) followed by olaparib maintenance treatment in patients (pts) with platinum-sensitive recurrent serous ovarian cancer (PSR SOC): a randomized, open-label phase II study [abstract]. J Clin Oncol 2012;30(Suppl):a5001.

24. Mabuchi S. The PI3K/AKT/mTOR pathway as a therapeutic target in ovarian can-cer. Gynecol Oncol 2015;137(1):173–9.

25. Haddadi N, Lin Y, Travis G, et al. PTEN/PTENP1: 'regulating the regulator of the RTK-dependent PI3K/Akt signalling', new targets for cancer therapy. Mol Cancer 2018;17(1):37.

26. Patrinos GP, Baker DJ, Al-Mulla F, et al. Genetic tests obtainable through pharmacies: the good, the bad, and the ugly. Hum Genomics 2013;7(1):17.
27. Storrs C. Patients armed with their own genetic data raise tough questions. Health Aff 2018;37:690–3.
28. Schnipper LE, Abel GA. Direct-to-consumer drug advertising in oncology is not beneficial to patients or public health. JAMA Oncol 2016;2(11):1397–8.
29. Kim H. Trouble spots in online direct-to-consumer prescription drug promotion: a content analysis of FDA warning letters. Int J Health Policy Manag 2015;4(12): 813–21.
30. Zhang L, Conejo-Garcia JR, Katsaros D, et al. Intratumoral T cells, recurrence, and survival in epithelial ovarian cancer. N Engl J Med 2003;348:203–13.
31. Adams SF, Levine DA, Cadungog MG, et al. Intraepithelial T cells and tumor proliferation: impact on the benefit from surgical cytoreduction in advanced serous ovarian cancer. Cancer 2009;115:2891–902.
32. Chu CS, Kim SH, June CH, et al. Immunotherapy opportunities in ovarian cancer. Expert Rev Anticancer Ther 2008;8:243–57.
33. Mantia-Smaldone G, Corr B, Chu CS, et al. Immunotherapy in ovarian cancer. Hum Vaccin Immunother 2012;8(9):1179–91.
34. Odunsi K, Qian F, Matsuzaki J, et al. Vaccination with an NY-ESO-1 peptide of HLA class I/II specificities induces integrated humoral and T cell responses in ovarian cancer. Proc Natl Acad Sci U S A 2007;104:12837–42.
35. Chiang CL, Kandalaft LE, Coukos G. Adjuvants for enhancing the immunogenicity of whole tumor cell vaccines. Int Rev Immunol 2011;30:150–82.
36. Santin AD, Hermonat PL, Ravaggi A, et al. In vitro induction of tumor-specific human lymphocyte antigen class I-restricted CD8 cytotoxic T lymphocytes by ovarian tumor antigen-pulsed autologous dendritic cells from patients with advanced ovarian cancer. Am J Obstet Gynecol 2000;183:601–9.
37. Tanyi JL, Bobisse S, Ophir E, et al. Personal cancer vaccine effectively mobilizes antitumor T cell immunity in ovarian cancer. Sci Transl Med 2018;10(436) [pii: eaao5931].

Gynecologic Cancer Survivorship

Elizabeth Lokich, MD

KEYWORDS

- Gynecologic cancer • Cancer survivorship • Quality of life • Surveillance
- Sexual health

KEY POINTS

- Cancer- and treatment-related effects in cancer survivors often include fatigue, cognitive impairment, neuropathy, lymphedema, psychological distress, menopausal symptoms, sexual dysfunction, and infertility.
- Surveillance for gynecologic cancer should be tailored based on stage and recurrence risk.
- Coordination of care following treatment is important.

OVERVIEW OF SURVIVORSHIP

Any woman diagnosed with cancer is considered a cancer survivor from the time of diagnosis through the rest of her life. Cancer survivorship includes the period of initial treatment, cancer-free survival, chronic or intermittent disease, and end of life care.[1]

In the United States, there are more than 1 million survivors of gynecologic malignancies, making up 10% of all cancer survivors.[2] The number of gynecologic cancer survivors is expected to increase by at least 33% over the next decade and addressing the needs of these women is a crucial part of cancer care.[3] In addition, women who have been diagnosed with a gynecologic cancer may face some unique challenges that should be addressed, including hormonal changes, sexual function, negative body image, and infertility.

The 2005 Institute of Medicine (IOM) report "From Cancer Patient to Cancer Survivor: Lost in Translation" addresses some of the particular needs and challenges for patients related to the effects of both cancer and treatment.[4] This report divides the components of survivorship care into 4 categories:

1. Prevention of new and recurrent cancer,
2. Surveillance for cancer spread or recurrence,

The author has no financial or commercial conflicts of interest.

Division of Gynecologic Oncology, Women and Infants Hospital, Warren Alpert Medical School at Brown University, 101 Dudley Street, Providence, RI 02905, USA

E-mail address: elokich@wihri.org

Obstet Gynecol Clin N Am 46 (2019) 165–178
https://doi.org/10.1016/j.ogc.2018.10.002
0889-8545/19/© 2018 Elsevier Inc. All rights reserved.

3. Evaluation of cancer and treatment side effects, and
4. Coordination of follow-up.[4]

This article addresses all 4 of these domains.

PREVENTION, RECURRENCE, AND SURVEILLANCE
Posttreatment Surveillance

Surveillance for recurrence is an important aspect of survivorship care. Surveillance should include practices that influence survival and are cost-effective. Surveillance practices are useful when there is effective treatment for recurrence and when monitoring for disease recurrence decreases treatment- and disease-related morbidity.[5] Patients also need to understand the potential benefits, limitations, and risks of surveillance including the potential for psychological morbidity.

Endometrial cancer

Surveillance recommendations for patients with a history of endometrial cancer are shown in **Table 1**.[5–7] More than three-quarters of endometrial cancer recurrences occur within the first 3 years and so more frequent surveillance is recommended during this time.[8,9] The most common location of recurrence is the vagina and the most common symptom is vaginal bleeding. A physical examination, including a speculum examination, as well as a history of symptoms detects most recurrences.[10,11] A pap test is not indicated for endometrial cancer surveillance.[5] Use of Ca125 testing and radiographic imaging is not routinely indicated; however when recurrence is suspected, these can be useful adjuncts.[5]

Ovarian cancer

Most patients with ovarian cancer are diagnosed with advanced disease. Even after achieving a complete clinical response following primary treatment, recurrence rates are as high as 25% in early stage patients, greater than 80% in advanced stage patients, and overall 5-year survival remains low at 47.4%.[12] The guidelines for surveillance for patients with epithelial ovarian cancer are shown in **Table 2**.[1,5,6] At each visit a bimanual and rectovaginal examination are recommended due to a high rate of pelvic recurrence.[13,14] In addition, 80% of epithelial ovarian cancers will have an elevated Ca125. Ca125 usually correlates with disease status and is often elevated 2 to 5 months before clinical detection of recurrence.[15] However, in the European Organization for Research and Treatment of Cancer trial published by Rustin and colleagues[16] in 2010, the outcome of patients who began treatment for recurrent ovarian cancer based on Ca125 alone was compared with the outcome of patients who began treatment only when recurrence was clinically detected. The investigators found that the overall survival did not differ between groups and they concluded that routine Ca125 measurement is not necessary for surveillance. Routine imaging

Table 1 Endometrial cancer surveillance				
Time from Completion of Treatment	Year 0–1	Year 1–2	Year 2–5	>5 y
Symptom review and examination				
Low risk (stage IA grade 1/2)	6 mo	6–12 mo	Yearly	Yearly
Intermediate risk (stage IB-II)	3 mo	6 mo	6 mo	Yearly
High risk (stage III/IV or high-risk histology)	3 mo	3 mo	6 mo	Yearly

Data from Refs.[5–7]

Table 2
Ovarian cancer surveillance

	0–1 y	1–2 y	2–3 y	3–5 y	>5 y
ROS and examination	Every 3 mo	Every 3 mo	Every 4–6 mo	Every 6 mo	Annually
Ca 125	Optional				
CT or PET	When recurrence suspected				

Abbreviation: CT, computed tomography.
Data from Refs.[1,5,6]

surveillance is not warranted but additional testing including imaging should be performed in symptomatic patients because common sites of recurrence such as lymph nodes and disease in the upper abdomen are not detectable on clinical examination.[5,6]

Cervical cancer

In the United States, 50% of cervical cancer cases are diagnosed at Stage I and 5-year survival is greater than 90%.[12] However, even in these patients, recurrence rates are as high as 10% to 20%.[17,18] Although local recurrences can potentially be cured with radiation or exenterative surgery, distant recurrences are rarely curable. Seventy five percent of recurrences occur within the first 2 to 3 years and thus, surveillance should be more frequent early on.[18–20] Recurrences are most commonly detected when patients present with symptoms such as abdominal, pelvic, and leg pain; lymphedema; vaginal bleeding or discharge; and urinary symptoms.[18] However, asymptomatic disease can be detected on physical examination, and therefore speculum, bimanual, and rectovaginal examinations are recommended at each surveillance visit.[5,6,18] In addition, because of the risk of other lower genital tract neoplasia mediated by human papillomavirus, an examination of the vulva, vagina, and perianal region is recommended. Although cytologic evaluation is not helpful in detecting recurrence, annual cytology may be useful in detecting other lower genital tract neoplasia.[18,21] Surveillance recommendations for women with a history of cervical cancer are shown in **Table 3**.[5,6,21]

Vulvar cancer

Vulvar cancer is rare, accounting for less than 1% of malignancies in women.[12] Early stage disease is usually curable with the most important prognostic factor being lymph node status. Although patients with negative inguinal lymph nodes have a 5-year

Table 3
Cervical and vulvar cancer surveillance

	0–1 y	1–2 y	2–3 y	3–5 y	>5 y
ROS and examination					
Low risk	Every 6 mo	Every 6 mo	Annually	Annually	Annually
High risk[a]	Every 3 mo	Every 3 mo	Every 6 mo	Every 6 mo	Annually
Cytology	Annually[b]				
CT or PET	When recurrence suspected				

[a] Advanced stage, treated with primary chemoradiation or surgery + adjuvant therapy.
[b] To detect other lower genital tract neoplasia.
Data from Refs.[5,6,21,23]

survival that exceeds 80%, this decreases to less than 50% in women with positive nodes and can be as low as 13% with 4 or more positive lymph nodes.[2,22] It is also important to recognize that many patients have later recurrences (>5 years) and thus, long-term surveillance is warranted.[5] Because of the rarity of this disease, no direct evidence for surveillance strategies is published. Surveillance strategies are largely extrapolated from cervical cancer. A careful examination of the vulva and groin as well as screening for other lower genital tract dysplasia is also recommended.[5,6,23] Surveillance recommendations for women with a history of vulvar cancer are shown in **Table 3**.[5,6,23]

ADDRESSING THE SIDE EFFECTS OF CANCER AND CANCER TREATMENT
Physical Exercise

Regular physical activity following cancer treatment has been shown to enhance recovery and reduce mortality in patients with cancer.[4,24–26] It helps treat many of the side effects of cancer treatment, including fatigue and mood disorders and can be helpful for patients with symptoms of cognitive dysfunction and lymphedema.[24] Few patients with cancer meet Acute Coronary Syndrome guidelines for physical activity. In one study of patients with endometrial cancer, only 12% met the minimum recommendation of 150 minutes of moderate exercise weekly.[27,28] Regular exercise, healthy diet, and weight management should be addressed with all cancer survivors.

Fatigue

Cancer-related fatigue is distressing, and persistent physical or emotional exhaustion related to cancer or cancer treatment is not proportional to activity and interferes with usual functioning.[24] It is one of the most prevalent long-term effects of cancer treatment.[4,24] Most women experience some fatigue during treatment and about one-third have persistent fatigue for years after treatment.[29] Cancer-related fatigue reduces overall quality of life (QoL) and is worsened by depression, pain, and sleep disturbances, which are all common in patients with cancer.[4]

The American Society of Clinical Oncology (ASCO) has published guidelines for the assessment and management of cancer-related fatigue.[29] They recommend following the NCCN guidelines for a focused assessment of fatigue.[24,29] This includes evaluating factors that could contribute to fatigue including cardiac or renal disease, medications, substance abuse, and laboratory testing with complete blood count, electrolytes, and thyroid-stimulating hormone.[24,29] Physical exercise has consistently shown benefit in reducing cancer-related fatigue and should be recommended to all patients.[4,24,29] Cognitive behavioral therapy (CBT) can be used if factors such as anxiety and poor coping skills are contributing.[29] Mindfulness-based exercises, yoga, and acupuncture also have benefit.[29] Stimulant medications, while effective in advanced-stage patients actively undergoing treatment, have not shown utility in patients who are disease free following treatment.[29]

Cognitive Dysfunction

There is increasing evidence for what is often referred to as "chemo brain" —short term memory deficits and decreased attention span and concentration.[4,30,31] Patients report that this is one of the most disruptive effects of cancer treatment and reduces QoL.[32,33]

Neuropsychological testing and brain imaging demonstrate abnormalities in patients who have had chemotherapy and there has been correlation between patient reports of cognitive dysfunction and objective deficits with testing.[24] There is limited evidence to guide management of cognitive impairment. Imaging and laboratory studies are not helpful except to rule out other reasons for cognitive deficits. It is important to screen and treat patients for things that can worsen cognitive impairment, including depression, anxiety, fatigue, pain, and sleep disturbances.[4,24]

Treatment of cancer-associated cognitive dysfunction is largely through lifestyle modifications. Teaching strategies such as using memory aids and reminder notes or alarms, doing the most cognitively demanding tasks at whatever time of day their energy levels are the highest, using stress reduction techniques such as meditation and yoga, as well as regular physical exercise can all be helpful.[24] Underlying comorbidities such as depression and pain should be addressed and substances that alter cognition and sleep such as alcohol should be avoided.[24]

Neuropathy

Chemotherapy-induced peripheral neuropathy is a common treatment-related adverse effect that consists predominantly of sensory symptoms, is dose dependen,t and adversely effects QoL.[34–36] Taxanes and platinums, commonly used in gynecologic malignancies, have a high risk of causing peripheral neuropathy. Paclitaxel-induced neuropathy improves in most patients in the months after completing treatment but in many patients continues to be a long-term problem.[35]

Decreasing dose and duration of treatment with chemotherapy agents that cause neuropathy or switching to a less neurotoxic alternative is the only proven strategy for mitigating long-term neuropathy in patients.[35]

There has been one large randomized trial of duloxetine for treatment of chemotherapy-induced painful neuropathy that showed a significant improvement in pain compared with placebo and therefore duloxetine, 30 to 60 mg, daily is recommended for patients with painful neuropathy.[35,37]

Many other agents have been studied and are commonly used in clinical practice, including tricyclic antidepressants, gabapentin, pregabalin, and a compounded gel containing baclofen, amitriptyline and ketamine. Although there is limited evidence that any of these have efficacy in chemotherapy-induced neuropathy, they have proven benefit in other forms of neuropathic pain, and thus, ASCO supports their use if duloxetine is not an option or is ineffective.[35]

Lymphedema

Lymphedema results from damage to the lymphatic system and occurs when lymph fluid accumulates in the interstitial tissue, causing swelling of the limb. It is characterized by swelling on the same side of the body as the cancer treatment. Women who have had surgery and/or radiation to the pelvic and inguinal lymph nodes are at risk for lower extremity lymphedema. A higher number of nodes removed increases the risk as do factors such as obesity, infection, and extent of initial disease.[24] Although sentinel lymph node biopsy may also increase the risk of lymphedema, it likely poses less risk than complete lymphadenectomy or radiation.

The Gynecologic Oncology Group (GOG) completed a study to determine the rates of lower extremity lymphedema in patients with vulvar, cervical, and endometrial cancers by obtaining serial leg volume measurements both before and at multiple time points after surgery[38(p244)]. **Table 4** shows the incidence of leg volume change (LVC) greater than 10%, greater than 15% and greater than 20% for each cancer. The peak incidence of LVC increase was 6 weeks postop but patients remained at risk throughout the 2 years of follow-up.[38]

Table 4
Percentage of patients with gynecologic cancer with changes in leg volume

Cancer Type	LVC >10%	LVC >15%	LVC >20%
Endometrial cancer (n = 733)	34%	19%	11%
Cervical cancer (n = 138)	35%	25%	12%
Vulvar cancer (n = 42)	43%	29%	14%

Data from Carlson JW, Kauderer J, Hutson A, et al. GOG 244, the lymphedema and gynecologic cancer (LEG) study: incidence and risk factors in newly diagnosed patients. Gynecol Oncol 2018;149(Supplement 1):6–7.

Detecting lymphedema early is important because in early stages lymphedema is reversible, but later stage is less responsive to treatment. Treatment is decongestive therapy with lymphedema therapists who specialize in treatment of patients with cancer.[24,39,40] Women with symptoms of lymphedema or at high risk for development of lymphedema should be promptly referred to a certified lymphedema therapist for manual lymphatic drainage and be fitted for compression garments.[24]

Patients should be educated about signs and symptoms of lymphedema and the importance of reporting this to their physician right away. Lymphedema increases the risk of localized infection that can require hospitalization and IV antibiotics. Women with lymphedema must be educated on infection prevention and signs of infection in the affected area and encouraged to seek prompt treatment.[24,41]

Depression and Anxiety

More than 85% of gynecologic cancer survivors report some level of psychological distress.[42] Significant distress is prevalent even in patients with early stage cancer as well as in patients remote from treatment.[43–45]

Depression and anxiety in cancer survivors is frequently due, in part, to fear of recurrence.[3] This is common for days to weeks before surveillance visits when women suffer from intrusive thoughts about cancer, irritability, and anxiety.[45] Although some fear of recurrence can be considered normal, it can also be severe enough to impair clinical care including avoidance of health care professionals and office visits, hypervigilance to changes in sensations, or excessive health care utilization and numerous outpatient or emergency room visits.[46,47]

ASCO has guidelines for the screening, assessment and care of anxiety, and depression in cancer survivors.[48] The Personal Health Questionnaire is a useful depression screening tool and has been validated in patients with cancer.[48,49]

It is important to identify and treat medical causes of depressive symptoms including pain and fatigue. Both pharmacologic interventions such as selective serotonin reuptake inhibitors (SSRIs) and nonpharmacologic interventions such as psychotherapy, CBT, and physical exercise can be used.[48]

Anxiety disorders often coexist with depression. In these cases, the mood disorder should be treated first.[48] Although there are many types of anxiety disorders, the most common is generalized anxiety disorder, which is characterized by multiple excessive worries that women may report as concerns or fears. Worry is disproportionate to the actual risk such as excessive fear of recurrence, concerns about multiple unrelated symptoms, and worries about noncancer-related topics.[48]

As with depressive symptoms, both pharmacologic and nonpharmacologic interventions can be helpful. SSRIs and anxiolytics can be useful in the short term and both individual and group psychotherapy can be helpful when appropriate.

Many patients with depression and/or anxiety have poor compliance with follow-up. Assessing compliance in these patients is an important part of treatment.

Menopausal Symptoms

Iatrogenic menopause is frequently a consequence of and can affect overall health and QoL.[50] Premature menopause puts women at risk for problems such as osteoporosis and heart disease.

Although hormone replacement therapy (HRT), including estrogen replacement therapy (ERT) and combined HRT, is not advised in women with granulosa cell tumors or endometrial stromal sarcomas, studies of women with a history of epithelial ovarian, endometrial, and cervical cancers have not shown any detrimental effects. Ovarian cancer survivors treated with HRT do not have an increased recurrence risk or worse overall survival (OS).[51,52] Eeles and colleagues[53] conducted a randomized controlled trial of women with a history of EOC assigned to HRT versus no HRT. Both OS and progression free survival were better in the group that received HRT. The women who took HRT had fewer deaths due to ovarian cancer, coronary heart disease, and thromboembolic disease.[53] Multiple other studies have shown no detrimental effects of HRT in ovarian cancer survivors who undergo premature menopause and who do not have other contraindications to HRT.

In young women with a history of low-risk endometrial cancer who undergo premature menopause due to treatment, HRT is considered first-line therapy for menopausal symptoms and also decreases long-term health consequences. A study performed by the GOG looked at more than 1200 endometrial cancer survivors who were randomly assigned to HRT or placebo and found no difference in recurrence between the 2 groups.[54] Vaginal estrogen can also safely be prescribed.[55]

In women with cervical cancer who have lost ovarian function due to the effects of primary pelvic radiation therapy, combined HRT with both estrogen and a progestin is necessary.

When nonhormonal treatment is preferred, both SSRIs and selective serotonin and norepinephrine reuptake inhibitors (SNRIs) can be used. SSRIs have been shown to be more effective than placebo in reducing vasomotor symptoms.[56] SNRIs have also been used to reduce hot flashes, anxiety, and sleep disturbance associated with menopausal symptoms.[56,57]

Sexual Health

Gynecologic malignancy and treatments including surgery, chemotherapy, and radiation directly affect the sexual organs and thus sexual morbidity can affect patients with gynecologic cancer in both the short- and longer-term survivorship.[58] Sexual dysfunction affects up to 90% of patients with gynecologic cancer.[59]

Sexual dysfunction is prevalent in women treated with simple hysterectomy.[59] After radical hysterectomy women are at higher risk due to the possibility of orgasmic problems from nerve damage, lymphedema, genital numbness, and vaginal shortening.[58]

Radiation therapy can affect sexual function by causing vaginal fibrosis and stenosis that limits capacity for vaginal intercourse. Both pelvic external beam radiation therapy (EBRT) and vaginal brachytherapy (VBT) can affect sexual function. In the QoL analysis of the PORTEC-2 trial, which randomized women with endometrial cancer to adjuvant EBRT to the whole pelvis versus VBT, both groups had a significant decrease in sexual functioning but there was no difference between patients who received EBRT versus VBT.[60] In patients with cervical cancer, both primary and adjuvant radiation therapy has been associated with greater sexual dysfunction than radical surgery alone.[61]

Multiple tools exist to assess sexual dysfunction in cancer survivors. The Female Sexual Function Index and the Patient Reported Outcomes Measurement Information System Sexual Function and Satisfaction Measures have been validated in patients with cancer and can be used to monitor patients over time.[62–64]

Many women are embarrassed to talk about sexual function so it is important to ask women about this and to provide anticipatory guidance before treatment.[65] Comorbidities such as hypertension, diabetes, depression, and social or partner stressors as well as medications such as beta blockers and SSRIs can impair sexual function and should be evaluated.[62] Pelvic examination can assess vaginal length, caliber, and severity of atrophy or stenosis.

The Diagnostic and Statistical Manual of Mental Disorders 5th edition defines 3 domains of sexual dysfunction (**Table 5**). All state that symptoms must be present for at least 6 months, cause clinically significant distress, and not be secondary to another cause.[66]

Consistent use of vaginal dilators and/or regular sexual activity both during and after radiation therapy is useful to prevent vaginal stenosis,[58] improve elasticity, and gain additional vaginal length and capacity.[58,65]

Fertility

Women can lose fertility either because surgery removes all of part of their reproductive organs or because of premature ovarian failure due to chemotherapy or radiation.

Table 5
Domains of sexual dysfunction

	Diagnostic Criteria	Treatment
Female sexual interest/arousal disorder	Must have 3 out of 4[66,a]: • Reduced interest in sexual activity • Reduced sexual/erotic thoughts/fantasies • Reduced initiation of sexual activity and unreceptive to a partners attempts • Reduced sexual excitement/pleasure	• Psychotherapy (individual or with partner)[58] • 5-HT1A and 5-HT2A antagonists (Flibanserin[b]) • Testosterone[62,b]
Female orgasmic disorder	Difficulty experiencing an orgasm and/or reduced intensity of orgasmic sensations[66,a]	• CBT[68] • Directed masturbation[68] • Stop SSRIs or switch to buproprion[58]
Genito-pelvic pain/penetration disorder[c]	Difficulty with any of the following[66]: • Penetration • Vulvovaginal or pelvic pain • Fear of pain in anticipation of, during, or as a result of vaginal penetration • Tension in vaginal floor muscles during attempted penetration[66]	• Daily moisturizers for vaginal dryness (polycarbophil-based, vitamin A or E)[58] • Vaginal estrogen (if appropriate)[65] • Topical lidocaine (for vulvodynia) • Lubrication during intercourse (water or silicone based)[58,61,d] • Vaginal dilators • Pelvic floor physical therapy[58] • Ospemifene

[a] In 75% to 100% of sexual encounters.[66]
[b] Never studied patients with cancer.
[c] Can be vulvovaginal atrophy, vaginismus, vulvodynia.
[d] Should be applied to both partners.

Infertility can be emotionally devastating, which can persist for a long time after cancer treatment.[67] In one study of gynecologic cancer survivors, the loss of fertility caused significant distress in 72%.[67] Women who already have children before treatment fair better.[67]

All women with cancer are entitled to consultation with an infertility specialist and should be informed of their fertility options. ASCO guidelines recommend addressing the possibility of infertility, referring patients who are interested or ambivalent to a fertility specialist and discussing options for fertility preservation before treatment starts and as early as possible because this ultimately reduces distress.[68,69]

Proven fertility preservation methods include embryo cryopreservation, oocyte cryopreservation, ovarian transposition, conservative surgery, and ovarian tissue cryopreservation.[68,70] Although GnRH agonists are frequently used by providers in hopes of reducing the likelihood of chemotherapy-induced ovarian failure, the current evidence does not support their use as a proven fertility preservation method.[68] However, when proven fertility preservation methods are not feasible these may be offered.[68]

The average cost in the United States for one fertility preservation cycle is $12,737 and most patients cite cost as the most significant factor in their decision not to pursue fertility preservation.[69] Recently, both Connecticut and Rhode Island became the first states to pass legislation requiring insurance coverage for fertility preservation in patients about to undergo a medical treatment that may have deleterious effects on the gonads.[69] However, for most patients in the United States outside of these 2 states, fertility treatment is cost-prohibitive.

Economic Impact of Cancer Treatment

Cancer survivors often face economic hardships during and after treatment. Cancer history can have an impact on employment opportunity and on ability to obtain and retain health and life insurance. This can also be worsened by the cost of some prescription drugs, medical supplies, and copayments. Some of these issues extend and pose financial burden to family members or caretakers.[4]

Most patients who were working at the time of their cancer diagnosis either continue to work through or return to work after treatment.[4] Despite the protections offered against being fired or denied benefits through the Americans with Disabilities Act, cancer survivors can face employment discrimination.[4,71]

Although most cancer survivors are covered by Medicare and protected from insurance discrimination, for those who are younger than 65 years and uninsured, the cost of cancer care can be financially devastating.[4] Furthermore, even those with health insurance can have trouble paying for prescription drugs. For patients with a history of cancer who are not eligible for Medicare, Medicaid, or other group coverage, a history of cancer can make purchasing individual health coverage too costly.[4] Helping patients to access financial assistance programs and other resources to cover costs of care is important.

COORDINATION OF FOLLOW-UP CARE

The Society of Gynecologic Oncology has developed survivorship care plan (SCP) templates for ovarian, cervical, vulvar, and endometrial cancers that provide information on a woman's treatment course, expected posttreatment side effects, and surveillance recommendations.

Although evidence of the effectiveness of SCPs is lacking,[72] a paradigm for coordination of care and communication between oncology providers, primary care providers (PCPs), and patients, following treatment for gynecologic cancer is necessary because there is often poor communication between the oncology team and the PCP. There is distinct benefit to involving patient's PCP and general gynecologists at the conclusion of cancer treatment because patients are more likely to receive recommended preventive care than if they are seen primarily by an oncologist.[73,74]

REFERENCES

1. National Comprehensive Cancer Network (NCCN). NCCN clinical practice guidelines in oncology: ovarian cancer including fallopian tube cancer and primary peritoneal cancer. Version 2.2018. March 2018. Available at: https://www.nccn.org/professionals/physician_gls/pdf/ovarian.pdf. Accessed May 5, 2018.
2. Gonzalez Bosquet J, Magrina JF, Gaffey TA, et al. Long-term survival and disease recurrence in patients with primary squamous cell carcinoma of the vulva. Gynecol Oncol 2005;97(3):828–33.
3. Salani R. Survivorship planning in gynecologic cancer patients. Gynecol Oncol 2013;130(2):389–97.
4. Hewitt M, Greenfield S, Stovall E, et al. From cancer patient to cancer survivor: lost in translation. Washington, DC: National Academies Press; 2005. Available at: http://www.nationalacademies.org/hmd/Reports/2005/From-Cancer-Patient-to-Cancer-Survivor-Lost-in-Transition.aspx.
5. Salani R, Backes FJ, Fung MFK, et al. Posttreatment surveillance and diagnosis of recurrence in women with gynecologic malignancies: Society of Gynecologic Oncologists recommendations. Am J Obstet Gynecol 2011;204(6):466–78.
6. Salani R, Khanna N, Frimer M, et al. An update on post-treatment surveillance and diagnosis of recurrence in women with gynecologic malignancies: Society of Gynecologic Oncology (SGO) recommendations. Gynecol Oncol 2017;146(1):3–10.
7. National Comprehensive Cancer Network (NCCN). NCCN clinical practice guidelines in oncology: uterine neoplasms. Version 1.2018. October 2017. Available at: https://www.nccn.org/professionals/physician_gls/pdf/uterine.pdf. Accessed May 5, 2018.
8. Keys HM, Roberts JA, Brunetto VL, et al. A phase III trial of surgery with or without adjunctive external pelvic radiation therapy in intermediate risk endometrial adenocarcinoma: a Gynecologic Oncology Group study. Gynecol Oncol 2004; 92(3):744–51.
9. Creutzberg CL, van Putten WLJ, Koper PC, et al. Survival after relapse in patients with endometrial cancer: results from a randomized trial. Gynecol Oncol 2003; 89(2):201–9.
10. Berchuck A, Anspach C, Evans AC, et al. Postsurgical surveillance of patients with FIGO stage I/II endometrial adenocarcinoma. Gynecol Oncol 1995;59(1):20–4.
11. Tjalma WA, van Dam PA, Makar AP, et al. The clinical value and the cost-effectiveness of follow-up in endometrial cancer patients. Int J Gynecol Cancer 2004;14(5):931–7.
12. Noone AM, Howlader N, Krapcho M, et al. SEER cancer statistics review, 1975-2015 - SEER Statistics. 2018. Available at: https://seer.cancer.gov/csr/1975_2015/. Accessed May 10, 2018.
13. Gadducci A, Cosio S, Zola P, et al. Surveillance procedures for patients treated for epithelial ovarian cancer: a review of the literature. Int J Gynecol Cancer 2007;17(1):21–31.
14. Trimbos JB, Parmar M, Vergote I, et al. International collaborative ovarian neoplasm trial 1 and adjuvant chemotherapy in ovarian neoplasm trial: two

parallel randomized phase III trials of adjuvant chemotherapy in patients with early-stage ovarian carcinoma. J Natl Cancer Inst 2003;95(2):105–12.

15. Fehm T, Heller F, Krämer S, et al. Evaluation of CA125, physical and radiological findings in follow-up of ovarian cancer patients. Anticancer Res 2005;25(3A):1551–4.

16. Rustin GJS, van der Burg MEL, Griffin CL, et al. Early versus delayed treatment of relapsed ovarian cancer (MRC OV05/EORTC 55955): a randomised trial. Lancet 2010;376(9747):1155–63.

17. Delgado G, Bundy B, Zaino R, et al. Prospective surgical-pathological study of disease-free interval in patients with stage IB squamous cell carcinoma of the cervix: a Gynecologic Oncology Group study. Gynecol Oncol 1990;38(3):352–7.

18. Elit L, Fyles AW, Oliver TK, et al, members of the Gynecology Cancer Disease Site Group of Cancer Care Ontario's Program in Evidence-Based Care. Follow-up for women after treatment for cervical cancer. Curr Oncol 2010;17(3):65–9.

19. Larson DM, Copeland LJ, Stringer CA, et al. Recurrent cervical carcinoma after radical hysterectomy. Gynecol Oncol 1988;30(3):381–7.

20. Greer BE, Koh W-J, Abu-Rustum NR, et al. Cervical cancer. J Natl Compr Canc Netw 2010;8(12):1388–416.

21. National Comprehensive Cancer Network (NCCN). NCCN clinical practice guidelines in oncology: cervical cancer. Version 1.2018. October 2017. Available at: https://www.nccn.org/professionals/physician_gls/pdf/cervical.pdf. Accessed May 5, 2018.

22. Beller U, Quinn MA, Benedet JL, et al. Carcinoma of the vulva. FIGO 26th annual report on the results of treatment in gynecological cancer. Int J Gynaecol Obstet 2006;95(Suppl 1):S7–27.

23. National Comprehensive Cancer Network (NCCN). NCCN clinical practice guidelines in oncology: vulvar cancer. Version I.2018. October 2017. Available at: https://www.nccn.org/professionals/physician_gls/pdf/vulvar.pdf. Accessed May 5, 2018.

24. National Comprehensive Cancer Network (NCCN). NCCN clinical practice guidelines in oncology: survivorship 3.2017. 2018. Available at: https://www.nccn.org/professionals/physician_gls/pdf/survivorship.pdf. Accessed May 5, 2018.

25. Calle EE, Rodriguez C, Walker-Thurmond K, et al. Overweight, obesity, and mortality from cancer in a prospectively studied cohort of U.S. adults. N Engl J Med 2003;348(17):1625–38.

26. McTiernan A, Irwin M, Vongruenigen V. Weight, physical activity, diet, and prognosis in breast and gynecologic cancers. J Clin Oncol 2010;28(26):4074–80.

27. von Gruenigen VE, Waggoner SE, Frasure HE, et al. Lifestyle challenges in endometrial cancer survivorship. Obstet Gynecol 2011;117(1):93–100.

28. The American Cancer Society medical and editorial content team. ACS guidelines for nutrition and physical activity. 2017. Available at: https://www.cancer.org/healthy/eat-healthy-get-active/acs-guidelines-nutrition-physical-activity-cancer-prevention/guidelines.html. Accessed May 5, 2018.

29. Bower JE, Bak K, Berger A, et al. Screening, assessment, and management of fatigue in adult survivors of cancer: an American Society of Clinical oncology clinical practice guideline adaptation. J Clin Oncol 2014;32(17):1840–50.

30. National Comprehensive Cancer Network (NCCN). NCCN clinical practice guidelines in oncology: genetic/familial high-risk assessment: colorectal 3.2017. 2017. Available at: https://www.nccn.org/professionals/physician_gls/pdf/genetics_colon.pdf.

31. Correa DD, Hess LM. Cognitive function and quality of life in ovarian cancer. Gynecol Oncol 2012;124(3):404–9.

32. Grover S, Hill-Kayser CE, Vachani C, et al. Patient reported late effects of gynecological cancer treatment. Gynecol Oncol 2012;124(3):399–403.

33. Hess LM, Chambers SK, Hatch K, et al. Pilot study of the prospective identification of changes in cognitive function during chemotherapy treatment for advanced ovarian cancer. J Support Oncol 2010;8(6):252–8.

34. Cavaletti G, Frigeni B, Lanzani F, et al. Chemotherapy-Induced Peripheral Neurotoxicity assessment: a critical revision of the currently available tools. Eur J Cancer 2010;46(3):479–94.

35. Hershman DL, Lacchetti C, Dworkin RH, et al. Prevention and management of chemotherapy-induced peripheral neuropathy in survivors of adult cancers: American Society of Clinical Oncology clinical practice guideline. J Clin Oncol 2014;32(18):1941–67.

36. Pachman DR, Barton DL, Watson JC, et al. Chemotherapy-induced peripheral neuropathy: prevention and treatment. Clin Pharmacol Ther 2011;90(3):377–87.

37. Smith EML, Pang H, Cirrincione C, et al. Effect of duloxetine on pain, function, and quality of life among patients with chemotherapy-induced painful peripheral neuropathy: a randomized clinical trial. JAMA 2013;309(13):1359–67.

38. Carlson JW, Kauderer J, Hutson A, et al. GOG 244; the lymphedema and gynecologic cancer (LEG) study: incidence and risk factors in newly diagnosed patients. Abstract presented at the: SGO Annual Meeting 2018; March 25, 2018; New Orleanse, LA.

39. International Society of Lymphology. The diagnosis and treatment of peripheral lymphedema: 2013 consensus document of the International Society of Lymphology. Lymphology 2013;46(1):1–11.

40. National Cancer Institute. National Cancer Institute Lymphedema (PDQ®)–Health Professional Version. July 2015. National Cancer Institute Lymphedema (PDQ®)–Health Professional Version. Available at: https://www.cancer.gov/about-cancer/treatment/side-effects/lymphedema/lymphedema-hp-pdf. Accessed May 13, 2018.

41. National Lymphedema Network. Position statement of the national lymphedema network. 2011. Available at: https://www.lymphnet.org/pdfDocs/position.papers/Risk.Reduction.pdf. Accessed May 13, 2018.

42. Hodgkinson K, Butow P, Fuchs A, et al. Long-term survival from gynecologic cancer: psychosocial outcomes, supportive care needs and positive outcomes. Gynecol Oncol 2007;104(2):381–9.

43. Wenzel LB, Donnelly JP, Fowler JM, et al. Resilience, reflection, and residual stress in ovarian cancer survivorship: a gynecologic oncology group study. Psychooncology 2002;11(2):142–53.

44. Simard S, Thewes B, Humphris G, et al. Fear of cancer recurrence in adult cancer survivors: a systematic review of quantitative studies. J Cancer Surviv 2013;7(3):300–22.

45. Ozga M, Aghajanian C, Myers-Virtue S, et al. A systematic review of ovarian cancer and fear of recurrence. Palliat Support Care 2015;13(6):1771–80.

46. Beckjord EB, Reynolds KA, van Londen GJ, et al. Population-level trends in posttreatment cancer survivors' concerns and associated receipt of care: results from the 2006 and 2010 LIVESTRONG surveys. J Psychosoc Oncol 2014;32(2):125–51.

47. Lebel S, Tomei C, Feldstain A, et al. Does fear of cancer recurrence predict cancer survivors' health care use? Support Care Cancer 2013;21(3):901–6.

48. Andersen BL, DeRubeis RJ, Berman BS, et al. Screening, assessment, and care of anxiety and depressive symptoms in adults with cancer: an American Society of Clinical Oncology guideline adaptation. J Clin Oncol 2014;32(15):1605–19.

49. Kroenke K, Spitzer RL, Williams JB. The PHQ-9: validity of a brief depression severity measure. J Gen Intern Med 2001;16(9):606–13.

50. Hinds L, Price J. Menopause, hormone replacement and gynaecological cancers. Menopause Int 2010;16(2):89–93.
51. Pergialiotis V, Pitsouni E, Prodromidou A, et al. Hormone therapy for ovarian cancer survivors: systematic review and meta-analysis. Menopause 2016;23(3): 335–42.
52. Li D, Ding C-Y, Qiu L-H. Postoperative hormone replacement therapy for epithelial ovarian cancer patients: a systematic review and meta-analysis. Gynecol Oncol 2015;139(2):355–62.
53. Eeles RA, Morden JP, Gore M, et al. Adjuvant hormone therapy may improve survival in epithelial ovarian cancer: results of the AHT randomized trial. J Clin Oncol 2015;33(35):4138–44.
54. Barakat RR, Bundy BN, Spirtos NM, et al, Gynecologic Oncology Group Study. Randomized double-blind trial of estrogen replacement therapy versus placebo in stage I or II endometrial cancer: a Gynecologic Oncology Group Study. J Clin Oncol 2006;24(4):587–92.
55. Committee on Gynecologic Practice. ACOG committee opinion. Hormone replacement therapy in women treated for endometrial cancer. Number 234, May 2000 (replaces number 126, August 1993). Int J Gynaecol Obstet 2001; 73(3):283–4.
56. Loprinzi CL, Kugler JW, Sloan JA, et al. Venlafaxine in management of hot flashes in survivors of breast cancer: a randomised controlled trial. Lancet 2000; 356(9247):2059–63.
57. Salani R, Andersen BL. Gynecologic care for breast cancer survivors: assisting in the transition to wellness. Am J Obstet Gynecol 2012;206(5):390–7.
58. Huffman LB, Hartenbach EM, Carter J, et al. Maintaining sexual health throughout gynecologic cancer survivorship: a comprehensive review and clinical guide. Gynecol Oncol 2016;140(2):359–68.
59. Onujiogu N, Johnson T, Seo S, et al. Survivors of endometrial cancer: who is at risk for sexual dysfunction? Gynecol Oncol 2011;123(2):356–9.
60. Nout RA, Putter H, Jürgenliemk-Schulz IM, et al. Five-year quality of life of endometrial cancer patients treated in the randomised post operative radiation therapy in endometrial cancer (PORTEC-2) trial and comparison with norm data. Eur J Cancer 2012;48(11):1638–48.
61. Frumovitz M, Sun CC, Schover LR, et al. Quality of life and sexual functioning in cervical cancer survivors. J Clin Oncol 2005;23(30):7428–36.
62. Dizon DS, Suzin D, McIlvenna S. Sexual health as a survivorship issue for female cancer survivors. Oncologist 2014;19(2):202–10.
63. Baser RE, Li Y, Carter J. Psychometric validation of the female sexual function index (FSFI) in cancer survivors. Cancer 2012;118(18):4606–18.
64. Flynn KE, Reeve BB, Lin L, et al. Construct validity of the PROMIS® sexual function and satisfaction measures in patients with cancer. Health Qual Life Outcomes 2013;11:40.
65. Falk SJ, Dizon DS. Sexual dysfunction in women with cancer. Fertil Steril 2013; 100(4):916–21.
66. A.P. Association. Diagnostic and statistical manual of mental disorders: DSM-5. 5th edition. Washington, DC: American Psychiatric Publishing; 2013.
67. Carter J, Chi DS, Brown CL, et al. Cancer-related infertility in survivorship. Int J Gynecol Cancer 2010;20(1):2–8.
68. Oktay K, Harvey BE, Partridge AH, et al. Fertility preservation in patients with cancer: ASCO clinical practice guideline update. J Clin Oncol 2018. https://doi.org/10.1200/JCO.2018.78.1914.

69. Cardozo ER, Huber WJ, Stuckey AR, et al. Mandating coverage for fertility preservation - a step in the right direction. N Engl J Med 2017;377(17):1607–9.

70. Donnez J, Dolmans M-M. Fertility preservation in women. N Engl J Med 2017; 377(17):1657–65.

71. The Americans with Disabilities Act of 1990. Available at: https://www.eeoc.gov/eeoc/history/35th/thelaw/ada.html. Accessed May 13, 2018.

72. Brothers BM, Easley A, Salani R, et al. Do survivorship care plans impact patients' evaluations of care? a randomized evaluation with gynecologic oncology patients. Gynecol Oncol 2013;129(3):554–8.

73. Earle CC, Burstein HJ, Winer EP, et al. Quality of non-breast cancer health maintenance among elderly breast cancer survivors. J Clin Oncol 2003;21(8): 1447–51.

74. Khan NF, Carpenter L, Watson E, et al. Cancer screening and preventative care among long-term cancer survivors in the United Kingdom. Br J Cancer 2010; 102(7):1085–90.

Palliative Care in Gynecologic Oncology

Mary M. Mullen, MD, James C. Cripe, MD, Premal H. Thaker, MD, MS*

KEYWORDS

- Palliative care • Palliative care economics • Palliative care barriers
- End-of-life symptom management

KEY POINTS

- Early palliative care is formally endorsed by the American Society of Clinical Oncology and the Society of Gynecologic Oncology.
- Palliative care and anticancer or disease-modifying treatment are not mutually exclusive and should occur concomitantly.
- The most efficient palliative care model consists of primary palliative care provided by the primary oncologist and secondary palliative care provided by a separate specialty palliative care team.
- Gynecologic oncologists should be well versed in common symptom management.
- The transition to hospice at end of life is an important aspect of palliative care and standard gynecologic oncology care for patients with advanced gynecologic malignancy.

INTRODUCTION

Palliative care is patient- and family-centered care that optimizes quality of life by anticipating, preventing, and treating suffering.[1] Improving quality of life of patients and their families should remain critically important for any serious diagnosis. The goals of palliative care are demonstrated by the nine domains outlined by the American Association of Hospice and Palliative Medicine. These domains include rapport and relationship building with patients and family caregivers, symptom distress and function status management, exploration of understanding and education of prognosis, clarification of treatment goals, assessment and support of coping, assistance with medical decision making, coordination with other providers, and provision of referrals to other providers.[2] These goals should be addressed near the time of

The authors have no commercial or financial conflicts of interest regarding this topic.
Funding Sources: None.
Division of Gynecologic Oncology, Department of Obstetrics and Gynecology, Washington University School of Medicine, Alvin J. Siteman Cancer Center, 660 South Euclid Avenue, Mail Stop 8064-37-905, St Louis, MO 63110, USA
* Corresponding author.
E-mail address: thakerp@wustl.edu

diagnosis as demonstrated by the quality of life and survival benefits in the landmark trial by Temel and colleagues[3] evaluating palliative care within 8 weeks of diagnosis with metastatic non–small cell lung cancer. The previously stated guidelines are supported and strongly endorsed by many oncologic professional societies. The American Society of Clinical Oncology (ASCO) is committed to facilitating the integration of palliative cancer care into existing health care systems worldwide to realize the vision of comprehensive cancer care by 2020. Additionally, the Society of Gynecologic Oncology (SGO) continues to make efforts promoting education and research in palliative care for trainees and providers.[4]

In 2016 ASCO released evidence-based recommendations regarding the incorporation of palliative care into standard gynecologic oncology care. Key recommendations include the following: "Patients with advanced cancer, whether inpatient or outpatient, should receive dedicated palliative care services, early in the disease course, concurrent with active treatment. Referring patients to interdisciplinary palliative care teams is optimal, and services may complement existing programs. Providers may refer caregivers of patients with early or advanced cancer to palliative care services." ASCO supports the delivery of services via interdisciplinary palliative care teams in any treatment setting.[5]

The SGO echoes these recommendations and states that the delivery of palliative care is essential in delivering quality care to women with gynecologic cancer.[6] The SGO has established 11 Principles of Palliative Care:

1. Express sensitivity to cultural differences and deliver palliative care with compassion, empathy, and respect for a woman as an individual.
2. Establish open communication with women and their families providing the information necessary to understand their condition, prognosis, and treatment options.
3. Alleviate pain and distressing symptoms, whether physical or emotional, maintaining hope and leading to an improvement in the woman's quality of life.
4. Recognize that a multidisciplinary approach using the services of professionals trained in psychological, social, and spiritual issues optimizes care and well-being.
5. Respect a woman's decision regarding acceptance or refusal of further treatment.
6. Recognize the practitioner's responsibility to fully inform women of treatments unlikely to achieve benefit or do harm.
7. Encourage women and families to consider hospice care as an option when appropriate.
8. Understand and support the woman's preferences regarding end-of-life care.
9. Maintain continuity of care for terminally ill women, avoiding feelings of isolation and abandonment for the woman and her family.
10. Acknowledge the effect that end-of-life care has on the family and provide emotional support including access to social and bereavement services.
11. Recognize that although providing palliative care is emotionally rewarding it is crucial to acknowledge the potential for compassion fatigue and the need to support each other including members of the multidisciplinary team to remain fully engaged.

DELIVERY OF PALLIATIVE CARE

Gynecologic oncologists deliver medical and surgical treatments of complex illnesses and through this process frequently treat patients from diagnosis to the end of life. Delivery of palliative care should be provided by the gynecologic oncologist managing the patient's illness (primary palliative care) and by providers with dedicated training in palliative care (specialty palliative care).[7] In 2006, Hospice and Palliative Medicine became a recognized specialty by the American Board of Medical Specialties, with the American Board of Obstetrics and Gynecology as one of the sponsoring boards. The unique relationship between the gynecologic oncologist and palliative care physician was further characterized in an in-depth qualitative interview study at six National Cancer Institute–designated cancer centers. Thirty-four gynecologic oncologists participated and two main themes were identified. Gynecologic oncologists value the palliative care clinician's communication skill and third-party perspective to increase prognostic awareness and help negotiate differences between patient preferences and provider recommendations. Additionally, they would prefer specialty palliative care services embedded within gynecologic oncology clinics.[8] Throughout the patient's cancer course, treatment with curative intent should be paired with palliative care for symptom relief, and ultimately, palliative care should be paired with hospice at the end of a disease course (**Fig. 1**).

BENEFITS OF PALLIATIVE CARE

When delivered in a timely fashion, palliative care offers benefits to patients and their families by improving symptom burden and quality of life. These benefits are associated with less aggressive care at the end of life, which limits overall costs, and interestingly, this shift in care may be associated with prolonged survival.[3]

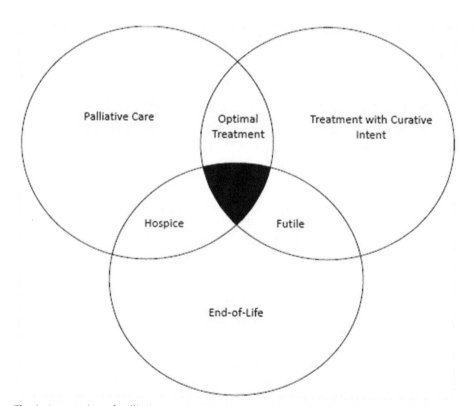

Fig. 1. Integration of palliative care into treatment with curative intent and end-of-life care.

Palliative care has been shown to improve symptom burden in other malignancies, most notably dyspnea in patients with lung cancer.[9] Symptom distress and functional status management is a complex problem in treating women with gynecologic malignancies; however, they also quickly benefit from specialty palliative care. A retrospective review of women with gynecologic malignancies admitted to hospital and had a palliative care consultation found improvement of symptom burden scored by the Edmonton Symptom Assessment System. They had statistically significant improvement in the frequency of moderate-to-severe symptoms in pain, anorexia, fatigue, and nausea from initial palliative care consultation to hospital discharge.[10] These benefits are not limited to inpatient admissions. In a similar study 78 women with gynecologic malignancies were followed in an outpatient palliative care clinic. Improvement in pain, fatigue, anxiety, depression, nausea, drowsiness, appetite, and shortness of breath were found to be statistically significant.[11]

End of Life and Hospice

Ultimately, to maximize survival, quality of life, and cost benefits of hospice, patients should transition to hospice when their life expectancy is less than 6 months. The literature, albeit limited, suggests 20% to 60% of gynecologic oncology patients die on hospice with a median length of stay in hospice only 19 to 25 days with 55% of patients enrolling less than 30 days before death.[12,13] Although patients may qualify for hospice, in a review of 268 gynecologic oncology patients admitted in the last 6 months of life, 70.5% were referred to hospice with a median time of enrollment to death of only 22 days suggesting earlier referral may be appropriate.[14] Per a 2010 study by Barbera and colleagues,[15] 51% of women with gynecologic cancer died in an acute care bed as an inpatient and according to two separate studies up to 60% of patients have an invasive procedure performed within the last 3 to 6 months of life.[16] End-of-life patients not managed on hospice are more likely to be inpatient, transferred to the intensive care unit, and receive invasive procedures without survival benefit.[17] Thus, to provide optimal end-of-life care, timely hospice referral is essential.

Although palliative care encompasses building rapport, clarification of goals, and improvement of patient understanding, which are most critical at the end of life, significant benefits of early introductions have been documented in the existing literature. Doll and colleagues[18] reviewed end-of-life discussions and found that when outpatient hospice discussions occurred, future admissions had a shorter length of stay and increased use of palliative care resources. Nevadunsky and colleagues[19] showed that specialty palliative care improved hospice use from 41% to 72%; however, if patients received specialty palliative care consultation within 14 days of death, there was no difference in aggressive measures or hospice use. Hospice enrollment was associated with a decrease in this rate to 3% of patients receiving a procedure, chemotherapy, or radiation within the last 6 months of life and a decrease in inpatient hospitalizations near end of life.[14]

Limiting futile chemotherapy, decreasing admissions, and increasing hospice use have a tremendous benefit of decreasing costs associated with end-of-life care. Lewin and colleagues[20] reviewed 84 women with ovarian cancer, 17 were enrolled in hospice and 67 were not. There was no significant difference in mean survival (32.4 vs 40.8 months; $P = .30$). However, nonhospice patients as compared with those enrolled in hospice consume significantly more resources in the last 60 days of life. These resource expenditures totaled $52,319 and $15,164, respectively. Most recently, Urban and colleagues[21] used the Surveillance, Epidemiology, and End Results Medicare database to review 5509 patients with ovarian cancer. On multivariate analysis, factors associated with increased cost in the last 90 days of life included medical comorbidity, chemotherapy, time spent admitted, and admissions associated with emergency room visits. They concluded reducing chemotherapy and increasing hospice services will aid in lowering costs. Time on hospice has a maximal cost benefit for oncology patients enrolled in hospice at least 58 days before death.[22]

Mechanisms must be identified to improve hospice use in the gynecologic oncology population to improve patient outcomes. Physicians are often the advocates to hospice enrollment and therefore it is critical that physicians partner with palliative care services and initiate end-of-life conversations before symptoms or a patient becoming unstable. Further research is necessary to determine how to improve hospice uptake in the patient population.

LOGISTICS OF EARLY INTEGRATION OF PALLIATIVE CARE
Barriers to Palliative Care

The benefits of early integration of palliative care into standard gynecologic oncologic care have been well established.[10,12,17,23–26] However, barriers to palliative care can make this integration extremely difficult. In fact, only 70.5% of gynecologic oncology patients are referred to hospice or palliative care before death and only 18% have palliative consultation within 30 days before death.[12] To determine methods to overcome these barriers it is important to first identify and define them.

Barriers to palliative care and/or hospice referral are multifactorial and include physician factors, patient factors, and institutional factors (**Box 1**).

Physician factors

Physicians are usually the gatekeepers of palliative care referral. Seventy percent of physicians report not fully understanding the benefits of palliative care and 73% of gynecologic oncologists report having fear that referral to palliative care will cause patients and families to feel abandoned, as if the physician has given up hope for the patient.[17,27,28] As a result, referral is often postponed until patients are symptomatic

---

Box 1
Barriers to the integration of palliative care into standard gynecologic oncology care

Physician Factors

Optimistic view of patient's life expectancy

Lack of awareness of palliative care/lack of training

Fear of upsetting patient

Admission of failure

Patient Factors

Optimistic view of patient's life expectancy

Lack of understanding of the meaning of palliative care

Fear of upsetting the physician

Institutional Factors

Inadequate resources

Poor reimbursement for palliative care services

Minimal formal training in palliative care for physicians

Late palliative care referrals

or until all anticancer treatments are exhausted.[29] Additionally, late palliative care or hospice referral often occurs as a result of a falsely hopeful view of the patient's remaining life expectancy.[17,30,31] Data demonstrate physicians regularly overestimate survival in terminally ill patients with cancer.[32]

Patient factors

Patient and family reluctance to palliative care enrollment is largely centered around the association of palliative care with death.[29] In fact, many patients and families consider palliative care to be equivalent to end-of-life care, and therefore assume it is discordant with oncologic therapy.[33] Because of an often overly optimistic view of a patient's or loved-one's prognosis palliative care is often forgone. Further reluctance occurs from fear of offending their physician by suggesting or using palliative care.[29] In a survey study of the SGO, 54% of respondents stated that unrealistic patient expectations were always or often a barrier to quality end-of-life care.[34]

Institutional factors

Institutional factors include limited resource availability and inadequate formal training of physicians. Palliative care services, specifically outpatient services, are common in most National Cancer Institute–designated cancer centers and academic settings, but are much less available in community hospitals and rural areas.[29,35] This is likely a result of poor reimbursement and limited institutional budgets for palliative care services.[17,35] Furthermore, unawareness of available resources and ignorance regarding how to use or provide these services creates additional barriers. Formal training in palliative care and hospice for oncologists is minimal with only 11% of gynecologic oncology fellows reporting palliative care training.[36] A total of 77% of gynecologic oncologists report additional training during fellowship would better prepare them to provide end-of life care.[37] As a result of these institutional barriers, referral often occurs late, on average only 30 to 60 days before death, limiting a palliative care program's maximum potential.[17,38]

Practical Models of Palliative Care

Establishing effective and practical models of palliative care will work to overcome known barriers. The National Comprehensive Cancer Network (NCCN) task force and ASCO and SGO recognize and emphasize that palliative care and anticancer or disease-modifying therapy are not mutually exclusive and should occur concomitantly. These professional organizations suggest palliative care should be provided from diagnosis to death in the form of bereavement support or to survivorship.[5,24,39] Simultaneously, the World Health Organization (WHO) definition of palliative care has evolved so the recipient of palliative care no longer needs to have an incurable illness.[40] The WHO emphasizes that palliative care is most effective in combination with other oncologic therapies. These contemporary definitions aim to integrate palliative care at a time during a patient's cancer when a cure is still a possibility.

The most efficient palliative care model consists of the oncologist and specialty palliative care, which allows the most relevant team to deliver care at the most appropriate time. The consulting palliative care teams are either independent or within the primary oncology clinic and should be present in the inpatient and outpatient setting to obtain maximum benefit.[29] Studies suggest the integration of consultants within the primary oncology clinic augments communication between the two teams and unifies a patient's care.[5] These palliative care teams should be interdisciplinary consisting of at least a palliative care physician and a palliative care nurse. They often also include social workers, physical therapists, occupational therapists, chaplains, counselors, and/or rehabilitation medicine physicians.[5,41]

The bow tie model of palliative care illustrates the priorities emphasized by the NCCN, ASCO, SGO, and the WHO (**Fig. 2**).[42] It demonstrates the dynamic need for varying balances of disease management and palliative care throughout a patient's illness. It also exhibits the gradual shift in focus as a patient's disease progresses. This model differs from archaic models in that palliative care is an integral part of early disease management and survivorship is included as a possible outcome. This allows patients to accept palliative care while cure is still a possibility, which is much less intimidating to patients.

This palliative care model can only work by establishing the roles of the different health care professionals involved in providing disease management and palliative care. Although it may seem ideal for palliative care specialists to provide all palliative facets of care, this is not sustainable. The increasing demand would certainly exhaust the supply of services. Furthermore, having a consultant provide all palliative services would likely fragment care and undercut oncologist-patient relationships.[43]

The oncologist should take responsibility for primary palliative care, and specialty palliative care should be carried out by consulting services.[43] Primary palliative care services include early management of pain, depression, anxiety, and other basic symptoms, and discussions about prognosis and goals of care. Specialty palliative care services are more complex and include management of refractory or multifaceted symptoms and conflict resolution between patients/families and treatment team. These services also are appropriate in addressing futile treatments and intricate end-of-life issues.[43] Once each health care worker recognizes and understands his/ her role, this palliative care paradigm can reach its full potential.[38] In this synchronized model the oncologist provides early and basic palliative care needs and consults the specialty palliative care team for more complex issues.[44] Once placed, a successful palliative care consultation should provide an initial and then ongoing assessment evaluating the patient's quality of life, symptom management, and goals of care.[3]

Timing of palliative care consultation
Only 18% of gynecologic oncology patients receive consultation greater than 30 days before death.[12] Although a gynecologic oncologist can provide primary palliative care it is likely that specialty services are needed as a patient progresses through her disease. Referral to specialty palliative care services should be made when "physical, social, psychological, or spiritual unmet needs" are not able to be effectively managed by the primary team.[29] Of note, this may be at a time when the goal of disease management is still curative. This implies that oncologists must regularly assess patient's and caregivers' needs to ensure timely referral to specialty palliative care services. Timely referral results in added benefits specifically in patients with advanced malignancies.[3,9] Of note, gynecologic oncologists often defer palliative care referral until patients have a high disease and symptom burden and are near the end of life. Erring on the side of earlier referral results in improved outcomes.[10] ASCO specifically recommends palliative care consultation within 8 weeks of the diagnosis of advanced or metastatic cancer.[3,5]

Palliative care reimbursement
Reimbursement specifically for primary palliative care services is minimal. It is only recently that reimbursement is available for primary palliative care services, such as advanced care planning discussions.[35] Regarding specialty palliative care services, palliative care is a board-certified specialty that is reimbursed similarly to other

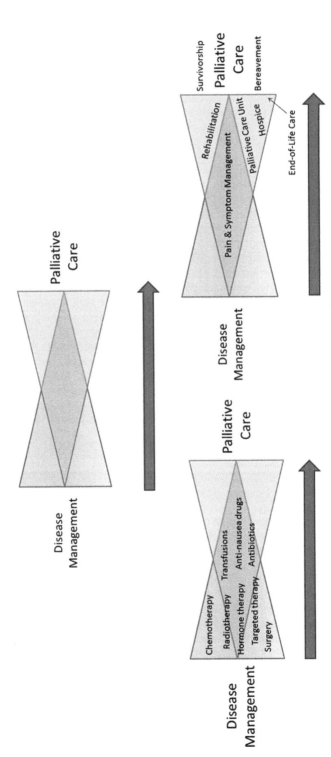

Fig. 2. The bow tie model of palliative care. (*From* Hawley PH. The bow tie model of 21st century palliative care. J Pain Symptom Manage 2014;47(1): e3–4; with permission.)

medical specialties with a unique Medicare billing identifier. Accordingly, a physician and/or a midlevel provider can bill for their time directly. However, other members of the interdisciplinary team, such as chaplains, social workers, and physical and occupational therapists, cannot. Therefore, other forms of compensation are made for these services.[41] Unfortunately, the enormous cost savings that occur as a result of patients receiving palliative care are not directly reallocated to support palliative care services.[29]

Disparities of Palliative Care

It has been established that minority patients with cancer unjustly experience increased comorbidities, are more likely to receive inferior quality of care, and are less like to be insured.[5] Although studies regarding disparities in palliative care are sparse, limited data suggest that, similar to other care, minority patients are less likely to receive equivalent palliative care. Studies document minorities have decreased satisfaction with palliative care and worse pain management when compared with their nonminority counterparts. In fact, compared with whites, minorities are more likely to be hospitalized and receive intensive care unit care in the last 6 months of life.[45] Medicaid patients are less likely to receive "quality-adherent palliative care" when compared with Medicare patients.[46] Furthermore, patients of minorities and low socioeconomic status are more likely to experience geographic disparities, such as living in an area that does not have access to palliative care services. White persons are overrepresented in all studies to date regarding palliative care outcomes, and further research is necessary to better understand disparities that exist within palliative care.[5]

STRATEGIES TO IMPROVE USE OF PALLIATIVE CARE

Despite the benefits, palliative care and hospice are grossly underused in gynecologic oncology, and it is important to understand strategies to improve use of palliative care and hospice. The strategies proposed would be most effective if used simultaneously.

Triggers to Referral

Many gynecologic oncologists do not have the training to complete a thorough primary palliative care assessment or to address palliative care needs once they are recognized. Therefore, identifying specific triggers for palliative care referral would likely improve the use of these services and quality outcomes. Adelson and colleagues[47] demonstrated that the standardized use of triggers for palliative care consultation among hospitalized patients resulted in decreased 30-day readmission rates, decreased chemotherapy after discharge, increased hospice referrals, and increased use of ancillary palliative care services on discharge. Similarly, in response to the need to better identify patients requiring specialized palliative care services, the Center to Advance Palliative Care assembled a consensus panel in 2010 to establish key triggers for palliative care referrals among hospitalized patients. These triggers include primary and secondary triggers. Primary triggers include frequent admissions, admission prompted by difficulty to control symptoms, complex care requirements, and decline in function. Secondary triggers include metastatic or incurable cancer, chronic oxygen use, admission from long-term care facility, and limited social support. Although these triggers were identified specifically for inpatients, these criteria are certainly pertinent to gynecologic oncology patients in the outpatient setting.[48] These triggers should be evaluated early and regularly in all gynecologic oncology patients regardless of diagnosis or symptoms to identify even patients with early stage disease who would benefit from these services. This approach considers the patient's disease, symptoms, and family variables objectively rather than using subjective thresholds for referral.[48]

Provider/Patient Education

It is imperative gynecologic oncologists provide primary palliative care services to maintain a sustainable model of palliative care. Despite these expectations, gynecologic oncologists actually receive minimal formal training in this arena. Although approximately 90% of gynecologic oncology fellows reported palliative care is integral to their training, only 11% actually had any formal training. Those who did receive formal training reported increased vigilance to deal with end-of-life issues.[36] A total of 77% of board-certified gynecologic oncologists stated that more training during fellowship would have been beneficial in practice.[16] In response, the SGO has made great efforts to improve education and promote collaboration with palliative care specialists.

Equally important is education of the public and patients regarding the role of palliative care and what services are provided. Palliative care is often mistaken for end-of-life or hospice care. Unlike end-of-life care, palliative care is delivered throughout the duration of treatment even when there is curative intent. This incorrect stigma comes from an often late introduction to palliative care. El-Sahwi and coworkers[49] surveyed gynecologic oncologists and noted that 53.9% deferred end-of-life discussions until the patient has sustained a major change in functional or medical status. The term "palliative care" was initially created as a more socially acceptable term in response to the historical association of hospice with dying. However, palliative care has now also become associated with end-of-life as hospice originally was.[35] Education is necessary to discredit misconceptions about the role of palliative care and the services it has to offer to improve implementation.[35] Early introduction to specialty palliative care may increase rapport with providers, dispel the negative association with end-of-life, enhance symptom control, and improve expectations.

Clinical Trials

Clinical trials provide innovative ways to increase palliative care uptake. Zander and colleagues[50] studied automatic palliative care consultation for patients with advanced, incurable cancer. As a result, 67% of oncologists believed patient care was improved and promoted discussion of patients end-of-life goals. Dalal and colleagues[51] trialed a name change of palliative care to supportive care and found an association with increased inpatient palliative care consultations and outpatient consultation. One health care system worked with an insurance supplier to change the model of payment; payment went from fee-for-service to pay-for-performance. Before the change in reimbursement, palliative care quality improvement metrics were selected including percentage of patients seen by the palliative care service who were deemed high-risk. After the intervention palliative care consultation rates tripled in high-risk groups.[52] Specifically in gynecologic oncology patients, Mullen and colleagues[53] demonstrated that the integration of palliative care and hospice resulted in increased hospice enrollment and increased time on hospice. Other clinical trials conducted within this patient population suggest that an established palliative care service well integrated into the gynecologic oncology service and with a constant presence/availability (someone on call 24 hours a day) improves consultation rates.[10,53] Although clinical trials suggest mechanisms to improve palliative care use, further research is necessary to understand how improved uptake of these interventions impacts all patients and practice settings.

MANAGEMENT OF COMMON SYMPTOMS

The SGO emphasizes providing comprehensive care to gynecologic oncology patients from the time of diagnosis to death.[4,54] Therefore, it is important to understand how to manage common symptoms that patients with advanced malignancies experience.[4]

Anorexia

- Address reversible causes (constipation, pain, medications, hypercalcemia, mucositis)
- Gastrokinetic agents (metoclopramide, domperidone)
- Low-dose corticosteroids (short term)
- Progesterone agents
- Cannabinoids (dronabinol and medical marijuana)
- Counsel patients and caregivers away from meeting nutrition goals to avoid suffering from forced feeding

Bone Metastasis

- External-beam radiation
- Opioids and analgesic nerve blocks for pain control
- Bisphosphonates (pamidronate, zoledronic acid)
- Denosumab (human monoclonal antibody to inhibit the receptor activator of nuclear factor-kappa B to diminish maturation of osteoclasts)
- Surgery or interventional radiology (to stabilize the skeleton by vertebroplasty)

Brain Metastasis

- Consult radiation oncology and neurosurgery
- Steroids (only if symptomatic, dexamethasone orally 4–8 mg/d up to 100 mg/d for severe symptoms)
  - If plan for radiation start 48 hours before treatment to prevent severe cerebral edema
- Whole-brain radiation (one to three lesions and widespread disease)
- Surgery (good prognosis) and/or stereotactic radiosurgery (multiple lesions, incompletely resected single lesion)[55]
- Antiepileptic drugs (only for patients with seizures)

Constipation

- Rule out bowel obstruction and fecal impaction
- Initiate bowel regimen immediately with opioid use
- Stool softeners (docusate sodium)
- Osmotic agents (magnesium hydroxide, lactulose, polyethylene glycol)
- Stimulants (senna, bisacodyl)
- Lubricants (glycerin suppositories)
- Enemas (mineral oil, soap suds)
- Opioid antagonist (methylnaltrexone)

Delirium

- Discontinue all high-risk medications, regularly reorient the patient, minimize stimulation, minimize use of restraints, encourage use of glasses/hearing aids
- Hyperactive delirium

○ Haloperidol (0.5–2 mg orally [PO]/intravenous [IV]/intramuscular [IM]/subcu-taneous [SC] every 2–12 hours as needed) or chlorpromazine (12.5–50 mg PO/IV/IM/SC/rectally every 4–6 hours as needed)
○ Olanzapine or risperidone (patients intolerant of haloperidol)
○ Lorazepam (for irreversible, hyperactive delirium)
- Hypoactive delirium
  ○ No pharmacologic interventions have been proven to be effective

Dyspnea

First Line:
- Relaxation or distraction techniques (music, guided imagery, cognitive behavioral therapy)
- Fan (facial cooling/air movement)
- Oxygen (even in patients without hypoxemia)
- Physiotherapy/chest wall percussion (helps mobilize secretions)

Second Line:
- Systemic opioids (opioid-naive morphine 2.5–5 mg PO every 4 hours; long-active opioid-increased baseline by 30% and adjust breakthrough)
- Benzodiazepine (lorazepam 0.5–1 mg PO every 4 hours as needed)
- Anticholinergics (glycopyrrolate 0.2–0.4 mg SC/sublingual/PO every 4– 8 hours)
- Interventions specific to etiology (**Table 1**)

Hemorrhage

- Volume resuscitation (blood transfusion case-by-case basis)
- Psychological support to patient and family
- Apply pressure
- Dark towels and suction
- Consider sedatives or narcotics (midazolam 2.5–5 mg IV or SQ every 10–15 minutes as needed)

Table 1
Management of dyspnea based on etiology

Disease Process	Possible Intervention
Pneumonia	Antibiotics, pulmonary toilet
Lymphangitic tumor	Diuretics, glucocorticoids
Pneumonitis, radiation or chemotherapy induced	Glucocorticoids
Venous thromboembolism	Anticoagulation, interior vena cava filter
Pleural effusion	Indwelling catheter, thoracentesis, video-assisted thoracoscopic surgery, pleurodesis
Airway obstruction by tumor or lymphadenopathy	Radiation therapy, glucocorticoids
Bronchoconstriction (chronic obstructive pulmonary disease, asthma)	Bronchodilators, glucocorticoids
Retained or excess secretions	Anticholinergic agents
Massive ascites	Drainage, including indwelling catheter
Anxiety, including hyperventilation	Anxiolytics, cognitive behavioral therapy

From Landrum LM, Blank S, Chen LM, et al. Comprehensive care in gynecologic oncology: the importance of palliative care. Gynecol Oncol 2015;137(2):194; with permission.

- Genitourinary
  - Packing (vaginal hemorrhage)
  - Bladder irrigation (bladder hemorrhage)
    - Cystoscopic coagulation > infusion of 1% alum
    - Administration of prostaglandin E_2 and silver nitrate
    - Formalin
  - External-beam radiotherapy (hypofractionation, 2 fractions over 2–3 days)
  - Arterial embolization by interventional radiology
- Gastrointestinal
  - Endoscopy
  - Surgical ligation or clipping of bleeding vessels

Hypercalcemia (Adjusted Total Serum Calcium >10.2)

- Hydration with intravenous normal saline
- Bisphosphonates (pamidronate or zoledronic acid)
  - Addition of calcitonin in patients with severe hypercalcemia

Intractable Symptoms at End of Life

- Palliative care consultation recommended
- Family meeting to verify goals of care/discuss sedation
- Midazolam, methotrimeprazine, propofol, phenobarbital

Malignant Ascites

- Maximize diuretics to decrease albumin loss
  - Furosemide (40–80 mg IV/PO twice a day) and spironolactone (50–200 mg PO twice a day)
- Paracentesis (immediate symptom relief)
- Permanent drains

Malignant Bowel Obstruction (Nonoperable)

- Conservative management with nasogastric tube
- Intravenous fluids
- Partial bowel obstruction
  - Prokinetic agent, metoclopramide
  - Steroid, dexamethasone
  - Antiemetic, haloperidol
  - Antispasmodic, hyoscine butylbromide
- Complete bowel obstruction
  - Avoid prokinetic agent if increased cramping/pain
  - Steroid, dexamethasone
  - Antiemetic, haloperidol
  - Octreotide to decrease secretions
  - Consider gastrostomy tube
  - Total parenteral nutrition (ONLY if possibility of surgery in the future)

Nausea/Vomiting

- Use optimal dosing/route (**Table 2**)
- Scheduled dosing
- Maximize primary agent and then add secondary (do not switch agents)
- Avoid drugs with similar toxicities (reduces side effects)

Table 2
Antiemetic agents, dosing, and adverse effects

Class	Drug	Principal Action	Route	Dose	Frequency	Major Adverse Events
Dopamine antagonist	Chlorpromazine	CTZ/vomiting center	PO/IM/IV	625 mg	Q 8 h	Dystonia, akathisia, sedation, postural hypotension
	Prochlorperazine	CTZ	PO	50–10 mg	Q 4–6 h	Dystonia, akathisia, sedation
			PR	25 mg		
			IM/IV	10–20 mg	Q 3–6 h	
	Metoclopramide	CTZ/GI cholinergic	PO/IV	10–20 mg	Q 2–4 h	Dystonia, akathisia, esophageal spasm, colic
	Haloperidol	CTZ	PO/IV	0.5–1 mg	Q 8 h	Dystonia and akathisia, anticholinergic, sedation
Anticholinergic	Scopolamine	Vestibular, vomiting center	Transdermal	1.5 mg	Q 3 d	Dry mouth, blurred vision, ileus, urinary retention, confusion
	Hydroxyzine	Periphery, GI tract	PO	6.25–25 mg	QHS	Dry mouth, sedation, dystonia
H₁ antihistamine	Diphenhydramine	Vomiting center	PO	50–75 mg	Q 4–6 h	Sedation, dry mouth, urinary retention
			IV/IM	25–50 mg		
	Promethazine	Upper GI tract, vomiting center	PO/IM	12.5–25 mg	Q 8 h	Dystonia, akathisia, sedation
5-HT3 antagonist	Ondansetron	Upper GI tract, CNS	PO/IV/SL	4–8 mg	Q 4–8 h	Headache, fatigue, constipation
	Dolasetron		PO	100 mg	Q 24 h	
	Granisetron		PO	2 mg PO	Q 24 h	
			IV	0.01 mg/kg	1 mg Q 24 h	
	Palonosetron		Transdermal	3.1 mg 24 h	Q 7 d	
			IV	0.25 mg	Q 24 h	
Steroids	Dexamethasone	Not known	PO/IV	4–24 mg	Q morning	Hyperglycemia, headache, oral candidiasis, peptic ulcer, insomnia, anxiety, psychosis
Cannabinoids	Dronabinol	Vomiting center	PO	7.5–15 mg	Q 3–4 h	Sedation, anticholinergic euphoria, dysphoria, tachycardia
Benzodiazepine	Lorazepam	Not known	IV, PO	0.5–2 mg	Q 4 h	Mild sedation, amnesia, confusion (avoid in elderly)

Abbreviations: CNS, central nervous system; CTZ, chemoreceptor trigger zone; GI, gastrointestinal; IM, intramuscular; IV, intravenous; PO, per os; PR, per rectum; SL, sublingual.

From Landrum LM, Blank S, Chen LM, et al. Comprehensive care in gynecologic oncology: the importance of palliative care. Gynecol Oncol 2015;137(2):196; with permission.

Table 3
Adjuvant pain medications

Class	Drug	Principal Action	Route	Starting Dose	Frequency	Major Adverse Events
Steroids	Dexamethasone	Inhibit prostaglandin synthesis	PO	1–2 mg	QD or BID	Hyperglycemia Headache Oral candidiasis
	Prednisone	Decrease inflammation	PO	7.5–10 mg	QD	Insomnia Anxiety Psychosis
Antidepressants	Desipramine	Tricyclic antidepressants, inhibit norepinephrine reuptake	PO	10–25 mg	QHS	Prolong QTc interval Sexual dysfunction Anticholinergic effects
	Nortriptyline		PO	10–25 mg (may increase to 50–150 mg QHS)	QHS	Lower seizure threshold
	Venlafaxine	Serotonin-norepinephrine reuptake inhibitor	PO	37.5 mg (may increase up to 37.5–112.5 mg BID)	QD	Nausea Sexual dysfunction Somnolence Hypertension
	Duloxetine		PO	30 mg (may increase up to 60 mg)	QD	
Anticonvulsants	Gabapentin	Inhibit depolarization of neurons	PO	100–300 mg (may increase up to 900–3600 mg in BID-TID doses)	QHS	Dizziness Somnolence
	Pregabalin		PO	50 mg (may increase to 100 mg TID)	TID	Mental cloudiness
Bisphosphonates	Pamidronate	Osteoclast inhibitors	IV	60 mg	Q month	Renal impairment
	Zoledronic acid		IV	4 mg	Q 21 d	Flulike syndrome with initiation of treatment

From Landrum LM, Blank S, Chen LM, et al. Comprehensive care in gynecologic oncology: the importance of palliative care. Gynecol Oncol 2015;137(2):199; with permission.

Pain Management

- Per the WHO analgesic ladder for pain management pain should be treated in a stepwise fashion first using nonopioids plus or minus adjunctive analgesics followed by opioid combinations including nonopioids and adjunctive analgesics (**Table 3**)[56]
- Long-active opioid and short-acting opioid for breakthrough pain if necessary
  - Dosage of long-acting opioid is based on 24-hour needs
  - Breakthrough is ~10% of 24-hour opioid dose
- Rotate opioid if unmanageable side effects
- Regularly monitor for opioid toxicity specifically in patients with renal dysfunction
- If pain decreased because of treatment, gradually decrease opioids to avoid oversedation
- Nonsteroidal anti-inflammatory drugs
- Neuraxial blocks

SUMMARY

The integration of palliative care into standard gynecologic care is undoubtedly associated with improved patient outcomes, enhanced quality of life, and financial benefits. As a result, it is strongly endorsed by the NCCN, ASCO, and SGO. However, use of these services by gynecologic oncology patients continues to be disappointing and to occur too late in the disease process to obtain maximum benefit. To optimize end-of-life care for patients, oncologists and palliative care providers must collaborate to concurrently provide palliative care and anticancer treatment throughout the disease course. Further research is necessary to identify interventions to increase hospice and palliative care uptake, to implement palliative care earlier in a patient's oncologic care, and to eliminate disparities.

REFERENCES

1. Meghani SH, Hinds PS. Policy brief: the Institute of Medicine report Dying in America: improving quality and honoring individual preferences near the end of life. Nurs Outlook 2015;63(1):51–9.
2. Ferrell BR, Temel JS, Temin S, et al. Integration of palliative care into standard oncology care: American Society of Clinical Oncology clinical practice guideline update. J Clin Oncol 2016;35(1):96–112.
3. Temel JS, Greer JA, Muzikansky A, et al. Early palliative care for patients with metastatic non-small-cell lung cancer. N Engl J Med 2010;363(8):733–42.
4. Landrum LM, Blank S, Chen LM, et al. Comprehensive care in gynecologic oncology: the importance of palliative care. Gynecol Oncol 2015;137(2): 193–202.
5. Ferrell BR, Temel JS, Temin S, et al. Integration of palliative care into standard oncology care: ASCO clinical practice guideline update summary. J Oncol Pract 2017;13(2):119–21.
6. Society of Gynecologic Oncology. Delivery of palliative care services. SGO Position Statements and Special Reports. 2010.
7. Lefkowits C, Solomon C. Palliative care in obstetrics and gynecology. Obstet Gynecol 2016;128(6):1403–20.
8. Hay CM, Lefkowits C, Crowley-Matoka M, et al. Gynecologic oncologist views influencing referral to outpatient specialty palliative care. Int J Gynecol Cancer 2017;27(3):588–96.

9. Zimmermann C, Swami N, Krzyzanowska M, et al. Early palliative care for patients with advanced cancer: a cluster-randomised controlled trial. Lancet 2014; 383(9930):1721–30.

10. Lefkowits C, Teuteberg W, Courtney-Brooks M, et al. Improvement in symptom burden within one day after palliative care consultation in a cohort of gynecologic oncology inpatients. Gynecol Oncol 2015;136(3):424–8.

11. Ruski RA I, Rabow M, Chen LM. Outpatient palliative care consultation is associated with a decrease in symptom burden for women with gynecologic malignancies. J Pain Symptom Manage 2014;47(2):394–5.

12. Nevadunsky NS, Gordon S, Spoozak L, et al. The role and timing of palliative medicine consultation for women with gynecologic malignancies: association with end of life interventions and direct hospital costs. Gynecol Oncol 2014; 132(1):3–7.

13. von Gruenigen VE, Daly BJ. Futility: clinical decisions at the end-of-life in women with ovarian cancer. Gynecol Oncol 2005;97(2):638–44.

14. Fauci J, Schneider K, Walters C, et al. The utilization of palliative care in gynecologic oncology patients near the end of life. Gynecol Oncol 2012;127(1):175–9.

15. Barbera L, Elit L, Krzyzanowska M, et al. End of life care for women with gynecologic cancers. Gynecol Oncol 2010;118(2):196–201.

16. Lopez-Acevedo M, Havrilesky LJ, Broadwater G, et al. Timing of end-of-life care discussion with performance on end-of-life quality indicators in ovarian cancer. Gynecol Oncol 2013;130(1):156–61.

17. Lopez-Acevedo M, Lowery WJ, Lowery AW, et al. Palliative and hospice care in gynecologic cancer: a review. Gynecol Oncol 2013;131(1):215–21.

18. Doll KM, Stine JE, Van Le L, et al. Outpatient end of life discussions shorten hospital admissions in gynecologic oncology patients. Gynecol Oncol 2013;130(1): 152–5.

19. Nevadunsky NS, Spoozak L, Gordon S, et al. End-of-life care of women with gynecologic malignances: a pilot study. Int J Gynecol Cancer 2013;23(3):546–52.

20. Lewin SN, Buttin BM, Powell MA, et al. Resource utilization for ovarian cancer patients at the end of life: how much is too much? Gynecol Oncol 2005;99(2):261–6.

21. Urban RR, He H, Alfonso R, et al. The end of life costs for Medicare patients with advanced ovarian cancer. Gynecol Oncol 2018;148(2):336–41.

22. Taylor DH Jr, Ostermann J, Van Houtven CH, et al. What length of hospice use maximizes reduction in medical expenditures near death in the US Medicare program? Soc Sci Med 2007;65(7):1466–78.

23. Keyser EA, Reed BG, Lowery WJ, et al. Hospice enrollment for terminally ill patients with gynecologic malignancies: impact on outcomes and interventions. Gynecol Oncol 2010;118(3):274–7.

24. Rimel BJ, Burke WM, Higgins RV, et al. Improving quality and decreasing cost in gynecologic oncology care. Society of Gynecologic Oncology recommendations for clinical practice. Gynecol Oncol 2015;137(2):280–4.

25. Smith TJ, Temin S, Alesi ER, et al. American Society of Clinical Oncology provisional clinical opinion: the integration of palliative care into standard oncology care. J Clin Oncol 2012;30(8):880–7.

26. Rugno FC, Paiva BS, Paiva CE. Early integration of palliative care facilitates the discontinuation of anticancer treatment in women with advanced breast or gynecologic cancers. Gynecol Oncol 2014;135(2):249–54.

27. Buckley de Meritens A, Margolis B, Blinderman C, et al. Practice patterns, attitudes, and barriers to palliative care consultation by gynecologic oncologists. J Oncol Pract 2017;13(9):e703–11.

28. Center to Advance Palliative Care. 2011 Public opinion research on palliative care: a report based on research by public opinion strategies. The American Cancer Society and the American Cancer Society Cancer Action Network; 2013.

29. Hawley PH. Barriers to access to palliative care. Palliat Care 2017;10. 1178224216688887.

30. Friedman BT, Harwood MK, Shields M. Barriers and enablers to hospice referrals: an expert overview. J Palliat Med 2002;5(1):73–84.

31. Massarotto A, Carter H, MacLeod R, et al. Hospital referrals to a hospice: timing of referrals, referrers' expectations, and the nature of referral information. J Palliat Care 2000;16(3):22–9.

32. Glare P, Virik K, Jones M, et al. A systematic review of physicians' survival predictions in terminally ill cancer patients. BMJ 2003;327(7408):195–8.

33. Bakitas M, Lyons KD, Hegel MT, et al. Oncologists' perspectives on concurrent palliative care in a National Cancer Institute-designated comprehensive cancer center. Palliat Support Care 2013;11(5):415–23.

34. Cripe JC, Mills KA, Kuroki LK, et al. Gynecologic oncologists' perceptions of palliative care and associated barriers: a survey of the society of gynecologic oncology. Gynecol Obstet Invest 2018. [Epub ahead of print].

35. Duska LR. Early integration of palliative care in the care of women with advanced epithelial ovarian cancer: the time is now. Front Oncol 2016;6:83.

36. Lesnock JL, Arnold RM, Meyn LA, et al. Palliative care education in gynecologic oncology: a survey of the fellows. Gynecol Oncol 2013;130(3):431–5.

37. Ramondetta LM, Tortolero-Luna G, Bodurka DC, et al. Approaches for end-of-life care in the field of gynecologic oncology: an exploratory study. Int J Gynecol Cancer 2004;14(4):580–8.

38. Biasco G, Tanzi S, Bruera E. "Early palliative care: how?" From a conference report to a consensus document, Bentivoglio, May 14, 2012. J Palliat Med 2013;16(5):466–70.

39. Levy MH, Adolph MD, Back A, et al. Palliative care. J Natl Compr Canc Netw 2012;10(10):1284–309.

40. World Health Organization. WHO definition of palliative care. 2016. Available at: http://www.who.int/cancer/palliative/definition/en/.

41. Ferrell B, Sun V, Hurria A, et al. Interdisciplinary palliative care for patients with lung cancer. J Pain Symptom Manage 2015;50(6):758–67.

42. Hawley PH. The bow tie model of 21st century palliative care. J Pain Symptom Manage 2014;47(1):e2–5.

43. Quill TE, Abernethy AP. Generalist plus specialist palliative care: creating a more sustainable model. N Engl J Med 2013;368(13):1173–5.

44. Hudson PTT, Kelly B, O'Connor M, et al. Reducing the psychological distress of family caregivers of home based palliative care patients: longer term effects from a andomized controlled trial. Psychooncology 2015;24(1):19–24.

45. Johnson K. Racial and ethnic disparities in palliative care. J Palliat Care Med 2013;16(11):1329–34.

46. Guadagnolo BA, Liao KP, Giordano SH, et al. Variation in intensity and costs of care by payer and race for patients dying of cancer in Texas: an analysis of registry-linked Medicaid, Medicare, and dually eligible claims data. Med Care 2015;53(7):591–8.

47. Adelson K, Paris J, Horton JR, et al. Standardized criteria for palliative care consultation on a solid tumor oncology service reduces downstream health care use. J Oncol Pract 2017;13(5):e431–40.

48. Weissman DE, Meier DE. Identifying patients in need of a palliative care assessment in the hospital setting: a consensus report from the Center to Advance Palliative Care. J Palliat Med 2011;14(1):17–23.

49. El-Sahwi KS, Illuzzi J, Varughese J, et al. A survey of gynecologic oncologists regarding the end-of-life discussion: a pilot study. Gynecol Oncol 2012;124(3): 471–3.

50. Zander MR, Rocque GB, Campbell TC, et al. Oncologist impressions of automatic palliative care consultation for inpatients with advanced cancer. J Clin Oncol 2014;32(15_suppl):e20541-e.

51. Dalal S, Palla S, Hui D, et al. Association between a name change from palliative to supportive care and the timing of patient referrals at a comprehensive cancer center. Oncologist 2011;16(1):105–11.

52. Bernacki RE, Ko DN, Higgins P, et al. Improving access to palliative care through an innovative quality improvement initiative: an opportunity for pay-for-performance. J Palliat Med 2012;15(2):192–9.

53. Mullen MM, Divine LM, Porcelli BP, et al. The effect of a multidisciplinary palliative care initiative on end of life care in gynecologic oncology patients. Gynecol Oncol 2017;147(2):460–4.

54. Rezk Y, Timmins PF 3rd, Smith HS. Review article: palliative care in gynecologic oncology. Am J Hosp Palliat Care 2011;28(5):356–74.

55. Tsao MN, Rades D, Wirth A, et al. Radiotherapeutic and surgical management for newly diagnosed brain metastasis(es): an American Society for Radiation Oncology evidence-based guideline. Pract Radiat Oncol 2012;2(3):210–25.

56. Jadad AR, Browman GP. The WHO analgesic ladder for cancer pain management. Stepping up the quality of its evaluation. JAMA 1995;274(23):1870–3.

Moving?

Make sure your subscription moves with you!

To notify us of your new address, find your **Clinics Account Number** (located on your mailing label above your name), and contact customer service at:

Email: journalscustomerservice-usa@elsevier.com

800-654-2452 (subscribers in the U.S. & Canada)
314-447-8871 (subscribers outside of the U.S. & Canada)

Fax number: 314-447-8029

Elsevier Health Sciences Division
Subscription Customer Service
3251 Riverport Lane
Maryland Heights, MO 63043

Printed and bound by CPI Group (UK) Ltd, Croydon, CR0 4YY

03/10/2024

01040480-0001